# Interventional Techniques in Uro-oncology

EDITED BY

## Hashim Uddin Ahmed, MRCS, BM, BCh(Oxon), BA(Hons)

Medical Research Council Clinical Research Fellow
Specialist Registrar in Urology
Division of Surgery and Interventional Science
University College London
University College London Hospitals NHS Foundation Trust,
London, UK

## Manit Arya, FRCS, FRCS(Urol)

Fellow in Laparoscopic and Minimally Invasive Surgery
King's College Hospital
London, UK

## Peter T. Scardino, MD

The David H. Koch Chair
Chair, Department of Surgery and Head of Prostate Cancer Program
Memorial Sloan-Kettering Cancer Center
New York, USA

## Mark Emberton, FRCS(Urol), FRCS(Eng), MBBS, BSc

Professor of Interventional Oncology and Honorary Consultant Urologist
Division of Surgery and Interventional Science
University College London Hospitals NHS Foundation Trust
London, UK

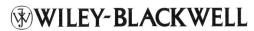

A John Wiley & Sons, Ltd., Publication

This edition first published 2011, © 2011 by Blackwell Publishing Ltd

Blackwell Publishing was acquired by John Wiley & Sons in February 2007. Blackwell's publishing program has been merged with Wiley's global Scientific, Technical and Medical business to form Wiley-Blackwell.

*Registered office:* John Wiley & Sons Ltd, The Atrium, Southern Gate, Chichester, West Sussex, PO19 8SQ, UK

*Editorial offices:* 9600 Garsington Road, Oxford, OX4 2DQ, UK
The Atrium, Southern Gate, Chichester, West Sussex, PO19 8SQ, UK
111 River Street, Hoboken, NJ 07030-5774, USA

For details of our global editorial offices, for customer services and for information about how to apply for permission to reuse the copyright material in this book please see our website at www.wiley.com/wiley-blackwell

The right of the author to be identified as the author of this work has been asserted in accordance with the UK Copyright, Designs and Patents Act 1988.

All rights reserved. No part of this publication may be reproduced, stored in a retrieval system, or transmitted, in any form or by any means, electronic, mechanical, photocopying, recording or otherwise, except as permitted by the UK Copyright, Designs and Patents Act 1988, without the prior permission of the publisher.

Designations used by companies to distinguish their products are often claimed as trademarks. All brand names and product names used in this book are trade names, service marks, trademarks or registered trademarks of their respective owners. The publisher is not associated with any product or vendor mentioned in this book. This publication is designed to provide accurate and authoritative information in regard to the subject matter covered. It is sold on the understanding that the publisher is not engaged in rendering professional services. If professional advice or other expert assistance is required, the services of a competent professional should be sought.

The contents of this work are intended to further general scientific research, understanding, and discussion only and are not intended and should not be relied upon as recommending or promoting a specific method, diagnosis, or treatment by physicians for any particular patient. The publisher and the author make no representations or warranties with respect to the accuracy or completeness of the contents of this work and specifically disclaim all warranties, including without limitation any implied warranties of fitness for a particular purpose. In view of ongoing research, equipment modifications, changes in governmental regulations, and the constant flow of information relating to the use of medicines, equipment, and devices, the reader is urged to review and evaluate the information provided in the package insert or instructions for each medicine, equipment, or device for, among other things, any changes in the instructions or indication of usage and for added warnings and precautions. Readers should consult with a specialist where appropriate. The fact that an organization or Website is referred to in this work as a citation and/or a potential source of further information does not mean that the author or the publisher endorses the information the organization or Website may provide or recommendations it may make. Further, readers should be aware that Internet Websites listed in this work may have changed or disappeared between when this work was written and when it is read. No warranty may be created or extended by any promotional statements for this work. Neither the publisher nor the author shall be liable for any damages arising herefrom.

*Library of Congress Cataloging-in-Publication Data*

Interventional techniques in uro-oncology / Edited by Hashim Uddin Ahmed . . . [et al]
    p. ; cm.
    Includes bibliographical references and index.
    ISBN 978-1-4051-9272-9 (hardback : alk. paper) – ISBN 978-1-4443-2990-2 (ePDF) –
    ISBN 978-1-4443-2989-6 (Wiley Online Library) – ISBN 978-1-4443-2991-9 (ePub)
  1. Genitourinary organs–Endoscopic surgery.  2. Laparoscopic surgery.  I. Ahmed, Hashim Uddin, editor.  II. Arya, Manit, editor.  III. Scardino, Peter T., 1945– editor.  IV. Emberton, Mark, editor.
    [DNLM: 1. Urologic Neoplasms–surgery.  2. Urologic Surgical Procedures–methods.
3. Surgical Procedures, Minimally Invasive–methods. WJ 160]
    RD572.I58 2011
    617.4′60597–dc22
                                                                    2010052263

A catalogue record for this book is available from the British Library.

This book is published in the following electronic formats: ePDF 9781444329902; Wiley Online Library 9781444329896; ePub 9781444329919

Set in 9/11.5 pt Sabon by Aptara®, Inc., New Delhi, India
Printed in Singapore by Ho Printing Singapore Pte Ltd

1  2011

# Contents

# Contributors

**Manit Arya**
Fellow
Laparoscopic and Minimally Invasive Surgery
King's College Hospital
London, UK

**Stephen G. Bown**
Professor of Laser Medicine and Surgery
National Medical Laser Center
University College London
London, UK

**Peter R. Carroll**
Professor and Chair, Department of Urology
Ken and Donna Derr–Chevron Distinguished
    Professor
Associate Dean, School of Medicine Director of
    Clinical Services and Strategic Planning
Helen Diller Family Comprehensive Cancer Center
University of California
San Francisco, CA, USA

**Matthew R. Cooperberg**
Assistant Professor
Department of Urology
Helen Diller Family Comprehensive Cancer Center
University of California
San Francisco, CA, USA

**Cole Davis**
Urologic Onconlogy Fellow
Department of Urology
Helen Diller Family Comprehensive Cancer Center
University of California
San Francisco, CA, USA

**Mark Emberton**
Professor of Interventional Oncology and Honorary
    Consultant Urologist
Division of Surgery and Interventional Science
University College London
London, UK

**Omid C. Farokhzad**
Associate Professor of Anesthesia
Department of Anesthesia
Brigham and Women's Hospital
Harvard Medical School
Boston, MA, USA

**Adam S. Feldman**
Assistant Processor of Surgery
Department of Urology
Massachusetts General Hospital
Harvard Medical School
Boston, MA, USA

**Jurgen J. Futterer**
Interventional Radiologist
Department of Interventional Radiology
Nijmegen Medical Center
Radboud University
Nijmegan, The Netherlands

**Stavros Gravas**
Department of Urology
University Hospital of Larissa
Larissa, Greece

**Peter Grimm**
Prostate Cancer Traetment Center
Seattle, WA, USA

**Stijn T.W.P.J. Heijmink**
Resident in Radiology
Department of Radiology
Nymegen Medical Center
Radboud University
Nymegen, The Netherlands

**Rowland Illing**
Department of Specialist Imaging
University College Hospital
London, UK

## Aaron E. Katz

Carl A. Olsson Professor and Vice Chairman of
    Urology
Director, Center for Holistic Urology
Columbia University Medical Center
NY Presbyterian Hospital
New York, USA

## Alex Kirkham

Department of Specialist Imaging
University College Hospital
London, UK

## Robert S. Langer

David H. Koch Institute Professor
Harvard-MIT Division of Health Science and
    Technology
MIT Department of Chemical Engineering
Cambridge, MA, USA

## Charalampos Mamoulakis

Urologist
Clinical Fellow in Endourology
Department of Urology
AMC University Hospital
Amsterdam, The Netherlands

## Michael Marberger

Professor and Chairman
Department of Urology
University of Vienna Medical School
Vienna, Austria

## Markus Margreiter

Department of urology
University of Vienna Medical School
Vienna, Austria

## W. Scott McDougal

Department of Urology
Harvard Medical School
Massachusetts General Hospital
Boston, MA, USA

## Caroline M. Moore

Clinical Lecturer in Urology
University College London and University College
    London Hospital Trust
London, UK

## Peter R. Mueller

Professor
Department of Radiology
Massachusetts General Hospital
Harvard Medical School
Boston, MA, USA

## Aleksandar F. Radovic-Moreno

Harvard-MIT Division of Health Sciences and
    Technology
MIT Department of Chemical Engineering
Cambridge, MA, USA

## Jorge Rioja

Department of Urology
AMC University Hospital
Amsterdam, The Netherlands

## Chad R. Ritch

Department of Urology
Columbia University Medical Center
NY Presbyterian Hospital
New York, USA

## Jean de la Rosette

Department of Urology
Academic Medical Center
University of Amsterdam
Amsterdam, The Netherlands

## Katsuto Shinohara

Professor
Department of Urology
Helen Diller Family Comprehensive Cancer Center
University of California
San Francisco, CA, USA

**John Sylvester**
Medical Director
Lakewood Ranch Oncology
  Center
Bradenton, FL, USA


**John Trachtenberg**
Professor
Department of Surgery
University of Toronto
Princess Margaret Hospital
Toronto, Canada

**Hashim U. Ahmed**
Medical Research Council Clinical Research Fellow
Specialist Registrar in Urology
Division of Surgery and Interventional Science
University College London
University College London Hospitals NHS
  Foundation Trust
London, UK

**Kai P. Yuet**
Harvard-MIT Division of Health Sciences and
  Technology
MIT Department of Chemical Engineering
Cambridge, MA, USA

# Preface to the First Edition

The face of urological cancers is changing. We are diagnosing disease earlier with the window of opportunity for cure that is much greater as a result. However, with such a change comes a shift in the pattern of malignancies with low-volume, low-risk disease increasingly found and treated. The need for refined interventions that carry accurate targeting through novel imaging, minimal side effects, and equal effectiveness to extirpative surgery is now more paramount than ever.

We have invited many eminent groups to write the chapters. These physicians not only practice the field they write about but are also endeavoring to forward the technologies and concepts within research programs that have patients with cancer at their heart. We are, indeed, very grateful to these experts.

This book provides a comprehensive review of the state-of-the-art in minimally invasive interventions. It is written for training and practicing oncologists, urologists, and radiologists as well as the general physician with a keen interest in cancer care. It is written to allow the nonexperts among this wider fraternity to understand what is available and whether a particular intervention is suitable for their patient in the clinic.

*Hashim Ahmed*
*Manit Arya*
*Peter Scardino*
*Mark Emberton*
*2011*

# 1 Rationale for minimally invasive interventional techniques in urological cancer

*Cole Davis, Matthew R. Cooperberg, Katsuto Shinohara, and Peter R. Carroll*
Department of Urology, Helen Diller Family Comprehensive Cancer Center, University of California, San Francisco, CA, USA

## Introduction

The goals of cancer therapy are either to cure or control disease while minimizing side effects to the patient. One must balance the number of life years gained (quantity) with the risk of morbidity and mortality of a given treatment technique (quality). The ultimate goal is to match treatment type with the biological aggressiveness of the disease in an individual patient. A difficult initial hurdle is predicting disease aggressiveness. Radiographic staging has been the cornerstone in renal cancer prediction, while nomograms incorporating multiple pathologic, laboratory, and clinical measures have become the basis for prostate cancer prediction. The predictions made from this information have, to a substantial extent, guided modern treatment. In modern urologic oncology practice, a continuing movement toward maximizing survival while minimizing morbidity has been seen.

This movement is seen clearly when examining the increasing use of laparoscopic and, more recently, robot-assisted laparoscopic techniques in the treatment of renal and prostate cancers as well as conformal and intensity-modulated radiation therapy (IMRT), cryotherapy, high-intensity focused ultrasound (HIFU), and brachytherapy in the treatment of prostate cancer. More recent interest in focal, percutaneous techniques (i.e., radiofrequency or cryotherapy) reflects this evolution in management.

Minimally invasive interventional techniques are attractive since the risks of local progression and thus metastasis are, in theory, decreased compared to surveillance, while the morbidity associated with radical (partial or complete) resection are also decreased. Other advantages regarding localized renal tumor management include technical ease compared to minimally invasive partial nephrectomy, no renal ischemia requirement, relative ease in locating endophytic lesions, the unique opportunity for retreatment with no significant increased morbidity of a second procedure and, finally, decreased convalescence.

The morbidity associated with radical prostatectomy and radiotherapy is well described and is primarily a result of treatment effects on adjacent structures [1]. Therefore, minimally invasive interventional techniques stand to have the greatest impact with respect to cavernosal nerve preservation, and limitation of extraprostatic radiation leading to advantages in erectile function preservation, improved continence, as well as hospital stay and return to normal daily activities and work. These techniques hold similar advantages to those for renal cell carcinoma with the added benefits of relatively easy access to the gland and discrete ablation that could facilitate less than whole-gland treatment.

Renal and prostate tumors are biologically unique and demand individual consideration for possible surveillance, local tumor treatment, or radical tumor

*Interventional Techniques in Uro-oncology*, First Edition. Edited by Hashim Uddin Ahmed, Manit Arya, Peter T. Scardino & Mark Emberton. © 2011 Blackwell Publishing Ltd. Published 2011 by Blackwell Publishing Ltd.

treatment. Select patients that would fall into each of these populations are now being considered for local tumor treatment with minimally invasive interventional techniques. The rationale for use of these modern techniques must be based on the following principles:

1)The technique offers similar *disease control* compared to the current standard.

2)The technique decreases *morbidity* compared to the current standard.

3)The technique offers *improved outcomes* compared to patients managed conservatively.

4)The technique is more *cost-effective* and, therefore, benefits healthcare services by reducing the overall healthcare financial burden.

## Renal cancer

### Disease control

With 54,390 newly diagnosed cases annually and 13,010 deaths in 2008, renal cell carcinoma is the most lethal of all genitourinary malignancies [2]. The majority (48%–66%) of new cases are diagnosed incidentally on imaging. Surgical resection remains the standard of care for clinically localized renal cell carcinoma with patients having pathologically small, localized tumors (pT1a) enjoying 5-year cancer-specific survival rates of $\geq$ 95% [3]. The importance of treatment for renal cell carcinoma localized to the kidney is heightened by the lack of adequate systemic therapy, once the disease has metastasized. This knowledge has historically led urologic surgical oncologists to follow Halsteadian principles of wide, enbloc excision. More recently the field has moved toward organ-sparing techniques. Partial nephrectomy has now become the procedure of choice at many institutions for small tumors due to its capacity for renal preservation and similar cancer-specific survival compared to radical nephrectomy for small, localized tumors [4] (Figure 1.1).

Radiofrequency ablation (RFA) and cryoablation remain the primary modes of ablative therapy for the management of renal masses, although investigation is underway using HIFU, laser interstitial thermal therapy, and microwave ablation. Cryoablation appears to be preferred by most urologists over RFA for renal tumors [5] due to its lower retreatment rate (0.9% vs.8.8%) [6], real-time monitoring, and excellent short-term oncologic outcomes with regard to local recurrence (4.6% vs.11.7%) or metastatic progression (1.2% vs.2.3%) [7]. Many series show encouraging, short-term results with ablation carrying a slightly higher risk of recurrence and persistence, but no change in the risk of metastasis as compared to partial nephrectomy.

A major problem with interpretation of data from these series is incomplete tissue staging making it difficult to compare outcomes to surgical extirpation. In most series, a successful ablation is defined as the absence of contrast enhancement [8]. A recent study shows a radiographic success rate of 85% for RFA and 90% for cryoablation at 6 months follow-up. Of the patients who underwent renal biopsy at 6 months, pathologic success (no cancer present) was found in 65% of those managed with RFA and 94% in those treated with cryoablation. This led the authors to conclude that radiographic outcomes were accurate and postoperative renal biopsy unnecessary in those managed with cryoablation [9].

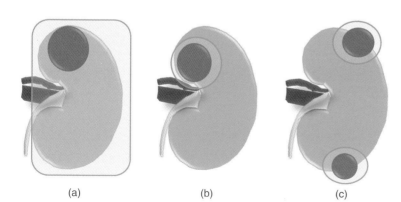

(a)          (b)          (c)

**Fig 1.1** Diagrammatic depiction of the changing paradigm in treatment of renal tumors from whole-kidney radical nephrectomy (a) to partial ablative therapy to one (b) or multiple renal tumors (c). In the latter case, multiple ablative procedures would be most suitable for a patient with Von Hippel-Lindau syndrome. (Images provided by Hashim U Ahmed, University College London, UK.)

Morbidity

The driving force behind the current trend toward more minimally invasive methods in treating localized renal cell carcinoma is an attempt to minimize the morbidity associated with open, radical, and partial nephrectomy. Laparoscopic and robot-assisted partial nephrectomy, although oncologically acceptable methods, remain technically difficult for many and can be associated with significant morbidity. The overall complication rate for laparoscopic partial nephrectomy was 19.7% in a large series from experts in the field at the Cleveland Clinic [10]. In select patients, ablative therapies have shown significant advantages with regard to complications. The overall complication rate of partial nephrectomy (majority open) in comparison to ablative techniques for tumors of similar size was found to be 16.3% vs. 2.2% for ablative procedures [11].

Complications have been primarily minor and few [12] in addition to minimal effects on renal function for both RFA and cryoablation [13]. Renal ablative therapies do carry further risk of complications due to the need for renal biopsy before and occasionally after the procedure. Image-guided renal biopsy complications include hematoma (1.3%), transfusion (1.7%), and pseudoaneurysm formation (0.7%) [14]. In addition, one must consider the risks, albeit small and difficult to quantify, associated with radiation exposure during the numerous follow-up studies that are required for proper monitoring postablation.

Comparison with conservative management

Active surveillance for small renal masses, including those that are malignant, has been assessed. Incidental radiographic detection of renal masses has resulted in stage migration downward and an increase in surgical intervention [15]. But is this significantly changing the natural history of small renal masses? Chawla et al have reported a median overall growth rate of 0.28 cm/year for masses ≤ 4 cm, and only a 1% rate of progression to metastatic disease at a median follow-up of 3 years [16]. Volpe and colleagues noted that approximately one-third of small masses progress on surveillance [17]. Most surveillance studies, however, are performed using retrospective data from elderly populations. Significant selection bias would be present in studies such as this comparing surveillance to surgical intervention.

Costs

Renal cancer treatment has been estimated to cost $40,176 per patient per year with a monthly cost of $3080 for patients diagnosed with localized disease. Inpatient hospitalization accounted for 42.1% of this cost [18]. Minimally invasive interventional techniques stand to decrease cost substantially by decreasing the hospital stay to 24 hours of observation and decreasing the cost of treating perioperative complications. In a detailed analysis, Panharipande et al concluded that RFA was more cost-effective than partial nephrectomy in the treatment of small renal masses, as long as the relative local recurrence rate remains only 48% greater than that of partial nephrectomy and the cost of partial nephrectomy did not drop more than $7500 [19]. Critical assessment of this study reveals that some series have reported a difference in local recurrence of 11.7% for RFA compared to 2.6% for partial nephrectomy (relative difference of nearly 450%) [7]. In addition, cost-effective analysis must include the rigorous imaging follow-up schedule after ablation, which currently includes CT or MRI scans 3–4 times during the first year based on retrospective data showing 70% of recurrent or residual disease identified within 3 months of initial treatment and 80% within the first year [20].

## Prostate cancer

Disease control

Approximately 94% of low-grade prostate cancer patients receive treatment in the modern era [21]. Widespread screening has led to an increasing prevalence of localized disease associated with an improved biochemical free survival [22]. Stage migration with an increased incidence of low-risk disease may allow for new treatment paradigms for low-risk, low-volume prostate cancer. Standard treatment whether surgery or radiation may not be needed in some of these patients. Many could potentially have been treated with a minimally invasive interventional technique or managed with active surveillance.

The earliest minimally invasive interventional technique introduced as prostate cancer treatment was radium brachytherapy, which first appeared in 1915 [23]. Since that time, brachytherapy has undergone profound refinements in implantation accuracy and dosimetry. Several potential advantages over radical prostatectomy and external beam radiotherapy have been noted. First, it is minimally invasive requiring no incisions and can be done under spinal anesthesia. Second, perioperative morbidity is limited and the procedure, when done using permanent seeds, is performed during a single outpatient visit. Third, recovery is generally rapid with most men returning to normal activities within 48 hours. Fourth, real-time imaging during implantation allows for accurate radiation delivery even during gland movement, preventing unwanted exposure. Oncologic outcomes for brachytherapy alone are associated with 8-year disease-free survival rates of 82% for low-risk and 70% for intermediate-risk disease [24]. Another study reported 12-year disease-free survival at 66% in a series with 80% cT2 patients [25].

Another percutaneous technique is whole-gland cryotherapy. It shares many of the same advantages noted with brachytherapy since its application is essentially identical. A significant advantage over brachytherapy is the creation of a discrete ablative lesion allowing for improved observation of the treatment effect in real time. Early outcomes using this modality were worrisome with major complications reported, such as urethrocutaneous and rectourethral fistula prior to refinement of the technique. Further refinements in monitoring, urethral warming, and probe technology have brought about resurgence of interest in this technique. A prospective randomized trial comparing cryoablation to external beam radiotherapy found near equivalent disease-free survival at 8 years, and a significantly higher negative biopsy rate

in the cryoablation arm [26]. The major disadvantage to whole-gland cryotherapy was the morbidity profile, most notably with respect to erectile dysfunction.

Other whole-gland interventional techniques have included HIFU and vascular targeted photodynamic therapy. The study with the longest follow-up for patients treated with HIFU reported an actuarial disease-free survival of 59% using the ASTRO-Phoenix definition of biochemical outcome at a mean follow-up of 6.4 years in patients with low- and intermediate-risk disease. Cancer-specific survival was reported at 98% and overall survival 83% [27]. By comparison, another series reported a biochemical disease-free survival of 78% at 5 years [28]. Photodynamic therapy (PDT) was first introduced in urology as treatment for superficial bladder cancer [29]. Although first described as a treatment for localized prostate cancer in 1990 [30]; there is renewed interest due to the introduction of novel photosensitizers. The therapeutic effect of these compounds is theoretically limited to the vascular bed and, therefore, should be thought of as vascular-targeted photodynamic therapy (VTP). Phase I/II studies are currently underway assessing the efficacy of this modality in patients who have failed radiation and in low-risk primary disease [31].

Currently, there is considerable interest in focal, rather than whole-gland therapy. Focal therapy involves the local application of therapy to a specific focus under real-time image guidance (Figure 1.2). Therapy can be applied ranging from a small focus to subtotal ablation thereby decreasing morbidity [32,33]. Several factors have to be considered before focal therapy can be considered as an option for early

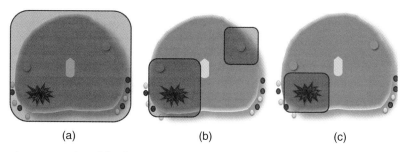

(a)          (b)          (c)

**Fig 1.2** Diagrammatic representation of the changing paradigm in treatment of prostate cancer from whole-gland radical therapy (a) (using surgery, radiation therapy, HIFU, cryotherapy) to focal therapy in which all lesions are targeted individually (b) (using HIFU, cryotherapy, photodynamic therapy, photothermal therapy) or the largest index lesion targeted (c). The avoidance of the neurovascular bundles, external sphincter, bladder neck, and rectal mucosa from the treatment zone is likely to lead to less impact on genitourinary function. (Images provided courtesy of Hashim U Ahmed, University College London, UK.)

stage prostate cancer. First, prostate cancer can be a multifocal disease. However, large studies have shown that between 10% and 44% of prostatectomy specimens harbor unilateral or unifocal tumor. There is growing evidence that the majority of progression is driven by the size ($>0.5$ cm$^3$) and grade (Gleason $\geq 7$) of the index tumor [34], and that 80% of multifocal tumors outside the index lesion have a volume of $<0.5$ cm$^3$, making their clinical significance questionable. Some have argued that tumors $<0.5$ cm$^3$ may not need immediate treatment [35], thus creating a large population of patients that could benefit from focal ablation of the index or unifocal tumor with subsequent surveillance of the smaller "insignificant" lesions if present. A recent study characterized 1000 RP specimens from men with early stage prostate cancer who had undergone surgery and found that 18% had unilateral disease. In those with unilateral disease, the largest focus of cancer (index lesion) contained 80% of the total cancer present and of the cases with extracapsular extension, 90% of the tumors outside the capsule were associated with the index lesion [36].

If focal therapy is to be considered, accurate localization of the index tumor is imperative. Both improved biopsy, as well as imaging techniques, may allow for clear localization. Small prostate masses ($<1$ cm) have in the past proven to be very difficult to accurately detect radiographically; forcing most clinicians to rely on prostate biopsy to derive location and volume information. This trend is rapidly changing as will be described in subsequent chapters (Figure 1.3). Crawford has described the use of transperineal-guided prostate biopsy at 5-mm intervals (mean of 80.7 cores/prostate) and has shown 95% sensitivity for detecting clinically significant ($\geq 0.5$ cm$^3$) cancers [37].

## Morbidity

Overall, each of the whole-gland radical treatments can be associated with significant morbidity. Radiotherapy causes short-term moderate bowel and/or urinary toxicity in almost 50% with most having limited toxicity [38]. Five to twenty percent of patients with bowel toxicity have long-term persistence. Select surgical series report as high as 27% risk of chronic urinary symptoms while both radiotherapy and surgery have a near 50% reduction in sexual function, though

the reports are widely variable [39]. In addition, newer techniques have shown very little change in the toxicity profiles [40,41]. A recent analysis evaluating outcomes from minimally invasive (laparoscopic and robotic) and open prostatectomy showed that incontinence and erectile dysfunction may be slightly higher in the minimally invasive group [42]. These and similar series should be the standard for which minimally invasive interventional techniques are compared.

## Comparison with conservative management

Prostate cancer has significant mortality worldwide [43], yet has an incidence-to-mortality ratio of 8.6 in the United States and 3.0 in the United Kingdom [44]. Such differences may reflect many factors, one of which is screening rates. This is supported by multiple autopsy series showing that 30%–40% of men suffering nonprostate cancer related deaths harbor prostate cancer [45]. Additionally, incidental prostate cancer is found in 23%–45% of men undergoing cystoprostatectomy for the management of bladder cancer [46]. Most recommend early treatment of prostate cancer, although the trend may be changing in recent years as more compelling data becomes available for surveillance.

Active surveillance with the potential for delayed therapy must incorporate several assumptions: (1) markers for disease progression are reliable, (2) patients are compliant, (3) the cancer will not progress at a speed exceeding follow-up windows, and (4) patients accept the potential anxiety associated with untreated cancer.

Surveillance, in lieu of immediate treatment, is likely to become a more popular option for many reasons. A meta-analysis including 828 patients on surveillance protocols found the risk of metastasis at 10 years after diagnosis in those with well-differentiated tumors to be 19% and cancer-specific mortality 13% [47]. Albertsen and colleagues assessed 767 patients managed conservatively and showed that those with Gleason 6 or less tumors, had a cancer-specific mortality of approximately 30% at 15 years [48]. This is a historical series based on biopsies using sextant cores, and so will have included many men with higher risk disease that was under-sampled. Another often-quoted study by Johansson et al used to justify active treatment showed that cancer-specific survival dropped from 79% to 54% as patients managed conservatively

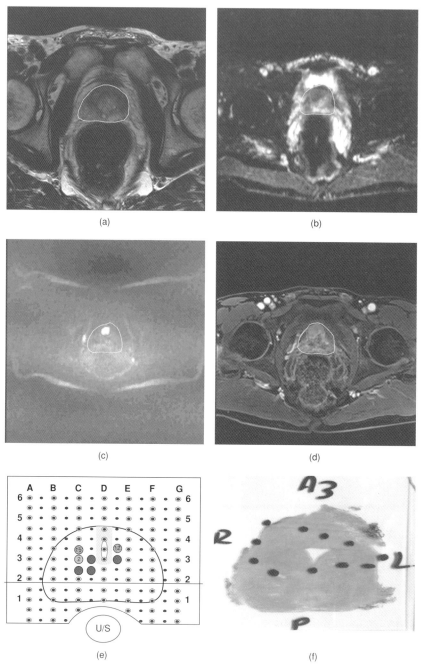

(a)

(b)

(c)

(d)

(e)

(f)

**Fig 1.3** Multiparametric MRI in a man with two previous negative prostate transrectal biopsies on a background of a rising PSA (3.6 ng/mL to5.8 ng/mL) and a positive family history. (a–d) All MRI sequences (T2W, ADC map and high *b*-value diffusion weighted, dynamic contrast enhancement) on a 1.5 T scanner demonstrate an anterior tumor. (e) This was confirmed on transperineal template biopsies (circles with lines and the circle with dots; numbers representing maximum cancer core length involvement). (f) The patient subsequently had surgery in which the tumor was again shown to be in the anterior transition zone. *See also plate 1.3.* (Images provided courtesy of Hashim U Ahmed, University College London, UK.)

were followed past 15 years [49]. Further evidence supporting active treatment is seen in a study describing 192 men who died of prostate cancer, 46% had early-stage tumors (T1–T2a) at the time of diagnosis, and 33% were Gleason ≤ 6 [50]. Finally, the Scandinavian Prostate Cancer Group conducted a randomized trial of patients with prostate cancer detected in the pre-PSA era treated by radical prostatectomy or watchful waiting, which revealed significant relative risk reductions in overall mortality, prostate cancer-specific mortality, metastasis, and local progression in the former group. Notably, only 12% had T1c and 20% had an initial PSA ≥ 20 [51].

A large population of patients are excluded from active surveillance protocols due to the following characteristics: PSA doubling time <3 years, PSA >10 ng/mL, tumor in >50% of any biopsy core, tumor present in >33% of all cores, and any pattern Gleason grade of 4 or 5. These strict criteria were relaxed in the Toronto active surveillance cohort of 229 men followed with intervention criteria for biopsy upgrading to Gleason grade ≥ 8 and /or PSA DT of ≤ 2 years. In this study 34% dropped out of surveillance due to: PSA DT ≤ 2 years (15%), histologic progression (4%), clinical progression (3%), and patient preference (12%) [42]. Furthermore, the PSA doubling time parameter in the Toronto protocol was changed to 3 years rather than 2 years in order to intervene earlier and because of concerns that more adverse PSA kinetics predicted poorer outcomes. The UCSF active surveillance series used more strict criteria and revealed a secondary treatment rate of 24% at 3-year median follow-up, though 37% met criteria for progression and 12% elected treatment without evidence of disease progression [52]. It must be noted however that of the patients in the Toronto active surveillance protocol only 3/331 (99% disease-specific survival) have died of their disease at a median follow-up of 7 years [53], and none have died of their disease in the UCSF series at a median follow-up of 3.6 years. Disease-specific survival remains 100% at 10-year follow-up in 42 patients.

Another consideration for those on active surveillance is the relatively large voluntary crossover rate in most series as exemplified by the 12% rate in the Toronto series, and another study finding 45% of men on a surveillance protocol seeking therapy prior to evidence of progression [54]. When strict criteria are applied to candidates for surveillance, Epstein et al found that pathologically indolent disease was present at prostatectomy in 79% of patients [55]. Unfortunately, when these same criteria were examined retrospectively in the large, community and university based cohort of the CaPSURE database, only 16.4% (310/1886) of patients met the criteria. And of those patients, only 9% (28/310) chose a surveillance strategy [56]. Thus, between the years 1999 and 2004, only 1.5% of patients in this cohort were actually undergoing surveillance in what appeared to be a very appropriate profile for such therapy.

## Cost

The cancer-attributable costs associated with the first 6 months of treatment in 1999 demonstrated the costs of radical prostatectomy to be $8113, external beam radiotherapy $6116, and brachytherapy $7596 [57]. Another study from the same time period found mean hospital charges of $5660 for radical prostatectomy compared to $4150 for cryotherapy. Most of the cost savings for cryotherapy exists in hospitalization costs of $2348 for radical prostatectomy and $682 for cryotherapy [58]. Most cost analyses do not take into account lost productivity from multiple treatment visits required for radiation therapy or postoperative visits and urethral catheter time associated with radical surgery. Cryotherapy, brachytherapy, and other forms of minimally invasive interventional techniques may have the advantage of being performed in a single, outpatient setting and could reduce treatment costs substantially.

## Conclusions

Due to widespread screening and imaging, many prostate and renal malignancies are smaller and more focal in nature. Given the stage and tumor volume migration that has occurred for these malignancies, functional as well as cancer-specific outcomes are being assessed. Minimally invasive interventional therapies provide an avenue for cancer control that may well fit the biologic aggressiveness of such early disease. Evidence is growing that novel techniques, when applied to appropriate patients, may offer similar disease control as the current "gold standards" while the treatment morbidity is considerably less in properly selected patients. Further development of minimally invasive interventional techniques is the next logical step in this progression. Refinement and longer term assessment of the techniques described (and new ones to be developed) are critical, if we are to better understand the role of such therapy in the management of patients with renal and prostate cancers. If minimally invasive interventional techniques prove efficacious in the long-term, they may very well be the preferred treatment modality for many patients. Given the rapid and impressive growth in our understanding of the biological processes unique to individual cancers and patients, targeted therapy, wether applied locallly, regionally or systemically will play an increasingly important role in the management of patients with a variety of cancers.

## References

1. Sandra MG et al (2008) Quality of life and satisfaction with outcome among prostate-cancer survivors. N Engl J Med 358: 1250.
2. American Cancer Society (2008) *Cancer Facts & Figures 2008*, Atlanta: American Cancer Society.
3. Frank I et al (2005) Independent validation of the 2002 American Joint Committee on cancer primary tumor classification for renal cell carcinoma using a large, single institution cohort. J Urol 173: 1889.
4. Gill IS et al (2007) Comparison of 1,800 laparoscopic and open partial nephrectomies for single renal tumors. J Urol 178: 41.
5. Bandi G, Hedican SP, Nakada SY (2008) Current practice patterns in the use of ablation technology for the management of small renal masses at academic centers in the United States. Urology 71: 113.
6. Park S, Cadeddu JA, Shingleton WB (2007) Oncologic outcomes for ablative therapy of kidney cancer. Curr Urol Rep 8: 31.
7. Kunkle DA, Egleston BL, Uzzo RG (2008) Excise, ablate or observe: the small renal mass dilemma – a meta-analysis and review. J Urol 179: 1227.
8. Smith S, Gillams A (2008) Imaging appearances following thermal ablation. Clin Radiol 63: 1.
9. Weight C et al (2008) Correlation of radiographic imaging and histopathology following cryoablation and radiofrequency ablation for renal tumors. J Urol 179: 1277.
10. Turna B et al (2008) Risk factor analysis of postoperative complications in laparoscopic partial nephrectomy. J Urol 179: 1289.
11. Desai MM, Aron M, Gill IS (2005) Laparoscopic partial nephrectomy versus laparoscopic cryoablation for the small renal tumor. Urology 66: 23.
12. Johnson DB et al (2004) Defining the complications of cryoablation and radio frequency ablation of small renal tumors: a multi-institutional review. J Urol 172: 874.
13. Lucas SM et al (2008) Renal function outcomes in patients treated for renal masses smaller than 4cm by ablative and extirpative techniques. J Urol 179: 75.
14. Somani BK et al (2007) Image guided biopsy diagnosed renal cell carcinoma. Critical appraisal of technique and long-term follow-up. Eur Urol 51: 1289.
15. Hollingsworth JM et al (2006) Rising incidence of small renal masses: a need to reassess treatment effect. J Natl Cancer Inst 98: 1331.
16. Chawla SN et al (2006) The natural history of observed enhancing renal masses: Meta-analysis and review of the world literature. J Urol 175: 425.
17. Volpe A et al (2004) The natural history of incidentally detected small renal masses. Cancer 100(4): 738.
18. Lang K et al (2007) The burden of illness associated with renal cell carcinoma in the United States. Urol Oncol 25: 368.
19. Pandharipande PV et al (2008) Radiofrequency ablation versus nephron-sparing surgery for small unilateral renal cell carcinoma: Cost-effectiveness analysis. Radiology 248(1): 169.
20. Matin SF et al (2006) Residual and recurrent disease following renal energy ablative therapy: a multi-institutional study. J Urol 176: 1973.
21. Cooperberg MR et al (2004) The changing face of low-risk prostate cancer: trends in clinical presentation and primary management. J Clin Oncol 22: 2141.
22. Mouraviev V et al (2007) Analysis of laterality and percentage of tumor involvement in 1386 prostatectomized specimens for selection of unilateral focal cryotherapy. Technol Cancer Res Treat 6: 91.
23. Barringer B (1917) Radium in the treatment of carcinoma of the bladder and prostate: review of one year's work. JAMA 68: 1227.
24. Zelefsky MJ et al (2007) Multi-institutional analysis of long-term outcome for stages T1-T2 prostate cancer treated with permanent seed implantation. Int J Radiation Oncology Biol Phys 67(2): 327.
25. Ragde H et al (2000) Modern prostate brachytherapy. CA-Cancer J Clin 50: 380.
26. Donnelly BJ et al (2010) A randomized trial of external beam radiotherapy versus cryoablation in patients with localized prostate cancer. Cancer. 116(2): 323–330.
27. Blana A et al (2008) First analysis of the long-term results with transrectal HIFU in patients with localized prostate cancer. Eur Urol 53(6): 1194.
28. Uchida T et al (2006) Five years experience of transrectal high-intensity focused ultrasound using the Sonablate device in the treatment of localized prostate cancer. Int J Urol 13: 228.

29. Pinthus JH et al (2006) Photodynamic therapy for urological malignancies: past and current approaches. J Urol 175: 1201.

30. Windahl T, Andersson SO, Lofgren L (1990) Photodynamic therapy of localized prostate cancer. Lancet 336: 1139.

31. Trachtenberg J et al (2008) Vascular-targeted photodynamic therapy (padoporfin, WST09) for recurrent prostate cancer after failure of external beam radiotherapy: a study of escalating light doses. BJU Int 102: 556.

32. Onik G et al (2008) The "male lumpectomy": Focal therapy for prostate cancer using cryoablation results in 48 patients with a least 2-year follow-up. Urol Oncol 26: 500.

33. Ahmed HU et al (2007) Will focal therapy become a standard of care for men with localized prostate cancer? Nat Clin Prac Oncol 4(11): 632.

34. Vis AN et al (2007) Should we replace the Gleason score with the amount of high-grade prostate cancer? Eur Urol 51: 931.

35. Ahmed HU (2009) The index lesion and the origin of prostate cancer. N Engl J Med 361(17): 1704–1706.

36. Polascik TJ, Mouraviev V (2008) Focal therapy for prostate cancer. Curr Opin Urol 18: 269.

37. Crawford ED et al (2005) Clinical staging of prostate cancer: a computer-simulated study of transperineal prostate biopsy. BJU Int 96(7): 999.

38. Giordano SH et al (2006) Late gastrointestinal toxicity after radiation of prostate cancer. Cancer 107: 423.

39. White WM et al (2008) Quality of life in men with locally advanced adenocarcinoma of the prostate: an exploratory analysis using data from the CaPSURE database. J Urol 180(6): 2409.

40. Hu JC et al (2009) Comparative effectiveness of minimally invasive vs open radical prostatectomy. JAMA 302(14): 1557–1564.

41. Khoo VS (2005) Radiotherapeutic techniques for prostate cancer, dose escalation and brachytherapy. Clin Oncol 17: 560.

42. Klotz L et al (2010) Clinical results of long-term follow-up of a large, active surveillance cohort with localized prostate cancer. J Clin Oncol 28(1): 126–131.

43. Marugame T, Mizuno S (2005) Comparison of prostate cancer mortality in five countries: France, Italy, Japan, UK and USA from the WHO mortality database (1960–2000). Jpn J Clin Oncol 35: 690.

44. Kamangar F, Dores GM, Anderson WF (2006) Patterns of cancer incidence, mortality, and prevalence across five continents: defining priorities to reduce cancer disparities in different geographic regions of the world. J Clin Oncol 24: 2137.

45. Sakr WA et al (1993) The frequency of carcinoma and intraepithelial neoplasia of the prostate in young male patients, J Urol 150: 379.

46. Revelo MP et al (2004) Incidence and location of prostate and urethral carcinoma in prostates from cystoprostatectomies: implications for possible apical sparing surgery. J Urol 171: 646.

47. Chodak GW et al (1994) Results of conservative management of clinically localized prostate cancer. N Engl J Med 330(4): 242.

48. Albertsen PC, Hanley JA, Fine J (2005) 20-year outcomes following conservative management of clinically localized prostate cancer. JAMA 293: 2095.

49. Johansson JE et al (2004) Natural history of early, localized prostate cancer. JAMA 291: 2713.

50. Thompson KE et al (2005) Prognostic features in men who died of prostate cancer. J Urol 174: 553.

51. Bill-Axelson A et al (2005) Radical prostatectomy vs. Watchful waiting in early prostate cancer. N Engl J Med 352: 1997.

52. Dall'Era MA et al (2008) Active surveillance for the management of prostate cancer in a contemporary cohort. Cancer 112(12): 2664.

53. Klotz L (2008) What is the best approach for screen-detected low volume cancers? – The case for observation. Urol Oncol 26: 495.

54. El-Geneidy M et al (2004) Delayed therapy with curative intent in a contemporary prostate cancer watchful-waiting cohort. BJU Int 93: 510.

55. Epstein JI, et al (1994) Pathologic and clinical findings to predict tumor extent of non-palpable (stage T1c) prostate cancer. JAMA 271: 368.

56. Barocas DA et al (2008) What percentage of patients with newly diagnosed carcinoma of the prostate are candidates for surveillance? An analysis of the CaPSURE database. J Urol 180: 1330.

57. Zeliadt SB et al (2007) Trends in treatment costs for localized prostate cancer: the healthy screenee effect. Med Care 45: 154.

58. Benoit RM, Cohen JK, Miller RJ Jr (1998) Comparison of the hospital costs for radical prostatectomy and cryosurgical ablation of the prostate. Urology 52(5): 820.

# 2 Brachytherapy for prostate cancer

*John Sylvester*[1] *and Peter Grimm*[2]
[1]Lakewood Ranch Oncology Center, Bradenton, FL, USA
[2]Prostate Cancer Treatment Center, Seattle, WA, USA

## Brief history

• In 1903 Alexander Graham Bell wrote, "... there is no reason why a tiny fragment of radium sealed in a fine glass tube should not be inserted into the very heart of the cancer, thus acting directly upon the disease material. Would it not be worthwhile making experiments along this line?"
• In 1910 Hugh Hampton Young (pioneer of the radical prostatectomy) used intraurethral-radium for the treatment of prostate cancer, with encouraging results. Although known for the perineal radical prostatectomy, he performed only 25 radical prostatectomies from 1906 to 1927. He performed approximately 500 prostate brachytherapy procedures from 1915 to 1927.
• In 1930 Flocks first injected radioactive gold into the prostate for the treatment of cancer.
• In the early 1970s Willet Whitmore and Basil Hilaris at Memorial Sloan-Kettering Cancer Center (MSKCC), New York, were the first physicians to perform I-125 prostate seed implants. An abdominal incision was used to implant the seeds directly into the exposed gland.
• In 1983 Hans Holm, University of Copenhagen, Denmark, was the first physician to perform the "closed" or "nonsurgical" implant method, which utilized transrectal ultrasound (TRUS).
• In 1985 Haakon Ragde, John Blasko, and Peter Grimm, further modified Holm's approach in Seattle, Washington.

• In 1989 John Blasko, Peter Grimm, Haakon Ragde, and John Sylvester started regular training programs in the Seattle technique at Northwest Hospital in Seattle.
• In the 1990s a dramatic increase in permanent seed implantation occurred in the United States. Significant advances occurred in dosimetry, patient selection, and implant technique including stranded and linked technologies.
• Seed implantation is linked with dosimetry and patient selection. The past 23 years have led to a continual refinement in patient selection, dosimetry, and technique.

## Introduction

Brachytherapy has been used as definitive treatment of prostate cancer since the early 1900s. One of the earliest reported experiences was a series of 100 patients treated by Denning in 1922 [1]. Due to inaccurate dosimetry in that era, complication rates were significant and cancer control rates poor. Brachytherapy lost ground to surgery as surgical and anesthetic technique advanced. During the 1960s to 1990s megavoltage external beam radiotherapy (EBRT) became more popular, as it had relatively fewer side effects than surgery and similar survival rates.

In the late 1960s Carlton and Scardino used permanent interstitial radioactive gold-198 combined with EBRT [2]. Memorial Sloan-Kettering Cancer Center

*Interventional Techniques in Uro-oncology*, First Edition. Edited by Hashim Uddin Ahmed, Manit Arya, Peter T. Scardino & Mark Emberton.  © 2011 Blackwell Publishing Ltd. Published 2011 by Blackwell Publishing Ltd.

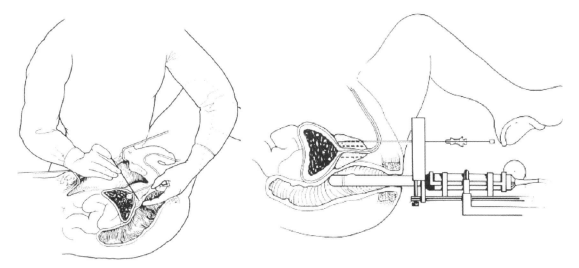

**Fig 2.1** Old open retropubic approach (a) and modern ultrasound-guided transperineal approach (b).

(MSKCC) pioneered the use of radioactive iodine-125 (I-125) seeds [3]. Using an open laparotomy retropubic approach, the seeds were placed directly into the surgically exposed prostate (Figure 2.1a). To achieve a uniform distribution of dose a nomogram table was used to calculate the appropriate number of seeds, of a given seed activity, for various prostate volumes. Those patients in whom orthogonal x-rays revealed a high-quality seed distribution and dose (matched peripheral dose of >140 Gy) achieved a local control rate of 60%. However, in those with a matched peripheral dose of <120 Gy the local control was only 20%. Hilaris and colleagues reported a 70% 15-year cause-specific survival in stage B1 patients treated with high-quality I-125 seed implantation [4–10]. These results were at least as good as the best contemporary surgical and EBRT series in that era. However, limited technology in the 1970s prevented this retropubic technique from consistently achieving high-quality implants. This inconsistency contributed to permanent seed brachytherapy falling out of favor.

The 1980s saw the introduction of multiple technologic advances that led to the rebirth of prostate brachytherapy [11]. Puthawala et al at Long Beach Memorial Hospital in Southern California, pioneered transperineal low-dose rate temporary interstitial brachytherapy (performed at time of open laparotomy) combined with EBRT [12]. Martinez et al used a transperineal applicator to guide the placement of the radioactive implant [13]. In 1983 Holm

and colleagues were the first to perform I-125 seed implantation via a transperineal approach using transrectal ultrasound guidance for the placement of the sources [14]. This technique allowed for more accurate placement of radioactive seeds. In 1985 Blasko, Grimm, and Ragde pioneered preplanned transrectal ultrasound, template-guided transperineal permanent I-125 seed implant in the United States. Using improved technologic advancements, patient selection due to prostate-specific antigen (PSA) screening, and improved radiation treatment planning systems (Figure 2.1b) the group demonstrated that consistently high-quality implantation was achievable with appropriately staged patients and appropriate doses of radiation based on the MSKCC experience.

## Patient selection

There are three key issues involved in the selection of patients for ultrasound-guided permanent prostate implant (PPI): oncologic issues, technical issues, and toxicity issues. The patient should be a good candidate in all three for PPI to be an ideal management option.

### Oncologic issues

Oncologic issues deal with the extent of disease: local, regional, and distant. Patients with proven lymph node involvement (N1) or distant metastatic disease

(M1) are not going to benefit from the local control of PPI because they will not have any legitimate chance for cure. For PPI, this would exclude biopsy-proven pelvic lymph node and distal seminal vesicle involvement from being candidates for brachytherapy as monotherapy. Extracapsular extension does not exclude a patient from brachytherapy, as the treatment includes a margin around the prostate. In palliative situations where local disease progression is causing symptoms, the role of brachytherapy for control of local symptoms of disease progression are limited and more easily treated (with less toxicity) by surgical procedures, such as transurethral resection of the prostate (TURP) or transurethral laser therapy, androgen ablation or external beam radiation therapy, or a combination of these.

The ideal candidate for I-125, palladium-103 (Pd-103) PPI, or cesium-131 (Cs-131) monotherapy is a patient with a low risk of microscopic extension beyond 1–3 mm. The risk of microscopic disease extension outside the prostate has been reported by Partin and colleagues [15–17]. The Partin tables correlate the risk of extraprostatic extension (EPE), seminal vesicle (SV) involvement, and lymph node (LN) involvement with the pretreatment biopsy Gleason score, clinical stage by rectal examination, and PSA level. The nomogram was based on the pathologic examination of 5730 radical prostatectomy specimens. The original work has recently been updated with results showing a reduced risk of extraprostatic disease extension for each of the categories, as a result of earlier disease detection in the current PSA era [18].

Some patients with documented EPE at radical prostatectomy have a low biochemical relapse free survival (BRFS) rate and others a high BRFS. Davis [19], Sohayda [20], and Chao [21] separately published the radial extension of disease outside of the prostate capsule, as measured in millimeters on postoperative radical prostatectomy specimens. They independently demonstrated that the risk of extension beyond 1–3 mm is low in the low- and low- to intermediate-risk cohorts. PPI monotherapy can be considered in these cases since the prescription dose margin of PPI is frequently on the order of 5–8 mm.

Epstein et al [22] showed that some radical prostatectomy patients with pathologically documented EPE had lower BRFS compared to those without EPE. The risk of failure was also correlated to the pathologic Gleason score, LN and SV status. Those with EPE and negative SV, negative LN, and Gleason score 2–6 had a 75% BRFS, whereas those with EPE and Gleason score 7 had only a 50% BRFS. Thus, some patients with EPE but favorable pathologic features (Gleason score 2–6) likely have less risk of disease beyond the surgical margin, and therefore are good candidates for local treatments.

A low-risk prostate cancer category can be defined as those with Gleason score 2–6, PSA ≤10 ng/mL, and stage cT1 a-cT2 a [23–25]. These patients have a low risk of significant EPE, and experience excellent BRFS with seed implantation monotherapy with either Pd-103 or I-125 [26–31]. Some physicians perform combined EBRT + PPI on all patients, even low-risk group patients, but the BRFS in these studies are not superior to those using PPI alone [32–33]. An exception to using PPI monotherapy in low-risk patients may involve patients with a high percentage of positive biopsies. D'Amico et al [34] demonstrated that low-risk patients undergoing radical prostatectomy, who had a high percentage of positive biopsy cores, suffered a significantly higher biochemical failure rate than those with a low percentage of positive biopsy cores. Whether this is an independent risk factor in PPI patients has yet to be proven.

Few studies have many patients in the high-risk group treated by monotherapy. The initial PPI experience of D'Amico at the Hospital of the University of Pennsylvania showed poor BRFS with the high-risk patients treated with monotherapy, but the quality of these initial implants is in question because of learning-curve issues, the relative lack of postoperative CT dosimetry, and surprisingly poorer results in their intermediate-risk patients, as compared to contemporary reports from the New York and Seattle groups [24,35]. Data from Seattle with Pd-103 monotherapy showed better results than those published with three-dimensional conformal therapy (3D-CRT) or surgery, but it was a small number of patients and has not yet been duplicated by others [25]. Data reported from Mount Sinai Medical Center demonstrated promising results with trimodality therapy, including neoadjuvant, concurrent, and adjuvant androgen deprivation therapy, external beam radiation therapy (seminal vesicles plus prostate), and seed implant boost [36]. The standard brachytherapy treatment of high-risk disease, at this time, is EBRT + seed implant boost with I-125, Pd-103, or Cs-131 with or without hormone therapy. Long-term (15-year) BRFS outcomes were published by Sylvester et al and showed a rate of 67.8% BRFS in high-risk patients treated by 45-Gy EBRT followed by Pd-103 or I-125 boost [37].

While monotherapy is generally recommended for low-risk patients and combined therapy for high-risk patients, the choice of mono versus combined therapy is more difficult for men with intermediate-risk disease. Some studies show excellent 5- and 10-year BRFS with PPI monotherapy, whereas others (usually involving implants carried out during the initial learning curve) have not [24,25,30,37–40]. The Seattle group previously reported the outcomes of their intermediate-risk patients treated with PPI, with or without EBRT. The data did not show any statistically significant difference between the two regimens, but the patients treated with combined therapy had worse pretreatment risk factors and longer follow-up, yet enjoyed a 4% better BRFS (not statistically significant) [41]. In a recently published series, they showed that 9-year BRFS outcomes for intermediate-risk disease treated from 1998 to 2000 of 91.9% in both the seed monotherapy and the combination EBRT + seed implant boost cohorts (80 patients in each). This was not a randomized trial and selection bias favored the monotherapy cohort [42].

The intermediate-risk group is heterogeneous. The current definition in Seattle of a favorable intermediate-group subset, or "Low-Intermediate Risk Group", includes those patients with Gleason 3 + 4 = 7, ≤1/3 core biopsies positive, PSA ≤10 or Gleason 6 and PSA 10–15 ng/mL. This group will tend to have high biochemical control rates with PPI monotherapy provided the quality of implant is high and lateral margins generous (~5 mm). [43] Intermediate-risk patients with worse prognostic factors such as a high percentage of positive biopsies may be served best by EBRT plus PPI, but the data are not yet conclusive for this patient-risk cohort. There is an open randomized RTOG trial (P-0232) to determine the role of supplemental EBRT in the intermediate-risk cohort. Figure 2.2 shows the current treatment guidelines recommended by Seattle, which are consistent with those advocated by the American Brachytherapy Society [23].

## Technical issues

Technical issues need to be evaluated before a patient becomes a candidate for PPI. The preoperative plan-

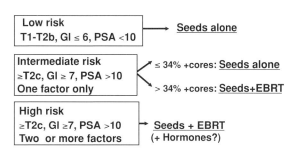

**Fig 2.2** Lakewood Ranch Oncology patient selection criteria.

ning TRUS prostate volume study can determine the gland volume and assess for the presence of pubic arch interference (PAI). If the prostate is much greater than 60 mL, the implant becomes technically more challenging. Large prostates also require more needles and seeds to achieve adequate dosimetric coverage. This increases the bleeding and trauma within and around the gland. Intraprostatic and periprostatic bleeding during the procedure can interfere with prostate visualization on ultrasound, and therefore negatively impact the quality of the implant. Prostate swelling and bleeding into the perineum can also move the prostate further away from the perineum and template, making it difficult to track the base position of the prostate. This can lead to underdosage of the base if one fails to adequately utilize sagittal imaging. In addition, the increase in trauma and swelling can increase the risk of acute urinary symptoms, including acute urinary retention. Thus, ideally the prostate should be less than 60–70 mL or reducible to this with androgen ablation, or a combination of an oral antiandrogen and a 5-alpha reductase inhibitor.

Significant PAI can prevent proper placement of needles, and therefore seeds, along the periphery of the gland. This in turn can decrease the margin of tissue treated anterior and laterally along the prostate capsule, and may underdose microscopic extracapsular extension. The technique for assessing this risk is discussed in the ultrasound-planning section. Evaluation of the pubic arch in every patient is necessary since occasionally a patient with an average size (30–40 mL) prostate will have significant PAI. If necessary, medical downsizing can be used. Traditionally, a combination of LHRH agonist depot and oral antiandrogen is used. Approximately 30%–40% volume downsizing effect can be seen after 3 months of total androgen deprivation therapy. Side effects include emotional lability, hot flashes, loss of libido, gynecomastia, fatigue, and weight gain. Merrick et al demonstrated that an antiandrogen and 5-alpha reductase inhibitor (bicalutamide and dutasteride in this case) can result in an approximate 33% volume reduction after 3 months of therapy, with less side effects than the LHRH agonist depot/antiandrogen combination [44].

A previous TURP may be a relative contraindication to PPI. Centers have noted higher rates of incontinence when TURP patients are treated with PPI [45,46,47]. This is especially true when a pure uniform loading dosimetric approach is used. The uniform loading dosimetric approach delivers a significantly higher dose to the urethra than the modern modified peripherally weighted dosimetry approach [48]. Some studies that report low incontinence rates in patients with a previous TURP suffer from short follow-up [48,49]. Some early series where this approach was taken showed that it took several years for incontinence to develop in TURP patients treated with the uniform loading dosimetry technique [46,50]. Therefore, patients with a history of a small TURP years ago should be counseled that their risk of incontinence may be higher than non-TURP patients. If an implant is performed in these patients the dosimetric plan should be more peripherally weighted. A large TURP defect is an absolute contraindication to PPI because there is not enough tissue to hold the radioactive sources for adequate dose delivery.

## Toxicity issues

Toxicity related risk factors are also important to consider before performing LDR brachytherapy. Patients with severe obstructive voiding symptoms, as defined by the international prostate symptom score (IPSS) questionnaire, urodynamic studies, and high postvoid residuals are at higher risk of experiencing greater acute urinary symptoms or temporary urinary retention postimplantation. Rarely, a TURP or urethrotomy may be required because of continued retention or obstructive symptoms. A TURP postimplantation can increase the risk for incontinence. Patients with high IPSS scores can become candidates for implantation if their urinary symptoms respond well to alpha-blockers alone or in combination with 5-alpha reductase inhibitors. If a patient is noted to have obstruction due to bladder neck contraction a transurethral

incision of the prostate (rather than resection) 6–12 weeks prior to implantation may decrease the risk of retention.

Inflammatory bowel disease historically has been considered a relative contraindication to radiation therapy, both for EBRT and brachytherapy. However, a retrospective study demonstrated that patients with Crohn's disease or ulcerative colitis did not have elevated rectal toxicity [51]. Nonetheless, patients with inflammatory bowel syndrome should undergo a colonoscopy to rule out active disease in the anterior rectum prior to implantation.

## Technique

### Dosimetry

The primary advantage of permanent seed implantation is the ability to deliver significantly higher doses of radiation to the prostate and the immediate margin laterally in a single outpatient setting. Multiple studies have reported that higher doses of radiation with different radiation modalities, delivered accurately to the prostate, result in superior BRFS [11,54–65,69]. While dose heterogeneity with brachytherapy is unavoidable due to the fact that individual radioactive sources (seeds) are emitting radiation separately, careful planning and execution can minimize hot or cold spots. Hot spots (areas of higher doses of radiation) occur when seeds are adjacent to each other, and cold spots occur if seeds are placed too far apart. The radiobiologic effective (RBE) dose of permanent seed implantation has been shown to be higher than EBRT approaches, such as 3D-CRT and intensity modulated radiation therapy (IMRT) [64,65,69]. Standardization of the prescription dose and careful planning is necessary to ensure reasonable dose distributions.

In the days of the retropubic implant, dose distribution was labeled a "matched peripheral dose" that described the dose delivered to a volume equal to an ellipsoid volume with the same average volume of the prostate being treated. This description was confusing. Treatment planning software has improved so that most radiation oncologists use minimal peripheral dose (MPD) to describe their prescription dose. The MPD describes the minimum dose delivered to the periphery of the target volume, which includes the prostate and a small margin of tissue. Most expert centers define the target volume to include an

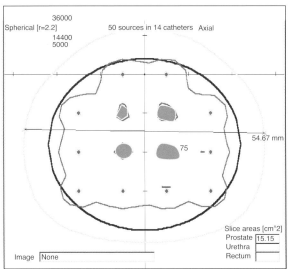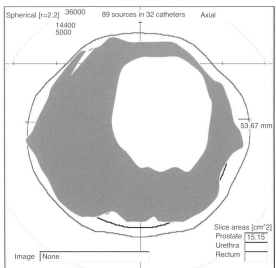

**Fig 2.3** Pure uniform loading (a) and pure peripheral loading (b). *See also plate 2.3.*

approximate 5-mm margin for low-risk disease, and slightly larger margin for more advanced cases.

The American Brachytherapy Society Prostate Low-Dose Rate Task Force recommends 145-Gy MPD for I-125 monotherapy implants and 125 Gy for Pd-103 monotherapy implants. In Lakewood Ranch Florida and Seattle, for I-125 145 Gy is used as monotherapy dose and 110 Gy for boost implants. For Pd-103 125 Gy as monotherapy and 90 Gy for boost implants. For 131-Cs 115 Gy as monotherapy and 84 Gy for boost implants. Due to inhomogeneity, two different centers may prescribe the same MPD but have significantly different internal isodose curve dosimetry. These variations are common because of philosophic differences from center to center in seed-loading patterns, seed activity, and dosimetry (uniform vs. peripheral vs. modified approaches).

From 1985 to 1991 the Seattle team used a pure uniform loading dosimetry approach. A relatively high number of low-activity seeds were evenly distributed throughout the prostate. Seed spacing was planned at 1 cm from seed center to seed center, and urethral visualization techniques were not employed. As a result, the central prostate doses were in excess of 150%–300% of the prescription dose (depending on gland size). Pure uniform loading had several drawbacks. There was a scalloping-in effect at the edges of the implant, which occasionally resulted in underdosing the edges of the gland, and there was an overdosing

of the central (urethral) portion of the gland (Figure 2.3a). These high central doses resulted in increased urinary morbidity in the patients who previously, or subsequently, underwent a TURP.

A pure peripheral loading implant in which the sources are placed just within the peripheral edge of the planning target volume was attempted by some centers to reduce the high dose to the urethra and reduce the overall number of seeds. This philosophy used a relatively lower number of higher activity seeds and, compared to uniform loading, had the advantage of delivering a lower dose to the urethra and thus less urinary toxicity (especially in TURP patients). However, it had significant disadvantages (Figure 2.3b) [48]. Even slight seed misplacement or migration of a few seeds resulted in hot spots in the rectum, neurovascular bundle, or urethra, risking greater complications, along with occasional cold areas within the peripheral zone of the prostate resulting in a higher risk of local and biochemical failure. Although using less seeds decreased the cost of the implant, these cases were more challenging technically. The early BRFS reports from centers using this technique were not as high as those achieved with the Seattle approach [40,51].

Modified uniform-peripheral loading or modified peripheral-uniform loading incorporates the advantages of both philosophies and minimizes the potential drawbacks. The vast majority of centers in

Derby Hospitals NHS Foundation Trust

Library and Knowledge Service

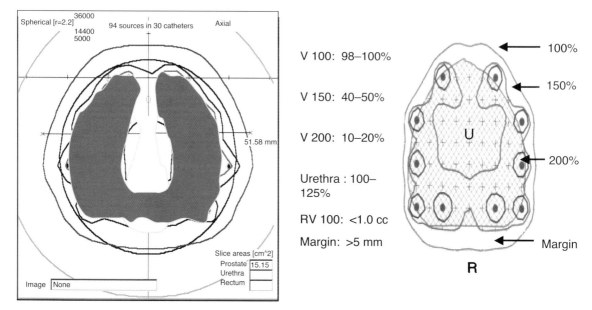

Fig 2.4 Modified uniform loading (a) and Seattle model (b). *See also plate 2.4.*

the United States currently use a modified uniform-peripheral loading approach [73]. This approach uses fewer seeds in the center of the gland and more in the periphery. Cold spots within the prostate are less likely than with a pure peripherally loaded implant, and the dose to the center of the gland is less than with a uniform loaded implant. The dosimetry outcomes are expected to result in less urethral toxicity and less local and biochemical failures, than a pure uniform or peripheral dosimetry approach, respectively (Figures 2.4a and 2.4b).

Clinical studies comparing dosimetric philosophies are lacking; and differences in skill from one brachytherapist to another, patient selection, and Gleason scoring from one center to the next also make it difficult to compare one dosimetric philosophy to another. Combining EBRT further complicates this analysis. While the vast majority of implant patients will fit into the modified peripheral loading philosophy, it is important to understand the anatomical relationship of the prostate and periprostatic structures, in addition to any predisposing conditions may have an effect on treatment planning. For example, a TURP patient with intermediate-risk disease for which a combination of EBRT and PPI may be planned, may require a more peripherally weighted implant. The addition of EBRT probably works as a "radia-

tion spackle" and fill in potential cold areas, with the peripheral loading decreasing the urethral dose and potentially reducing the risk of urethral and urinary complications.

When a brachytherapist speaks of "urethral sparing" he/she really means avoiding urethral "over-dosage" rather than "sparing" the urethra from the prescription dose. The dose the urethra typically receives when urethral "sparing" is used is 100%–140% of the prescription dose. Currently, most centers use TRUS ultrasound preplanning (in the clinic or the operating room [OR]), and a fusion of the Manchester (peripheral loading) and Quimby (uniform loading) systems to develop a modified uniform-peripheral loaded implant plan, and then reproduce that plan in the OR under ultrasound guidance [74]. This is consistent with the ABS recommendations [23].

Some centers have documented difficulties in achieving excellent postoperative dosimetry with the preplan technique, yet have done well with the real-time technique [74]. Sylvester and Grimm recently reported on 1131 consecutive patients using a preplan, preloaded needle approach. They demonstrated excellent coverage of the prostate in all but one patient with no rectal overdoses (RV 100 >1.0 cc) [75]. Reported improvement in dosimetry with the real-time technique may be the result of a learning curve effect, quality of the preplanning TRUS volume study or individual physician strengths or weaknesses in performing the procedure rather than a true technique effect. It is probably true to say that there is no one "right" way to perform prostate brachytherapy. Some will excel with the "preplan" technique, others with the "real-time" technique, and yet others with a hybrid between the two. All centers should have adequate postimplant quality assurance evaluation programs to evaluate their techniques and planning philosophies. Virtually all centers currently use ultrasound to guide needle placement in the OR, and postoperative CT or MRI for postoperative dosimetry. This allows one to evaluate the quality of the implants, thus optimizing and improving subsequent implant quality.

## Isotope selection

Recognizing that Pd-103, I-125 , and Cs-131have different photon energies, activities, and half-lives, different prescription doses are used in order to achieve similar radiobiologic effects. Much is written about isotope selection because of these differences, but Pd-103, I-125, and Cs-131 isotopes are all very low energy level sources (21 keV, 28 keV, and 30 keV, respectively). They are all prescribed to a very high biological effective dose compared to 3D-CRT and IMRT. Not surprisingly, since the prescription doses are designed to be radiobiologically identical, there is no convincing clinical evidence that one isotope is superior to the other in terms of RFS or toxicity. The Seattle team usually use I-125 for monotherapy cases (ABS Low-Risk Group), and Pd-103 90-Gy implant with 45-Gy IMRT with gold fiducial or Calypso™ 4D real-time Image Guided Radiation Therapy (IGRT) tracking for intermediate- and high-risk patients. In Lakewood Ranch Sylvester currently used IMRT with cone-beam CT guidance, and a 108Gy I-125 boost, in patients receiving combined therapy. I-125, Pd-103, or Cs-131 can be used for monotherapy or in combination with EBRT. There is no significant data showing one isotope to be superior to another in terms of RFS or long-term toxicity.

The method of modified peripheral loading incorporates a plan for a significant percentage of seeds (20%–40% depending on prostate size) being placed outside the prostate, especially at the base and apex. EPE is usually on the order of 1–3 mm for low-risk and favorable intermediate-risk disease. The treatment

**Table 2.1** Day 1 postoperative CT dosimetry results.

| Isotope | Monotherapy | Boost |
|---------|-------------|-------|
| I-125 | 0.326–0.414 mCi | 0.27–0.326 mCi |
| Pd-103 | 1.5–1.8 mCi | 1.0–1.2 mCi |
| Cs-131 | 1.9–2.0 U | 1.5–1.6 U |
| | (1.5–1.6 mCi) | (1.18–1.26 mCi) |

margin typically encompasses the prostate, the proximal 1 cm of the seminal vesicles plus 4–8 mm of periprostatic tissue laterally and anteriorly. For unfavorable intermediate-risk patients, 45-Gy EBRT will aid in covering the periprostatic tissue, and importantly, the seminal vesicles. The typical seed activity used at the Lakewood Ranch Oncology Center is described in Table 2.1. A higher activity could be used if less seeds and needles are required to minimize trauma to the gland.

## Transrectal ultrasound volume study

Patients undergo a TRUS study just prior to or after initial consultation. A high-quality TRUS at 5-mm transverse images from base to apex allows for accurate dosimetric planning. Important elements also include obtaining a clear sagittal image that simultaneously shows the base and the apex in order to measure the midsagittal length of the prostate. This allows for an accurate determination of the length of the gland, which in turn determines the number of seeds in each centrally placed preloaded needle. The transverse image of the prostate is centered on the brachytherapy grid in midgland with the posterior row ~1–2 mm anterior to the posterior capsule of the prostate. The base is identified in transverse and sagittal imaging planes. Then individual transverse images are obtained from the base to the apex in 5-mm increments. The total number of images obtained will be equal to the length of the prostate in centimeters times 2, plus 1. For example, a 4.0 cm long gland will have 9 (= 4 × 2 + 1) transverse images.

It is ideal to obtain these images without distorting the shape of the prostate with the ultrasound probe. Planning with a distorted gland will result in incorrect needle coordinates and/or incorrect numbers of seeds per needle on the dosimetric preplan. One needs to apply sufficient pressure on the gland with the ultrasound probe to obtain a clear image of the gland

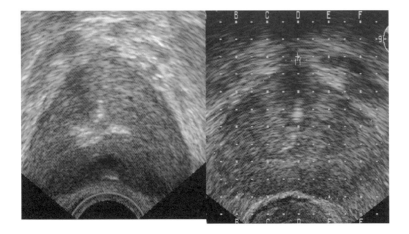

Fig 2.5 Distorted versus undistorted.

without distorting it with too much pressure (Figure 2.5). A gel-filled or water-filled condom can provide adequate contact with the rectal surface to obtain good, consistent images.

The angle of the probe at the TRUS is usually set at 10–15 degrees. If it is too steep, PAI at time of implant can occur. PAI can be evaluated during the TRUS by first scanning the pubic arch caudal to the apex of the gland, then outlining the arch on the ultrasound monitor with a dry-erase marker. Scanning at the largest transverse image of the prostate will demonstrate whether the pubic arch will interfere with needle placement (noticed as prostate tissue extending anterior to the drawn pubic arch). If interference exists, it may sometimes be overcome by altering the ultrasound probe angle to a flatter, lower angle (Figure 2.6). After the images are obtained (by the radiation oncologist, urologist, or ultrasound technician) the radiation oncologist should outline the target volume for dosimetry planning.

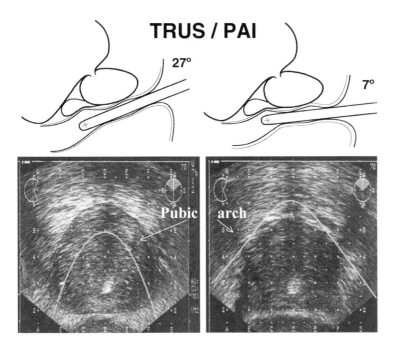

Fig 2.6 Adjustment for pubic arch.

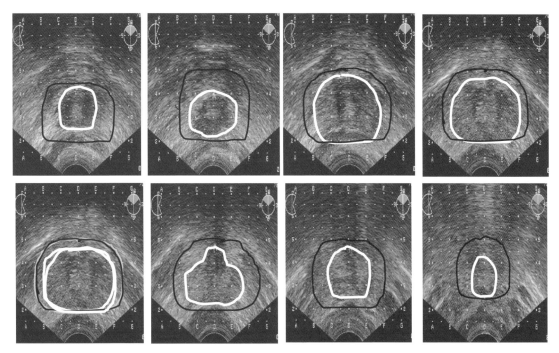

**Fig 2.7** Transrectal ultrasound volume study and target volumes.

## Target volumes

Target volumes include the prostate plus a margin. Target volumes are larger than the prostate to allow coverage of EPE and for slight prostate or seed movement. EPE is common and usually <3 mm. A ~5 mm posterolateral margin in the area of the neurovascular bundle (NVB) [19–22] can be drawn in all patients, as radical prostatectomy specimens have demonstrated most EPE occurring at or near the NVB. Margins are tighter posteriorly by the rectum and anteriorly at the dorsal venous plexus (Figure 2.7). Margins at the base and apex are typically wider to accommodate slight prostate movement or seed placement.

The dosimetry process involves creating a preplan that is simple and easy to reproduce in the OR. The number of needles that contain only 2 seeds can be limited to a minimum, and plans that have needle(s) with only 1 seed/needle should be avoided. The plans are typically symmetrical mirror images, from the left side of the prostate to the right. Special loading with a reduced number of seeds in the few centrally placed needles helps avoid overdosage to the urethra.

The learning curve generally favors initially using a higher number of seeds with a relatively low ac-

tivity per seed. As experience grows, one can gradually increase the activity per seed to a more moderate level. The combination of planning from an undistorted TRUS, a symmetrical plan that limits the number of needles, an approximate 5-mm PTV (laterally), and higher numbers of lower-activity seeds creates a preplan that is easy to reproduce in the OR.

This planning philosophy is robust enough that minor or moderate adjustments or changes in needle position in the OR will not negatively affect the quality of the postimplant CT dosimetry. For example, in January 2002, Sylvester altered the insert coordinate of the periurethral needles in an attempt to decrease the dose to the apical urethra. Moving the central needles from the preplanned positions of c3 to C3 and d3 to E3 kept the mean urethral dose to well under 150% of prescription dose without lowering the V100 or D90 (Table 2.2).

## Implant procedure

Anesthesia can be spinal or general. Spinal anesthesia is usually performed at large ambulatory centers, and general anesthesia at urology private offices in

| Year of treatment | 2000–2001<br>Needles in c3 and d3 | 2002–2003<br>Needles in C3 and E3 |
|---|---|---|
| Mean V100 | 92.6% | 91.8% |
| Mean D90 | 106.3% | 104.4% |
| Mean V150 | 57.1% | 50.7% $p<0.001$ |
| Number of images where urethra received > 150% of prescription dose | 331 | 38 $p<0.001$ |

Table 2.2 Day 1 postoperative CT dosimetry results.

outlying communities. Following anesthesia, the patient undergoes a perineal prep and ~200 cc of sterile water is instilled into the bladder. This expands the bladder and improves the contrast and visualization between the base of the prostate and the bladder on sagittal imaging. A 16 French gauge red Robinson catheter is attached to a syringe filled with aerated surgical lubrication jelly and then inserted a short distance into the membranous urethra. This aerated jelly is used intraoperatively to visualize the urethra.

The transrectal ultrasound probe is then inserted into the rectum at approximately the same angle and with the same pressure, as during the TRUS volume study. In transverse imaging the prostate is aligned in the center of the grid and the base and apex identified, and the length double checked. The template grid device is secured 1–2 finger widths away from the perineum.

The implant begins with insertion of needles into the anterior coordinates in transverse imaging. Individual preloaded needles (preloaded by the manufacturer or their preloading partner) are inserted into the prostate one row at a time. The transverse imaging plane 1.0 cm or 1.5 cm from the prostate base is used for initial targeting during these needle insertions. Insertion at this plane allows easier identification of the needle and avoids bladder trauma as well as recognition of prostate drift (due to small amounts of swelling and/or bleeding) (Figure 2.8).

After the needles are inserted into their planned x and y coordinates according to the preplan, the stepper is advanced to the planned needle insertion depth. The needle coordinate positions are then reconfirmed and adjusted, if necessary a few millimeters one direction or another to match the plan. The prostate shape can vary slightly from the preplan and the urethra may not be in the precise center row of the prostate (D row) requiring slight adjustments to avoid the urethra and

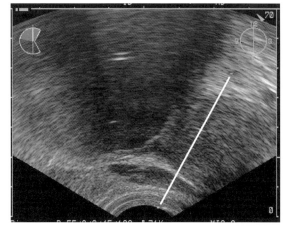

Fig 2.8 Insert needles while 1–1.5 cm from base.

assure placement to cover the prostate. The needles are oriented such that they are spaced in an even line at appropriate distances from each other (Figure 2.9). Rotating the probe and positioning the central on the first coordinate on the patient's right allows for imaging in the sagittal mode. The final millimeter or 2 of insertion depth is adjusted under sagittal imaging. A ruler measurement from the template to the needle hub is used to verify the depth (even when the needle is well visualized). This reference depth is recorded and may be used later if the needle visualization is difficult.

The seeds are deployed into the prostate by first advancing the needle to the proper depth and then advancing the first seed to the bevel of the needle. The proper depth of the stylet is determined by the number of seeds within the needle, shown on the preplan. For example, the stylet hub in a needle with 4 seeds will extend approximately 4.5 cm from the needle hub, and will need to be advanced to approximately 4 cm

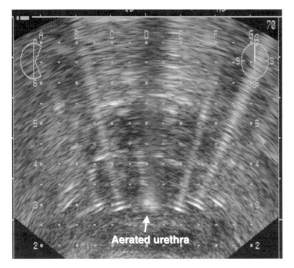

**Fig 2.9** Insert entire row of needles.

prior to insertion of the seeds. With the needle at correct depth and seed advanced to the tip of the needle deployment of the stranded, linked, or free seeds is carried out (Figure 2.10) under sagittal imaging. The seed closest to the base is imaged and verified to be at the proper depth by visualization on ultrasound. The probe is then rotated clockwise until the adjacent needle is seen and the process repeated.

Before moving to the next row of needles, the prostate position is checked and adjusted, so that the prostate position within the grid matches its pre-plan position. The next row of needles is inserted in the transverse image plane and seeds are deposited in the sagittal image plane as described. With each row, the ultrasound image seed position is compared to the preplanned needle positions (Figure 2.11). The seeds, linked or stranded, typically visualize well because the seeds orient more consistently than free seeds horizontally to the ultrasound plane, offering a large surface area for the ultrasound waves to interact with.

When inserting the periurethral needles, care is taken to keep these needles >5 mm from the urethra as visualized with the aid of aerated surgical lubrication jelly. The aerated jelly allows accurate visualization of the urethra, outlines the verumontanum and allows visualization of needles directly anterior to the urethra (Figure 2.12). The most posterior row of needles near the rectum require special attention to ensure adequate margin of tissue from the rectum. Typically the needles

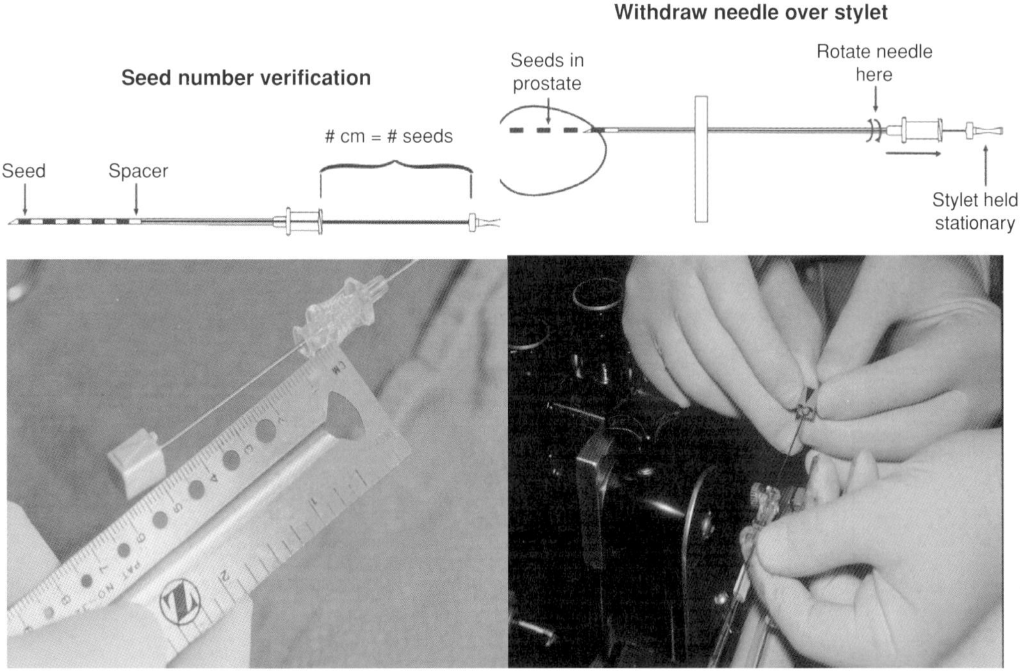

**Fig 2.10** Needle and seed stylet.

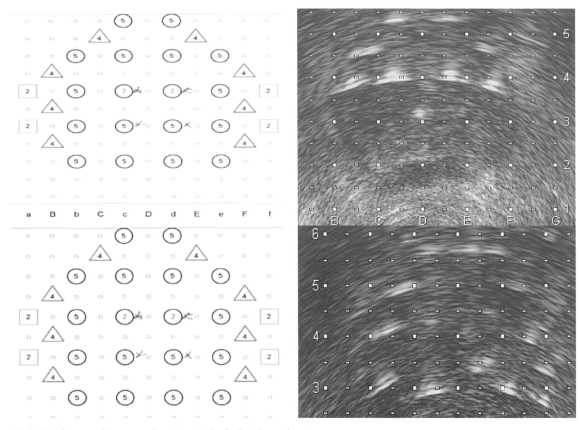

Fig 2.11 Ultrasound image seed position is checked with preplanning set-up.

are placed in their planned coordinates and directed 2–4 mm anterior to the posterior prostate capsule. This needle position is checked on both transverse and sagittal imaging. On sagittal imaging, the ultrasound probe is retracted from base to apex before deploying seeds to verify that no seeds will be posterior to the prostate or too close to the rectum. If the needle is too close to the rectum on sagittal imaging, the needle will be inserted into the template at a row 0.5 cm to 1.0 cm anterior to the planned coordinate and direct the needle to allow for a margin of tissue. This minor adjustment is quicker than repositioning the probe

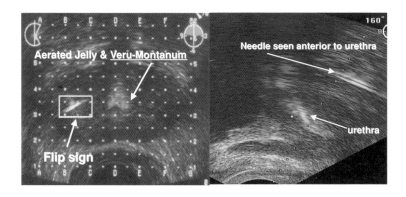

Fig 2.12 Urethral visualization: aerated KY$^{TM}$ Jelly.

angle or patient leg position, and has resulted in 100% success at limiting the RV100 to <1.0 cc without any underdosage of the posterior wall of the prostate [75].

At the end of the procedure, a fluoroscopic image for seed verification purposes is taken. An ultrasound survey from base to apex to identify any potential "cold" areas is performed between rows and at the end of the procedure. "Bonus" seeds are very rarely required with connected seeds. Postimplant radiation exposure measurements are taken in the OR. These measurements are of the radiation exposure at the anterior pelvic surface, and at 100 cm from the patient's surface. The OR room including staff, Foley catheter, and drainage bag are surveyed to avoid loss of radioactive seeds. A 3-way catheter can be placed for bladder irrigation until the anesthesia wears off. The catheter is removed prior to discharge. The following day the postoperative dosimetry CT scan is done. Some centers perform this at day 28. A chest x-ray can be performed to rule out migratory seed(s).

## Postoperative dosimetry evaluation

Orthogonal film dosimetry was used in the past for postoperative implant quality evaluation. Unfortunately this technique does not evaluate source position within the prostate. Thus, studies that report high-quality implants based on postoperative orthogonal film dosimetry may not have truly achieved high-quality implants. Modern postoperative implant quality evaluation uses CT and/or MRI-based dosimetry. These show the radioactive sources in cross-sectional images where they lie within the prostate. Dose volume histograms (DVH) and isodose curves can then be derived with the aid of computer treatment planning software (Figure 2.13). Problems with CT-based dosimetry involve artifact caused by the seeds, by artificial hips, difficulty in identifying the apex of the gland, and difficulty in distinguishing the prostate capsule from the periprostatic vascular structures. These latter factors can result in the CT scan overestimating the size of the prostate as opposed to ultrasound, MRI, or operative measurements [75–77]. These factors can make it challenging to outline the prostate margin accurately on postoperative CT scans. To help overcome inconsistencies and physician bias in prostate contouring, some centers use the preoperative TRUS to outline the prostate contour on the CT (correct magnification factor adjustment). Multiple studies have

documented that prostate swelling after implantation is approximately 20%, and can be as high as 50% [77–82]. Serial CT scans show continual shrinkage of the gland over time. The initial swelling can cause the seeds to move further apart. As the seeds lose their radioactivity the prostate swelling resolves, and the seeds move closer together. This can affect the postoperative dosimetry isodose curves especially if a tight margin or no margin is given. Therefore, even if one accurately outlines the prostate contour on the postoperative CT scan, the DVH from one center to another may vary depending on how many days or weeks postoperatively the CT scan was performed. This complicates comparisons of implant quality from one center to the next.

At 1 month after implant, most of the prostate swelling has resolved. Performing postoperative dosimetry at this time is reasonable if the logistics work out with the patient population [78,79,82]. At centers where the patients travel large distances, postoperative dosimetry performed on postoperative day zero or day one may be more practical. Qualitative evaluation with orthogonal films or CT scans without DVH analysis has indicated superior quality implants with modern PPI techniques, as compared with retropubic techniques of the 1970s [14,80,83–87,90–92]. Modern CT scan derived DVH analysis further documents the superiority of the modern PPI technique [92,93]. Stock et al [51] documented better BRFS in those patients treated with I-125 monotherapy who received a D90 of greater than 140 Gy, than those with a D90 less than 140 Gy. Potters et al [96] reported significantly better BRFS in monotherapy PPI (I-125 or Pd-103) in which postoperative D90 of greater than 90% was achieved. Grimm and colleagues [30] have shown that the initial Seattle I-125 monotherapy patients treated from 1986 to 1987 achieved significantly worse BRFS than I-125 monotherapy patients treated at the same institution, by the same physicians, from 1988 to 1990. It should be noted that these two cohorts of I-125 monotherapy patients had equivalent follow-up and were treated in the same era. These implants were performed before the availability of DVH analysis, but it is likely that the patients treated from 1988 to 1990 received higher quality implants than the initial *discovery-curve* patients treated from 1986 to 1987. These studies clearly demonstrate that higher quality implants result in better BRFS in monotherapy PPI.

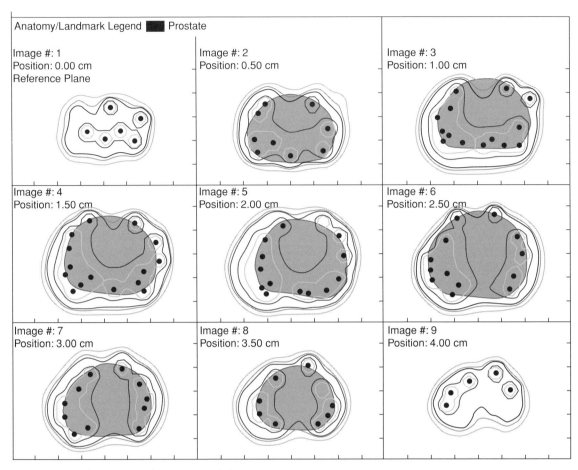

**Fig 2.13** Cover the prostate with margin, avoid the rectum.

Postoperative dosimetry provides important immediate feedback on the individual patient's implant. If there is a significant region of underdosing, it can be addressed with supplemental EBRT, HDR, or further strategically placed seeds at a second PPI procedure. Postoperative dosimetry can also reveal an individual brachytherapist's dosimetry trends. If consistent underdosing of the base or overdosing of the anterior wall of the rectum is noted, the brachytherapist should alter his or her implant technique. Currently, the ABS recommends CT scan-based postoperative dosimetry and that it be reported when PPI results are published [97]. Postoperative DVH analysis should be performed on each patient. Ideally, it should be performed on approximately the same postoperative day or within 30 days of the procedure. It should include isodose curves overlaid on the prostate and should document the D90, V100, V150, RV100, and urethral doses. Some centers are looking at doses to the bulb of the penis as well [99].

### Dosimetric goals

The goal of prostate brachytherapy is to achieve biochemical control while avoiding overdosage of critical surrounding structures. To date multiple studies have shown excellent correlation with postoperative dosimetry and BRFS and radiation proctitis. High-quality implants, as documented by D90 of greater than 90% of prescription dose or >140 Gy for I-125 monotherapy implants, or by a V100 of >80% or 90%, correlates well with BRFS [51,96,97,99,100].

**Table 2.3** Seattle dosimetry: median values (1131 consecutive patients 1998–2000).

| 1131 patients | V100 | %D90 | V150 | RV100 |
|---|---|---|---|---|
| I-125 Mono | 95 | 106 | 47 | 0.30 |
| Pd-103 Mono | 91 | 102 | 55 | 0.13 |
| Cs-131 Mono | 97 | 112 | 47 | 0.38 |
| I-125 Boost | 91 | 101 | 40 | 0.16 |
| Pd-103 Boost | 92 | 104 | 57 | 0.14 |

RV100 ranges <0.1 cc – 0.92 cc.

Other studies reveal that the incidence of radiation proctitis increases as the rectal volume receiving 100% of the prescribed dose (RV100) increases, especially >1.0 cc on day 1 dosimetry and >1.3 cc on day 30 postoperative dosimetry [101–104]. Current goals should center on achieving a consistently high V100 and a consistently low RV100 on postoperative dosimetry in order to maximize BRFS and minimize the incidence of radiation proctitis. Modern implants on 1131 consecutive patients performed by the Sylvester, Blasko and Grimm, while in Seattle, from 2005 to 2007 resulted in only 3 patients with D90 <87% prescription dose and zero patients with an RV100 >1.0 cc on day 1 dosimetry [75] (Tables 2.3 and 2.4).

## Toxicity

Major acute operative morbidity is virtually unheard of. Severe bleeding requiring transfusions or admission to intensive care for any postoperative acute events and or death have not been reported. In the Seattle experience, with over 11,000 PPI procedures no serious intraoperative or postoperative morbidity was noted. Acute postoperative side effects are common and are primarily Radiation Therapy Oncology Group (RTOG) grade 1–2 irritative and obstructive lower urinary symptoms, including increased frequency, urgency, dysuria, and poor stream. Alpha blockers are routinely started a few days prior to the implant, and continue until urinary obstructive symptoms subside [109,110,112–114]. The symptoms are at their worst during weeks 2 to 6 postoperatively, but typically are bothersome for 2 to 9 months. Short term (<3 weeks) acute urinary retention occurs in approximately 10% of patients. Several factors have been implicated in single institution univariate analysis, including large gland size, high pretreatment urinary symptom score, and pretreatment with androgen ablation. On multivariate analysis most of these risk factors drop out or are not reproducible between various institutions [118–122].

In the small percentage of patients that experience retention of more than a few weeks duration, self-catheterization is taught or a suprapubic catheter is placed until the swelling and retention spontaneously resolve. If retention does not resolve, surgical intervention with a transurethral urethrotomy or a minimal TURP is usually indicated. It must be emphasized that these procedures should not be performed until at least 9 months (preferably >12 months) after PPI due to risk of incontinence [119]. Occasionally, a staged procedure can minimize risk of incontinence.

Chronic bladder complications include cystitis and overactive bladder. These occur with ~2% incidence, and can be managed with medication. Intravesical therapy using a xylocaine-based cocktail can be used to treat moderately severe cystitis. Urinary incontinence with PPI can occur, but is rare (~1%). Late urinary retention due to urethral stricture occurs with a 5%–10% incidence. This can be corrected in ~90% of patients with dilation or urethrotomy [119].

A temporary increase in bowel frequency and urgency occasionally occurs and usually responds to diet modification or antidiarrheal medication. Chronic or delayed rectal bleeding occurs with a 2%–10% incidence [112–121]. Multiple studies have correlated this and other rectal complications with the postimplant dosimetric parameter of the rectal volume receiving 100% of the prescribed dose (RV100) [46,121–126].

**Table 2.4** Post-implant dosimetry on 1131 patients: only 3/1,131 had %D90 < 90%.

| | V100 | %D90 | Boost? | notes |
|---|---|---|---|---|
| 1 | 84 | 91 | N | |
| 2 | 82 | 92 | N | |
| 3 | 84 | 93 | N | |
| 4 | 83 | 92 | N | |
| 5 | 84 | 91 | N | |
| 6 | 82 | 91 | Y | "Boost case" |
| 7 | 82 | 87 | N | De-escalation trial |
| 8 | 81 | 85 | N | TURP |
| 9 | 75 | 75 | N | Different than usual technique |

Proctitis may be conservatively managed with dietary changes, steroids, suppositories, and sucralfate enemas. Significant rectal bleeding should be investigated with colonoscopy or flexible sigmoidoscopy. Biopsy or electrocautery of the anterior rectum following PPI should be avoided, due to risk of acquired rectourethral fistula (RUF) or nonhealing rectal ulcer. If a patient is due for colonoscopy within a couple of years for other reasons, then this should be performed immediately prior to PPI. This may eliminate the need for subsequent biopsies to rule out rectal malignancy. If necessary, chemical cautery with dilute formalin or minimal argon plasma coagulation of the rectal mucosa can be considered for rectal bleeding. A recent multi-institutional randomized study demonstrated the benefit of hyperbaric oxygen in radiation induced, medically refractory proctitis. One caveat is that prostate patients made up a small proportion of those in the study [127]. Less than 1% of RUFs are caused by PPI directly [128–132]. Fecal diversion is typically required to manage severe rectal symptoms. This can be followed by resection of the fistula, graciloplasty, and hyperbaric oxygen therapy in selected patients. A small proportion of patients manage to have the fecal diversion reversed.

Hematuria and hematospermia are to be expected for at least a few days following PPI. One third of sexually active patients will experience some level of pain with orgasm; this can persist for weeks to months and is usually mild typically responding to nonsteroidal anti-inflammatory drugs. The prostatic and seminal vesicle fluid components ($\sim$90%) of the ejaculate will decrease dramatically following PPI, but sperm can still be present. Whether or not the sperm is significantly damaged by the radiation exposure is unknown, but birth control measures are recommended for those couples who are still fertile. Ejaculation of a seed is rarely reported. The Seattle team is aware of less than five patients who have noted this event over the past 15 years.

Erectile dysfunction (ED) occurs at a considerable rate with all prostate cancer treatments. Data is difficult to interpret because of subjectivity of patient questionnaires, reliability of patients answering the questions, and most importantly the age and health of the patient pretreatment. A meta-analysis comparing EBRT, PPI, EBRT+PPI, nerve-sparing RP, and non-nerve-sparing RP showed no significant difference between PPI and RP in terms of ED rates [124]. In these studies the surgical patients were significantly younger and healthier pretreatment than the brachytherapy or EBRT patients. Most studies show surgery to result in significantly higher rates of ED than brachytherapy treated patients, despite the younger age of surgical patients. Cesarettie and Stock reported that 92% of patients who were in their 50s at the time of PPI and had a pretreatment Sexual Health Inventory for Men (SHIM) score of >20 maintained the ability for erections adequate for intercourse 7 years after PPI [125]. Although data from EBRT treated patients supports a dose correlate with the penile bulb, analysis from PPI does not hold similar [126]. Pretreatment function is the most significant predictor of ED. New data is emerging on the use of continuous low dose, prophylactic PDE-5 inhibitors to prevent ED after prostate treatment [127].

The topic of second malignancies arises when the use of therapeutic radiation is discussed, especially with younger men opting for PPI. Luiaw and Sylvester reported the only large single institution study with long follow-up on this topic. They showed no increase in secondary malignancy when PPI monotherapy was used compared with age matched cohorts [128]. A small increase was associated with those receiving combination EBRT and PPI, but that could also be attributed to preexisting risk factors and smoking histories in those individuals. A SEER database analysis by Tward et al confirmed this finding [129].

## Cancer control

BRFS is used as the endpoint for disease control due to the long natural history of prostate cancer, which results in a large portion of patients (even those exhibiting biochemical failure after primary radical treatment) dying of causes other than prostate cancer. The earlier American Society of Therapeutic Radiology and Oncology (ASTRO) definition of biochemical failure (3 consecutive PSA rises above nadir) has been recently replaced by the ASTRO-Phoenix definition, which requires a PSA of nadir +2 ng/mL to document failure.

Most BRFS reports from the Seattle group concern patients diagnosed and treated in the late 1980s and early 1990s. These patients are from a different era than those currently treated with modern radical prostatectomy, 3D-CRT, IMRT, and HDR brachytherapy. Multiple studies from the surgical and

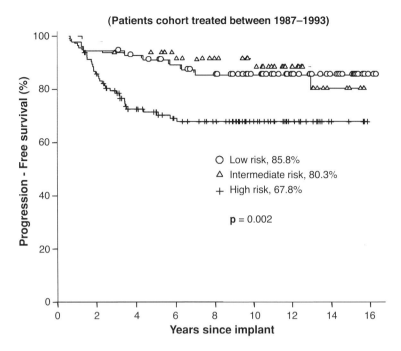

**(Patients cohort treated between 1987–1993)**

○ Low risk, 85.8%
△ Intermediate risk, 80.3%
+ High risk, 67.8%

**p** = 0.002

**Fig 2.14** Seattle long-term BRFS outcomes EBRT + seeds.

radiotherapy literature show that patients treated a decade ago do more poorly in terms of BRFS, and cause specific survival than modern patients. This is due to a variety of factors, such as improved Gleason scoring, stage migration, improved imaging, improved treatment techniques, and PSA screening effects. Thus, it is impressive that the results of seed implantation in these patients from 1987 to 1994 (many of whom were Gleason underscored, had no postoperative CT dosimetry, were treated without sagittal imaging, and with reusable needles) compare so favorably to more recent surgical and EBRT series. The undergrading phenomenon has been reported in the urologic literature [105].

Sylvester reported the 15-year (Seattle) experience with combined EBRT and PPI without androgen ablation [37]. Patients were analyzed based on two different risk group stratification systems defined by MSKCC and D'Amico. A modification of the ASTRO definition of BRFS was used where only two rises in PSA were needed to define a failure instead of the old ASTRO criteria of three consecutive rises. Most patients were treated with a total dose of 45 Gy EBRT to a "limited pelvis" followed by either a 90-Gy Pd-103 or 110-Gy I-125 PPI boost. Two hundred and twenty-three patients had a median follow-up of 9.43 years.

Current 15-year BRFS results by the D'Amico risk grouping system are low-risk 85.8%, intermediate-risk 80.3%, and high-risk 67.8% (Figure 2.14).

Grimm reported the long-term Seattle experience with I-125 monotherapy. From 1988 to 1990 a total of 125 patients were consecutively treated with I-125 implant to a dose of 144 Gy [30]. The average follow-up of the nondeceased patients was 94.5 months. The local control rate by digital rectal examination and biopsy was 97%. The metastatic disease rate was 3%. The low- and intermediate-risk patients experienced a 10-year BRFS of 87% and 76%, respectively. Sylvester updated the 15-year BRFS outcomes of I-125 monotherapy patients treated from 1988 to 1992. The median follow-up was 11.7 years for the entire cohort, and 15.4 years for the patients who had no biochemical evidence of disease. The low-, intermediate-, and high-risk patients achieved a BRFS of 85.9%, 79.9%, and 62.2%, respectively [107] (Figure 2.15).

Blasko et al reported the Seattle experience with Pd-103 monotherapy [108]. These patients had higher Gleason Scores than the patients treated with I-125 monotherapy that Grimm et al had reported. A total of 232 patients were treated with Pd-103 monotherapy from 1989 to 1995, with an average follow-up

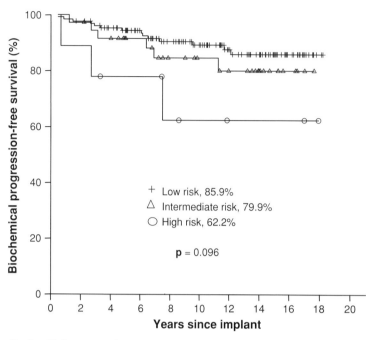

·Kaplan-Meier curves for biochemical progression-free survival using the Nadir +2 definition,

· stratified by group using the D'Amico method of risk classification.

·I-125 monotherapy patients treated form 1988–1992.

Fig 2.15 Seattle long-term BRFS outcomes I-125 alone.

of 49 months. The local control rate was also 97%. The metastatic disease rate was 6%. The 5-year BRFS for the low-, intermediate-, and high-risk patients was 94%, 82%, and 65%, respectively, although only a small number of high-risk patients were treated with Pd-103 monotherapy. Those patients with Gleason score 7–10 and a PSA ≤10 ng/mL experienced a 5-year BRFS of 80%. None of the patients in the above reports by Blasko, Grimm, or Sylvester received any androgen ablation therapy.

Modern series from multiple institutions have shown outstanding BRFS rates with 5- and 7-year results of 97%–98% BRFS for low-risk patients [31,65,69,74]. Sylvester recently reported a cohort of intermediate-risk patients treated from 1998 to 2000 showing a 91.9% BRFS at 9 years with or without supplemental EBRT or androgen ablation [42]. Excellent BRFS results in modern low-, intermediate-, and high-risk patients treated by low dose rate seed implant brachytherapy at centers of excellence are shown in Table 2.5 [42,109,110,112–116]. Grimm and Sylvester have recently reviewed over 15,000 prostate cancer articles published in the peer reviewed medical literature from 2000 to 2009. Those articles that reported on BRFS using commonly accepted risk grouping (NCCN, D'Amico, MSKCC), had a median follow-up of at least 5 years, had at least 100 patients per risk group, and did not exclude patients due to postoperative pathologic findings, were accepted into the final outcomes charts [117].

## Future directions

Edema of the prostate due to needle trauma or radiation can cause urinary obstructive symptoms including acute urinary retention. Studies implicating needle trauma specifically include those analyzing number of needles required for the implant and the number of needle punctures [130]. Prostate gland edema seen on postimplant CT is predictive of urinary retention, but also may play a role in dose distribution and impotence. A new seed called "Thin-Strand", which is 40% thinner than the standard seeds

**Table 2.5** Brachytherapy series.

| BRFS seed implant (Modern era) | Follow-up | Low-risk | Intermediate-risk | High-risk |
|---|---|---|---|---|
| Memorial Sloan Kettering Cancer Center New York City [109] | 7-years | 98% | 93% | |
| Multicenter pooled data (all patients had Gleason 8–10) [110] | 5-years | – | – | 86% |
| Institute Curie. Paris [112] | 5-year | 97% | 94% | |
| Cleveland Clinic [113] | 5-years | 95% | 85% | |
| Mt Sinai, New York City [114] | 10-years | 94% | 89.5% | 78% |
| M.D. Anderson, Houston [115] | 5-years | 96% | 100% | |
| Seattle [42] Sylvester et al | 9-years | | 91.9% | |
| British Columbia Cancer Center, Vancouver Canada [116] | 5-years | >94% | <95% | |

currently in use and delivered through a 20-gauge needle, may be able to positively impact toxicity. Early dosimetric and health-related quality of life outcome measures are encouraging [131].

Minimizing the rectal dosage is also something that requires further investigation. A Spanish group has published a report of perirectal injection of hyaluronic acid to create a spatial buffer between the prostate and the rectum for this very purpose. In a small prospective study, they demonstrated a reduced risk of visualized rectal mucosa injury and a lower risk of rectal bleeding [132]. Hyaluronic acid is not currently approved for this use in the United States.

## Conclusions

Brachytherapy is now a standard treatment for low- to intermediate-risk prostate cancer. It can be carried out in an ambulatory care setting with minimal acute toxicity, early recovery to normal activities, and acceptable genitourinary side effects. The cancer control of brachytherapy demonstrates that it is at least as effective as external beam radiation therapy and surgery. Further technological improvements in seed delivery and protection of the rectal mucosa should reduce toxicity of this procedure further.

## References

1. Denning CL (1922) Carcinoma of the prostate seminal vesicles treated with radium. Surg Gynecol Obstet 34: 99–118.
2. Scardino P, Carlton C (1983) Combined interstitial and external irradiation for prostate cancer. In: N Javadpour (ed.) *Principles and Management of Urologic Cancer*. Baltimore: Williams & Wilkins, pp. 392–408.
3. Whitmore WF Jr, Hilaris B, Grabstald H (1972) Retropubic implantation to iodine125 in the treatment of prostatic cancer. J Urol 108: 918–920.
4. DeLaney TP et al (1986) Preoperative irradiation, lymphadenectomy, and 125iodine implantation for patients with localized carcinoma of the prostate. Int J Radiat Oncol Biol Phys 12: 1779–1785.
5. Fuks Z et al (1991) The effect of local control on metastatic dissemination in carcinoma of the prostate: long-term results in patients treated with 125I implantation. Int J Radiat Oncol Biol Phys 21: 537–547.
6. Giles GM, Brady LW (1986) 125-Iodine implantation after lymphadenectomy in early carcinoma of the prostate. Int J Radiat Oncol Biol Phys 12: 2117–2125.
7. Kuban DA, el-Mahdi AM, Schellhammer PF (1989) I-125 interstitial implantation for prostate cancer. What have we learned 10 years later? Cancer 63: 2415–2420.
8. Schellhammer PF et al (1989) Morbidity and mortality of local failure after definitive therapy for prostate cancer. J Urol 141: 567–571.
9. Kovacs G et al (1999) Prostate preservation by combined external beam and HDR brachytherapy in nodal negative prostate cancer. Strahlenther Onkol 175(suppl. 2): 87–88.
10. Hilaris B et al (1991) Interstitial irradiation in prostatic cancer: Report of 10-year results. In: S Rolf (ed.) *Interventional Radiation Therapy Techniques/Brachytherapy*. Berlin: Springer, p. 235.
11. Sylvester J et al (1997) Interstitial implantation techniques in prostate cancer. J Surg Oncol 66: 65–75.
12. Puthawala A, Syed A, Tansey L (1985) Temporary iridium implant in the management of carcinoma of the prostate. Endocurie Hypertherm Oncol 1: 25–33.
13. Martinez A et al (1985) Combination of external beam irradiation and multiple-site perineal applicator (MUPIT) for treatment of locally advanced or recurrent prostatic, anorectal, and gynecologic malignancies. Int J Radiat Oncol Biol Phys 11: 391–398.

14. Holm HH et al (1983) Transperineal 125-iodine seed implantation in prostatic cancer guided by transrectal ultrasonography. J Urol 130: 283–286.

15. Partin AW et al (1993) The use of prostate specific antigen, clinical stage and Gleason score to predict pathological stage in men with localized prostate cancer. J Urol 150: 110–114.

16. Partin AW et al (1997) Combination of prostate-specific antigen, clinical stage, and Gleason score to predict pathological stage of localized prostate cancer. A multi-institutional update. JAMA 277: 1445–1451.

17. Partin AW et al (2001) Contemporary update of prostate cancer staging nomograms (Partin Tables) for the new millennium. Urology 58: 843–848.

18. Makarov D et al (2007) Updated nomogram to predict pathologic stage of prostate cancer given prostate-specific antigen level, clinical stage, and biopsy Gleason score (Partin tables) based on cases from 2000–2005. Urology 69: 1095–1101.

19. Davis BJ et al (1999) The radial distance of extraprostatic extension of prostate carcinoma: implications for prostate brachytherapy. Cancer 85: 2630–2737.

20. Sohayda C et al (2000) Extent of extracapsular extension in localized prostate cancer. Urology 55: 382–386.

21. Chao KK et al (2006) Clinicopathologic analysis of extracapsular extension in prostate cancer: should the clinical target volume be expanded posterolaterally to account for microscopic extension? Int J Radiat Oncol Biol Phys 65: 999–1007.

22. Epstein JI et al (1993) Influence of capsular penetration on progression following radical prostatectomy: a study of 196 cases with long-term followup. J Urol 150: 135–141.

23. Nag S et al (1999) American Brachytherapy Society (ABS) recommendations for transperineal permanent brachytherapy of prostate cancer. Int J Radiat Oncol Biol Phys 44: 789–799.

24. D'Amico AV et al (1998) Biochemical outcome after radical prostatectomy, external beam radiation therapy, or interstitial radiation therapy for clinically localized prostate cancer. JAMA 280: 969–974.

25. Blasko JC, Grimm PD, Ragde H (1994) External beam irradiation with palladium-103 implantation for prostate carcinoma. Int J Radiat Oncol Biol Phys 30(suppl.): 219.

26. Wallner K (1991) I-125 brachytherapy for early stage prostate cancer: new techniques may achieve better results. Oncology 5: 115–126.

27. Wallner K, Roy J, Harrison L (1996) Tumor control and morbidity following transperineal iodine 125 implantation for stage T1/T2 prostatic carcinoma. J Clin Oncol 14: 449–453.

28. Schellhammer PF, Ladaga LE, El-Mahdi A (1980) Histological characteristics of prostatic biopsies after l25 iodine implantation. J Urol 123: 700–705.

29. Prestidge BR et al (1997) Posttreatment biopsy results following interstitial brachytherapy in early-stage prostate cancer. Int J Radiat Oncol Biol Phys 37: 31–39.

30. Grimm P et al (2001) 10-year biochemical (prostate-specific antigen) control of prostate cancer with 125-I brachytherapy. Int J Radiat Oncol Biol Phys 51: 31–40.

31. Merrick GS et al (2001) Five-year biochemical outcome following permanent interstitial brachytherapy for clinical Tl-T3 prostate cancer. Int J Radiat Oncol Biol Phys 51: 41–48.

32. Roy JN et al (1996) Determining source strength and source distribution for a transperineal prostate implant. Endocurie/Hyperthermia Oncol: 12: 35–41.

33. Lederman GS et al (2001) Retrospective stratification of a consecutive cohort of prostate cancer patients treated with a combined regimen of external-beam radiotherapy and brachytherapy. Int J Radiat Oncol Biol Phys 49: 1297–3003.

34. D'Amico AV et al (2000) Clinical utility of the percentage of positive prostate biopsies in defining biochemical outcome after radical prostatectomy for patients with clinically localized prostate cancer. J Clin Oncol 18; 1164–1172.

35. Grimm P (1998) Clinical results of prostate brachytherapy. Presented at: 84th Annual Radiological Society of North of America Meeting, Chicago, IL.

36. Stock RG et al (2006) Changing the pattern of failure for high risk prostate cancer patients by optimizing local control. Int J Radiat Oncol Biol Phys 66: 389–394.

37. Sylvester JE et al (2007) 15-year biochemical relapse free survival in clinical stage T1-T3 prostate cancer following combined external beam radiotherapy and brachytherapy; Seattle experience. Int J Radiat Oncol Biol Phys 67: 57–64.

38. Sylvester JE, Blasko J, Grimm P (2001) Brachytherapy as monotherapy. In: P Kantoff, PC Carroll, AV D'Amico (eds.) Prostate Cancer: Principles and Practice. Philadelphia, PA: Lippincot Williams and Wilkins, pp. 336–357.

39. Beyer DC, Priestley JB (1995) Biochemical disease-free survival following I-125 prostate implantation [Abstract]. Int J Radiat Oncol Biol Phys 32(suppl.): 254.

40. Wallner K et al (1994) Short-term freedom from disease progression after 1–125 prostate implantation. Int Radiat Oncot Biol Phys 30: 405–409.

41. Kaye KW, Olson DJ, Payne JT (1995) Detailed preliminary analysis of l25iodine implantation for localized prostate cancer using percutaneous approach. J Urol 153: 1020–1025.

42. Sylvester JE et al (2009) Prostate Brachytherapy biochemical relapse free survival outcomes in intermediate risk prostate cancer patients [Abstract]. Brachytherapy 8(2): 140.

43. Sylvester JE (2001) Modern permanent prostate brachytherapy. In: American Society of Therapeutic Radiation Oncology 43rd Annual Meeting, San Francisco.

44. Merrick GS et al (2006) Efficacy of neoadjuvant bicalutamide and dutasteride as a cytoreductive regimen prior to prostate brachytherapy. Urology 68: 116–120.

45. Blasko JC et al (1996) Should brachytherapy be considered a therapeutic option in localized prostate cancer?. Urol Clin North Am 23: 633–649.

46. Blasko JC, Ragde H, Grimm PD (1991) Transperineal ultrasound-guided implantation of the prostate: morbidity and complications. Scand J Urol Nephrol Suppl 137: 113–118.

47. Talcott JA et al (2001) Long-term treatment related complications of brachytherapy for early prostate cancer: a survey of patients previously treated. J Urol 166: 494–499.

48. Wallner K et al (1997) Low risk of urinary incontinence following prostate brachytherapy in patients with a prior transurethral prostate resection. Int J Radiat Oncol Biol Phys 37: 565–569.

49. Stone NN, Ratnow ER, Stock RG (2000) Prior transurethral resection does not increase morbidity following real-time ultrasound-guided prostate seed implantation. Technique Urol 6: 123–127.

50. Peters CA et al (2006) Low-dose rate prostate brachytherapy is well tolerated in patients with a history of inflammatory bowel disease. Int J Radiat Oncol Biol Phys 66: 424–429.

51. Stock RG et al (1998) A dose-response study for I-125 prostate implants. Int Radiat Oncol Biol Phys 41: 101–108.

53. Potters L et al (2001) A comprehensive review of CT-based dosimetry parameters and biochemical control in patients treated with permanent prostate brachytherapy. Int J Radiat Oncol Biol Phys 50: 605–614.

54. Zelefsky MJ et al (1998) Dose escalation with three-dimensional conformal radiation therapy affects the outcome in prostate cancer. Int J Radiat Oncol Biol Phys 41: 491–500.

55. Kupelian PA et al (2000) Higher than standard radiation doses (>or = 72 Gy) with or without androgen deprivation in the treatment of localized prostate cancer. Int J Radiat Oncol Biol Phys 46: 567–574.

56. Hanks GE et al (1998) Dose escalation with 3D conformal treatment: five year outcomes, treatment optimization, and future directions. Int J Radiat Oncol Biol Phys 41: 501–510.

57. Kupelian PA, Reddy CA, Klein CA (1999) Factors associated with biochemical relapse after either low-dose external beam radiation, high-dose external beam radiation, or radical prostatectomy for localized prostate cancer: 8 year results [Abstract]. Int Radiat Oncol Biol Phys 45(suppl.): 219.

58. Pollack A, Zagars GK (1997) External beam radiotherapy dose response of prostate cancer. Int J Radiat Oncol Biol Phys 39: 1011–1018.

59. Kupelian P A et al (2008) Effect of increasing radiation doses on local and distant failures in patients with localized prostate cancer. Int J Radiat Oncol Biol Phys 71: 16–22.

60. Pollack A et al (2002) Prostate cancer radiation dose response, results of the MD Anderson phase III randomized trial. Int J Radiat Oncol Biol Phys 53: 1097–1105.

61. Dearnaley D P et al (2005) Phase III pilot study of dose escalation using conformal radiotherapy in prostate cancer: PSA control and side effects. Br J Cancer 92: 488–498.

62. Zietman A L et al (2005) Comparison of conventional-dose vs. high-dose conformal radiation therapy in clinically localized adenocarcinoma of the prostate: a randomized controlled trial. JAMA 294: 1233–1239.

63. Ho A Y et al (2009) Radiation dose predicts biochemical control in intermediate-risk prostate cancer patients treated with low-dose-rate brachytherapy. Int J Radiat Oncol Biol Phys 75(1): 16–22.

64. Stock RJ et al (2006) Biological effective dose values for prostate brachytherapy: effects on PSA failure and posttreatment biopsy results. Int J Radiat Oncol Biol Phys 64: 527–533.

65. Stone NN et al (2009) Multicenter analysis of effect of high biologic effective dose on biochemical failure and survival outcomes in patients with Gleason score 7–10 prostate cancer treated with permanent prostate brachytherapy. Int J Radiat Oncol Biol Phys: 73: 341–346.

69. Prestidge BR et al (1998) A survey of current clinical practice of permanent prostate brachytherapy in the United States. Int J Radiat Oncol Biol Phys 40: 461–465.

70. Zelefsky MJ et al (2007) Intraoperative real-time planned conformal prostate brachytherapy: post-implantation dosimetric outcome and clinical implication. Radiother Oncol 84: 185–189.

71. Sylvester JE et al (2009) Permanent prostate brachytherapy preplanned technique: the modern seattle method step by step and dosimetric outcomes. Brachytherapy 8(1): 34–39.

72. Hastak SM, Gammelgaard J, Holm HH (1982) Transrectal ultrasonic volume determination of the prostate: a preoperative and postoperative study. J Urol 127; 1115–1118.

73. Hricak H et al (1987) Evaluation of prostate size: a comparison of ultrasound and magnetic resonance imaging. Urol Radiol 9: 1–8.

74. Waterman FM et al (1997) Effect of edema on the post-implant dosimetry of an I-125 prostate implant: a case study. Int J Radiat Oncol Biol Phys 38: 335–339.

75. Prestidge BR et al (1998) Timing of computed tomography-based postimplant assessment following permanent transperineal prostate brachytherapy . Int J Radiat Oncol Biol Phys 40: 1111–1115.

76. Moerland MA et al (1997) Evaluation of permanent I-125 prostate implants using radiography and magnetic resonance imaging. Int J Radiat Oncol Biol Phys 37: 927–933.

77. Narayana V et al (1997) Impact of differences in ultrasound and computed tomography volumes on treatment planning of permanent prostate implants. Int J Radiat Oncol Biol Phys 37: 1181–1185.

78. Merrick GS et al (1998) Influence of timing on the dosimetric analysis of transperineal ultrasound-guided, prostatic conformal brachytherapy. Radiat Oncol Investig 6: 182–190.

79. Blasko IC, Grimm PD, Ragde H (1993) Brachytherapy and organ preservation in the management of carcinoma of the prostate. Semin Radiat Oncol 3: 240–249.

80. Blasko JC, Radge H, Schumacher D (1987) Transperineal percutaneous iodine-125 implantation for prostatic carcinoma using transrectal ultrasound and template guidance. Endocuriether Hyperthermia Oncol 3: 131–139.

81. Wallner K et al (1991) An improved method for computerized tomography-planned transperineal 125iodine prostate implants. J Urol 146; 90–95.

82. Stock RG et al (1995) A modified technique allowing interactive ultrasound-guided three-dimensional transperineal prostate implantation. Int J Radiat Oncol Biol Phys 32: 219–225.

83. Wallner K et al (1994) Fluoroscopic visualization of the prostatic urethra to guide transperineal prostate implantation. Int J Radiat Oncol Biol Phys 29: 863–867.

84. Kaye KW et al (1992) Improved technique for prostate seed implantation: combined ultrasound and fluoroscopic guidance. J Endourol 6: 61–66.

85. Ragde H et al (1989) Use of transrectal ultrasound in transperineal I-125 seeding for prostate cancer: methodology. J Endourol 3: 209–218.

86. Roy JN et al (1991) CT-based optimized planning for transperineal prostate implant with customized template. Int Radiat Oncol Biol Phys 21: 483–489.

87. Stock RG et al (1996) Prostate specific antigen findings and biopsy results following interactive ultrasound guided transperineal brachytherapy for early stage prostate carcinoma. Cancer 77: 2386–2392.

90. Nag S et al (2000) The American Brachytherapy Society recommendations for permanent prostate brachytherapy postimplant dosimetric analysis. Int J Radiat Oncol Biol Phys 46: 221–230.

91. Merrick OS et al (2001) A comparison of radiation dose to the bulb of the penis in men with and without prostate brachytherapy-induced erectile dysfunction. Int J Radiat Oncol Biol Phys 50: 597–604.

92. Choi S et al (2004) Treatment margins predict biochemical outcomes after prostate brachytherapy. Cancer J 10: 175–180.

93. Snyder KM et al (2001) Defining the risk of grade 2 proctitis following 125I prostate brachytherapy using a rectal dose-volume histogram analysis. Int J Radiat Oncol Biol Phys 50: 335–341.

95. Waterman FM, Dicker AP (2003) Probability of late rectal morbidity in 125I prostate brachytherapy. Int J Radiat Oncol Biol Phys 53: 342–353.

96. Sherertz T et al (2004) Factors predictive of rectal bleeding after 103 Pd and supplemental beam radiation for prostate cancer. Brachytherapy 3: 130–135.

97. Allsbrook WC Jr et al (2001) Interobserver reproducibility of Gleason grading of prostatic carcinoma: urologic pathologists. Hum Pathol 32: 74–80.

99. Sylvester JE et al (2009) 15 year biochemical relapse free survival following 125-I prostate brachytherapy in clinically localized prostate cancer: Seattle experience [Abstract]. 51st American Society for Radiation Oncology Annual Meeting, Chicago, IL.

100. Blasko JC et al (2000) Palladium-103 brachytherapy for prostate carcinoma. Int J Radiat Oncol Biol Phys 46: 839–850.

101. Zelefsky MJ et al (2007) Comparison of 7-year outcomes between LDR brachytherapy and high dose IMRT for patients with clinically localized prostate cancer. Int J Radiat Oncol Biol Phys 69:S178.

102. Stone NN et al (2009) Multicenter analysis of impact of high biologically effective dose (BED) on biochemical failure (Phoenix definition) and survival outcomes in patients with Gleason score 7–10 prostate cancer treated by permanent prostate brachytherapy. Int J Radiat Oncol Biol Phys 73(2): 341–346.

103. Cosset JM et al (2008) Selecting patients for exclusive permanent implant prostate brachytherapy: The experience of the Paris Institute Curie/Cochin Hospital/Necker Hospital Group on 809 patients. Int J Radiat Oncol Biol Phys 71(4): 1042–1048.

104. Kupelian PA et al (2007) Hypofractioanted intensity-modulated radiotherapy (70 Gy at 2.5 Gy per fraction) for localized prostate cancer: Cleveland Calinic experience. Int J Radiat Oncol Biol Phys 68(5): 1424–1430.

105. Stock RG et al. (2006) Biologically Effective Dose Values For prostate Brachytherapy: Effects On PSA Failure

And Posttreatment Biopsy Results". Int J Radiat Oncol Biol Phys 64(2); 527–533106.

106. Frank SJ et al (2008) Prostate brachytherapy- The M.D. Anderson Cancer Center Experience. Proceedings from the American Urology Association Annual meeting, Orlando, FL. May 2008.

107. Morris WJ et al (2009) Evaluation of dosimetric parameters and disease response after $I^{125}$ iodine transperineal brachytherapy for low and intermediate risk prostate cancer. Int J Radiat Oncol Biol Phys 73(5): 1432–1438.

108. Grimm PD et al (2009) Low and intermediate risk prostate cancer- comparative effectiveness of brachytherapy, cryotherapy, external beam radio therapy, HIFU, proton therapy, radical prostatectomy and robot assisted radical prostatectomy [Abstract]. 51st ASTRO Annual Meeting, Chicago, IL.

109. Arterbery VE et al (1993) Short-term morbidity from CT-planned transperineal I-125 prostate implants. Int Radiat Oncol Biol Phys 25: 661–667.

110. Grier D (2001) Complications of permanent seed implantation. J Brachytherapy Int 17; 205–210.

112. Shah SA et al (2004) Rectal complications after prostate brachytherapy. Dis Col Rec 47: 1487–1492.

113. Kao J et al (2008) (125)I monotherapy using D90 implant doses of 180 Gy or greater. Int J Radiat Oncol Biol Phys 70: 96–101.

114. Herstein A et al (2005) I-125 versus Pd-103 for low-risk prostate cancer: long-term morbidity outcomes from a prospective randomized multicenter controlled trial. Cancer J 11: 385–389.

115. Kang SK et al (2002) Gastrointestinal toxicity of transperineal interstitial prostate brachytherapy. Int J Radiat Oncol Biol Phys 53: 99–103.

116. Martin AG et al (2007) Permanent prostate implant using high activity seeds and inverse planning with fast simulated annealing algorithm: a 12-year Canadian experience. Int J Radiat Oncol Biol Phys 67: 334–341.

117. Anderson JF et al (2009) Urinary side effects and complications after permanent prostate brachytherapy: the MD Anderson Cancer Center experience. Urology 74(3): 601–605.

118. Clarke RE. et al (2008) Hyperbaric oxygen treatment of chronic refractory radiation proctitis: a randomized and controlled double-blind crossover trial with long-term follow-up. Int J Radiat Oncol Biol Phys 72(1): 134–143.

119. Theodorescu D, Gillenwater JY, Koutrouvelis PG (2000) Prostatourethral-rectal fistula after prostate brachytherapy. Cancer 89: 2085–2091.

120. Shakespeare D et al (2007) Recto-urethral fistula following brachytherapy for localized prostate cancer. Colorectal Dis 9: 328–331.

121. Gelblum DY, Potters L (2000) Rectal complications associated with transperineal interstitial brachytherapy for prostate cancer. Int J Radiat Oncol Biol Phys 48: 119–124.

122. Shah JN, Ennis RD (2006) Rectal toxicity profile after transperineal interstitial permanent prostate brachytherapy: use of a comprehensive toxicity scoring system and identification of rectal dosimetric toxicity predictors. Int J Radiat Oncol Biol Phys 64: 817–824.

123. Tran A et al (2005) Rectal fistulas after prostate brachytherapy. Int J Radiat Oncol Biol Phys 63: 150–154.

124. Robinson JW, Moritz S, Fung T (2002) Meta-analysis of rates of erectile function after treatment of localized prostate carcinoma. Int J Radiat Oncol Biol Phys 54: 1063–1068.

125. Cesaretti JA et al (2007) Effect of low dose-rate prostate brachytherapy on the sexual health of men with optimal sexual function before treatment: analysis at > or = 7 years of follow up. BJU Int 100(2): 362–367.

126. Solan AN et al (2009) There is no correlation between erectile dysfunction and dose to penile bulb and neurovascular bundles following real-time low-dose-rate prostate brachytherapy. Int J Radiat Oncol Biol Phys 73: 1468–1474.

127. Potters L et al (2001) Potency after permanent prostate brachytherapy for localized prostate cancer. Int J Radiat Oncol Biol Phys 50: 1235–1242.

128. Liauw SL et al (2006) Second malignancies after prostate brachytherapy: incidence of bladder and colorectal cancers in patients with 15 years of potential follow-up. Int J Radiat Oncol Biol Phys 66: 669–673.

129. Tward JD et al (2008) The risk of second primary malignancies following brachytherapy monotherapy, external beam plus brachytherapy, or radical prostatectomy for prostate cancer. Int J Radiat Oncol Biol Phys 72: S94.

130. Eapen L et al (2004) Correlating the degree of needle trauma during prostate brachytherapy and the development of acute urinary toxicity. Int J Radiat Oncol Biol Phys 59: 1392–1394.

131. Wong J et al (2009) First report on the use of a thinner I125 radioactive seed that fits into 20 gauge needles for permanent seed prostate brachytherapy: A report on post-implant dosimetry and acute toxicity [Abstract]. 51st ASTRO Annual Meeting, Chicago, IL.

132. Prada PJ et al (2009) Transperineal injection of hyaluronic acid in the anterior perirectal fat to decrease rectal toxicity from radiation delivered with low-dose-rate brachytherapy for prostate cancer patients. Brachytherapy 8: 210–217.

# 3

# High-intensity focused ultrasound

*Markus Margreiter and Michael Marberger*
Department of urology, University of Vienna Medical School, Vienna, Austria

## Introduction

In 1950 Frey and Lochmann first described the use of ultrasound for ablating malignant tumors in animals [1,2]. Several groups picked up this revolutionary idea, and only a few years later Burov demonstrated that high-intensity ultrasound could be used to destroy cancer cells in humans [3]. The early work on this technique was limited by the lack of devices with adequate performance and accuracy. By 1990 more advanced systems became available, and detailed experimental studies to treat malignant tumors were performed. High-intensity focused ultrasound (HIFU) was introduced in oncology to destroy a variety of malignant lesions, including tumors of the liver, pancreas, bone, rectum, and breast [4,5].

In 1992 Chapelon et al used HIFU to create local tumor necrosis in prostatic adenocarcinoma in an animal model [6]. Subsequently, Gelet and Chapelon reported the first clinical studies to evaluate the efficacy of transrectal HIFU for the treatment of localized, low-grade prostate cancer in humans [7]. By 1995 Madersbacher et al reported the successful use of this technique to destroy entire cancer lesions in the human prostate [8]. This was the first systematic study to evaluate the extent and location of the intraprostatic necrosis by planimetry analysis of whole-mount prostate sections in patients who underwent radical retropubic prostatectomy after HIFU treatment. To date, prostate cancer [9] as well as renal [10], bladder [11], and testicular tumors [12] have been treated with HIFU, and clinical results are now available [13].

## Basic science

HIFU relies on the same principles as conventional ultrasound. Ultrasound is acoustic energy in the form of longitudinal waves. These sound waves are transmitted as alternating series of compressions and rarefactions. As the waves propagate through nonhomogeneous media such as biologic tissue, particles are forced to oscillate back and forth from their original rest positions, and as they do so, some of the mechanical ultrasound energy is converted to heat [8, 14]. With conventional diagnostic ultrasonography, the change in temperature is minimal, and therefore, the insonicated tissue is not altered. If the ultrasound waves are focused at a precisely defined location to achieve higher site intensity (i.e., HIFU), heat sufficient for thermal destruction of all biologic tissues can be achieved [15]. A higher level of site intensity can lead to cavitation processes, with microbubble formation and implosion, and ultimately mechanical disruption of tissues within the focal area [6,15].

The thermal effect of ultrasound depends on several factors, including the absorption coefficient of the insonicated tissue, the site intensity achieved, the duration of insonication, and the conduction of heat throughout the targeted structures [14]. Irreversible

*Interventional Techniques in Uro-oncology*, First Edition. Edited by Hashim Uddin Ahmed, Manit Arya, Peter T. Scardino & Mark Emberton.  © 2011 Blackwell Publishing Ltd. Published 2011 by Blackwell Publishing Ltd.

cell destruction of biologic tissues occurs rapidly above a threshold of 60°C, resulting in coagulative necrosis. At site intensities above 1200 W/cm$^2$, these temperatures are reached at the focal point within seconds. As a result, heat losses by conduction near larger vessels impact ablation efficacy significantly less than with other thermal ablation techniques, which are based on slower heat generation. The size of the lesion created by HIFU is proportional to the duration of insonication. It can be controlled by modulating the energy administered and also with an on/off mode to avoid overheating and potential cavitation. To achieve larger lesions, the focus is moved during the off phase by moving the transducer. Alternatively, tissue can be insonicated continuously, and the focus is moved during insonication (*painting*). The lesion is created at the focus, but then it always grows toward the transducer [8].

If energy at the focal point increases above a threshold of approximately 2000 W/cm$^3$, microbubbles form within the insonicated tissues because of the negative pressure of the ultrasound wave [15,16]. These microbubbles increase in size to the point at which resonance is achieved. When the bubbles suddenly collapse, mechanical disruption of tissues occurs, resulting in a cavitation process. This process mainly depends upon energy, pulse length, frequency, and tissue factors. As a natural consequence of thermal ablation, this is a process that is difficult to control [17]. Moreover, microbubble formation reflects incoming ultrasound waves so that the area of tissue damage grows rapidly outside the focal area (i.e., the intended target) toward the transducer, with the risk of damaging nontarget structures [15,18].

In contrast to thermal ablation, cavitation causes more rapid tissue destruction, which can be visualized with real-time ultrasonography [19]. Cavitation is produced by administering very short (20 microseconds) pulses composed of 10−15 waves that show similar morphology to shock waves, which are repeated at a rate of 100 Hz. This process essentially eliminates thermal ultrasound effects [20]. Lake et al studied this technique in vivo in canine models using an annular 18-element, 750-kHz, phased-array ultrasound system. Histological evaluation showed well-demarcated cavities containing liquefied material with a sharply delineated rim to morphologically intact cells [21,22]. Beyond this margin, no tissue damage was apparent. This technique, termed histotripsy, ap-pears promising, but the transition to clinical utilization has not yet occurred.

When utilizing energy ablative techniques to destroy malignant tumors, it is essential that systemic spread of tumor cells with metastatic potential is avoided. Experimental studies have clearly shown that this is not a risk with *thermal* HIFU ablation [6]. However, this has not been shown conclusively in techniques specifically targeting tissue with the aim of causing cavitation. The tissue effect of cavitation is mainly due to mechanical disruption, which, at least theoretically, could propagate systemic dispersion of living cells. There are similarities between cavitation and shock-wave lithotripsy (SWL), and early studies with SWL suggest that the spread of tumors with a high metastatic potential might be enhanced by shock-wave exposure [23].

## HIFU devices

For clinical use, an effective HIFU system must combine focused ultrasound with an integrated imaging device. Early HIFU systems were derived from piezo-electric lithotriptors. A number of piezoceramic elements were mounted on a concave dish and directed at a joint focal point [11]. To change the position of the focus the entire dish had to be moved. Although used in phase II clinical studies, the approach was rapidly abandoned because of the unreliable focusing and difficult manipulation of the very large generator. The current generation of HIFU systems mainly uses single, spherical transducers (Figure 3.1). They either have a fixed focus defined by the transducer shape and frequency [8,9,15,24], or the energy of a transducer is focused with acoustical lenses [25–27]. The latter system has the advantage of variable focal distances. The latest HIFU devices are based on phased-array systems. They are constructed with a multitude of different focal length transducers, so that focal depth and size can be changed rapidly in real time without having to reposition probes. Phased-array systems are more efficient and accurate than single element transducers, and permit contouring of the focal region to the target area three dimensionally [28]. Tissues are insonicated continuously and hence ablation is faster [28–30]. The systems can be miniaturized to allow placement into small cavities, such as the urethra [30].

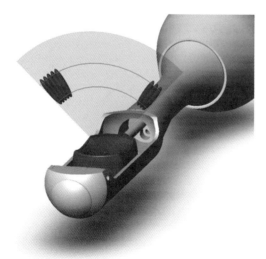

Fig 3.1 High-intensity focused ultrasound (HIFU) probe. (Reproduced with permission from Focus Surgery, Inc.)

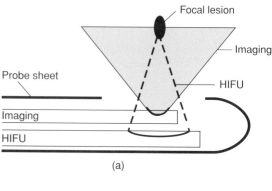

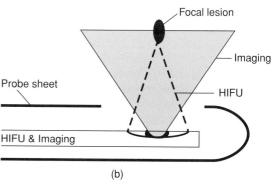

Fig 3.2 Transrectal (HIFU) probe. (a) Two separate transducers for imaging and therapy. (b) The same transducer is used for imaging and therapy. (Reproduced with permission from Margreiter, MD)

Ultrasonography has been the traditional imaging modality to direct HIFU. In single transducer systems, the central zone of the transducer can be used for imaging and the peripheral zone for HIFU. This permits real-time monitoring of the treatment zone, but as the same frequency used for ablation is used for imaging, this technique negatively impacts on image quality [8,10,31,32]. Alternatively, a therapeutic transducer may be coupled with a separate imaging transducer [9,27,33,34]. Imaging is then at optimal frequency and quality, but can only be performed intermittently (Figure 3.2).

One of the decisive drawbacks of HIFU is the difficulty of monitoring the tissue effect during treatment. As thermocouples interfere with insonication, traditional thermometry cannot be used. Attempts to utilize complex ultrasonography techniques such as elastography have not proven practical [35,36]. In general, HIFU ablation therefore follows treatment algorithms based on clinical experience and the scant data available from histological studies of tissues after HIFU [8,10,26,37]. Microbubble formation emerging near the cavitation threshold is of course easily visualized. Some authors have defined this as a sign of adequate energy deposition [31,38], and recommend "visually" directing HIFU by treating tissues until this occurs [39]. Although this achieves more thorough tissue ablation, it comes at higher morbidity and significantly longer treatment time [40]. Recently, there

has emerged an ultrasound-based thermometry for a transrectal HIFU device (Sonablate 500) for prostate ablation that may reduce the need for visually directed HIFU, although the method does need to be validated.

MRI thermometry appears at present to be the only reliable approach to real-time thermometry during HIFU. Temperature dependent tissue changes can be defined most precisely by field changes, so that temperatures can be monitored in vivo virtually in real time [41,42]. A prerequisite for precise MRI thermometry is the complete absence of movement of the target during measurement since a change in position by 1–3 mm may result in errors on the magnitude of 10–20°C. Mobile organs such as the prostate can be stabilized with a transrectal or transurethral device. With this configuration, automated 3D MRI treatment modeling combined with MRI thermometry for real-time monitoring of the HIFU effect appears promising. New phased-array HIFU systems integrated into

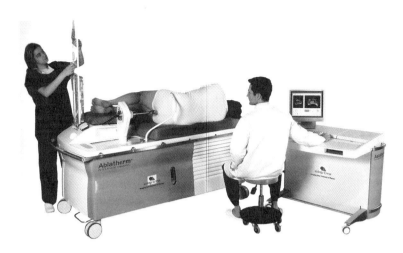

**Fig 3.3** Ablatherm HIFU system. Treatment module (left). Control module (right). (Reproduced with permission from EDAP-TMS, France) *See also plate 3.3.*

open access MRI scanners for transurethral (Profound Medical, Toronto, Canada) or transrectal (InSightec, Tel Aviv, Israel) ablation of prostate cancer are presently going into phase I clinical testing.

## Prostate cancer

As a minimally invasive procedure, HIFU promises lower overall morbidity, particularly with respect to continence and erectile function and comparable cancer control outcomes in the medium to long term.

### Transrectal HIFU devices

Currently two systems are commercially available and in clinical use. The Ablatherm® system (EDAP-TMS, Lyon, France) consists of a treatment and a control module (Figure 3.3). The treatment module includes a bed for positioning the patient, the HIFU generator, the HIFU probe with an integrated cooling system, and a robotic positioning system for the probe. Integrated in the HIFU probe are a separate 3-MHz treatment transducer and a 7.5-MHz imaging transducer. The treatment probe is focused at 45 mm from the crystal, which permits ablation to a maximum depth of 25 mm within the prostate. Depending on the treatment protocol pulses of 4–5-second insonication are delivered in an automated manner interrupted by 4–7-second intervals. One to four overlapping target areas are defined and treated from the apex to the bladder neck, starting 5–6 mm proximal to the external sphincter. To reduce the risk of rectal injury the "safety distance"

between the rectal mucosa and the posterior border of the prostate is defined as 3–6 mm.

The Sonablate 500® system (Focus Surgery, Indianapolis, Indiana, USA) consists of a console, a HIFU probe with an articulated arm and an integrated rectal wall cooling device (Figure 3.4). The HIFU probe has two 4-MHz transducers with focal distances of 3 cm and 4 cm, which are mounted back to back.

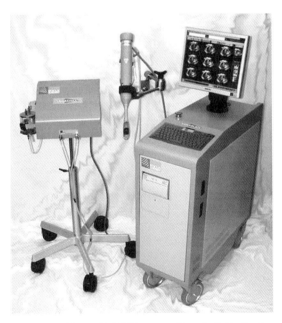

**Fig 3.4** Sonablate 500 HIFU system. Console (left). Cooling device (right). HIFU probe with articulated arm (Top right). (Reproduced with permission from Focus Surgery, Inc.) *See also plate 3.4.*

They can be used alternatively by rotating the treatment head 180° within the probe depending on the prostate penetration depth required. Each transducer has a dual function, with the center segment being used for confocal real-time imaging and the periphery for treatment. Pulse duration is routinely 3 seconds interrupted by 6-second intervals, although the off time can be reduced to 3 seconds. Depending on prostate size and shape, treatment is performed in segments covering the entire prostate, using the 4-cm transducer for the anterior and the 3-cm transducer for the posterior parts of the gland. As safety features the temperature at the rectal wall and the distance to the rectal wall are monitored continuously, with an automatic shut-off if safety limits are violated.

For HIFU of the prostate, the HIFU probe is inserted into the rectum, with the patient in the dorsal lithotomy position (Sonablate 500) or in a lateral position (Ablatherm). The transducer is covered by a condom, through which degassed, cooled water is circulated, cooling the rectal wall and eliminating acoustic interference between the transducer and the rectal mucosa. Multiple images of the prostate are taken and the treatment zones are defined (Figure 3.5). Large glands cannot be treated with the upper limit usually set at 40 mL, although the ultimate determining factor is the focal length of the probe. With the Ablatherm system, the maximum distance from the rectal wall to the most anterior part of the prostate can only be 25 mm, whereas the focal length of the Sonablate 500

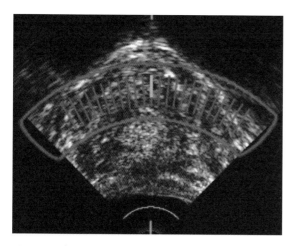

**Fig 3.5** Defining and monitoring treatment zones during the HIFU treatment of prostate cancer. (Reproduced with permission from Focus Surgery, Inc.)

can be up to 4 cm. The procedure is monitored continuously by ultrasonography and takes between 1 and 3 hours. It can potentially be performed as an outpatient procedure but requires epidural or general anesthesia to reduce patient movement. Due to swelling of the prostate secondary to the thermal effects a urethral or suprapubic catheter is placed into the bladder and left in place for 1 to 2 weeks. If a transurethral resection of the prostate (TURP) is performed prior to the HIFU treatment the catheters can usually be removed after 2 to 3 days.

### Primary prostate cancer

Morbidity of primary HIFU with curative intent is generally low (Table 3.1). In a multicenter trial of 402 patients treated with the Ablatherm system, catheters could be removed after a median period of 5 days, but 12.2% of patients had prolonged retention or urethral strictures requiring interventions [43]. Uchida et al performed HIFU with the Sonablate system for curative therapy in 181 patients with organ-confined disease [44]. In this single-center experience only 0.6% of patients required TURP for urinary retention, but 22% of patients needed urethral dilatation or urethrotomy for a urethral stricture. Other morbidities observed in these two series were rectourethral fistula in 1.2% and 1% of patients and temporary grade I stress incontinence in 10.6% and 0.6%, respectively. HIFU was repeated for positive biopsies in 28% and 13% of patients, respectively. Retreatment clearly increased the risk for complications. In a more recent series of 223 patients treated with the Ablatherm system, Blana et al found urinary tract infection in 0.4%, chronic pelvic pain in 0.9%, infravesical obstruction needing TURP or urethrotomy in 19.7%, and stress incontinence in 7.6% (7.2% grade I, 0.4% grade II) after the first treatment. In 49 patients needing a second HIFU treatment for positive biopsies or biochemical progression, the cumulative incontinence rate increased to 12.2%. Ahmed et al demonstrated a high stricture rate with use of a urethral catheter, but this dropped significantly when their practice changed to using a suprapubic catheter. They had no rectourethral fistula out of 172 men treated with a very high and encouraging pad-free rate of 99.4% [70].

The effect of HIFU on erectile function is poorly documented due to poor reporting of function, usually without the use of validated questionnaire measures.

**Table 3.1** Morbidity of hifu for the treatment of localized prostate cancer.

| Study | Complications | | | | |
| --- | --- | --- | --- | --- | --- |
| | Incontinence | Erectile dysfunction | Fistulae | Stricture | Urinary tract infection/dysuria |
| Ahmed et al [53,64] | 7.0% (grade I leak, no pads) 0.6% (pads) | 30% IIEF-15 decreased from 33.8 to 28.1 | 0 | 15% (suprapubic catheter) 44% (urethral catheter) | 24% |
| Mearini et al [65] | 16% (grade I) 0.6% (grade III) | IIEF decreased from 16 to 12 | 0.6% | 15% | – |
| Uchida et al [31,44] | 2% (grade I) | 17% | 2% | 24% | – |
| Uchida et al [31,44] | 0.5% (grade I) | 13% | 1% | 22% | 6% |
| Blana et al [13,37] | 6.1% (grade I) 1.8% (grade II) 0 (grade III) | 45% | 0 | 25% | 8% |
| Blana et al [13,37] | 5.8% (grade I) No grade II/III | 53% | 0.6% | 12% | 4% |
| Poissonnier et al [45] | 12% (grade I–II) 1% (grade III) | 39% | 0 | 12% | 2% |
| Ficarra et al (2006) | 7% (no grade) | – | 0 | 10% | 16% |
| Vallancien et al [24] | 3% (no grade) | 32% | 0 | 6% (retention) | 10% |
| Blana et al [56] | 5% (grade I) 0.7% (grade II) | 43% | 0 | 14% (urinary obstruction) | 7% |
| Thüroff et al [43] | 11% (grade I) 2.5% (grade II) 1.5% (grade III) | – | 1% | 3.6% 9% (retention) | 14% |
| Chaussy and Thüroff [63] | 15.4% (pre-HIFU TURP) 6.9% (HIFU only) | – | – | – | UTI (47.9% pre-HIFU TURP versus 11.4% HIFU only) |

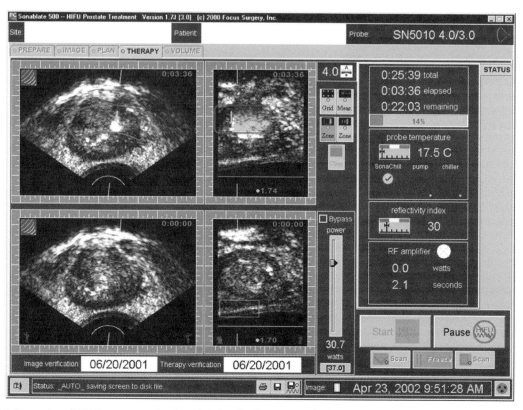

**Fig 3.6** Screenshot of HIFU treatment planning with visualized neurovascular bundles. (Reproduced with permission from Focus Surgery, Inc.)

Poissonnier et al reported complete loss of potency in 39% of 41 previously potent patients [45]. If the presumed location of the neurovascular bundles was not treated ("nerve-sparing HIFU"), erections were preserved in 18 (69%) of 26 patients (Figure 3.6). Blana et al reported a 49.8% impotence rate after one HIFU treatment and a cumulative rate of 55% after a second HIFU [46]. The UK series reported by Ahmed et al showed 30% impotence rate, although this was based on a minority of men who filled in validated questionnaires [64].

Table 3.2 summarizes published data on the therapeutic efficacy of HIFU, which is usually based on posttherapy PSA values and inconsistently on follow-up biopsies. The majority of patients in these series had low- to intermediate-risk cancers. If stratified according to preoperative PSA, Poissonnier et al reported a disease-free survival rate (defined as negative biopsy and absence of biochemical progression by ASTRO criteria) at 5 years of 90% in patients with a preop-

erative PSA <4 ng/mL, 57% for PSA 4.1–9.9 ng/mL and 61% for PSA >10 ng/mL [45]. Blana et al recently reported long-term outcomes after HIFU in 163 patients with low- to intermediate-risk prostate cancer. Using the Phoenix definition (PSA nadir + 2 ng/mL) the 5-year disease-free survival rate was 66% [13]. The use of the Phoenix definition in the setting of HIFU might, however, be misleading since the Phoenix definition was designed to define biochemical failure following external beam radiotherapy. In contrast to all forms of radiotherapy, the PSA nadir is reached within 6 months after HIFU. The nadir has been found to correlate significantly with treatment outcome. Ganzer et al evaluated the impact of the PSA nadir achieved within 8 weeks of treatment: <0.2 ng/mL (20 patients), 0.21–1.0 ng/mL (25 patients), and >1 ng/mL (18 patients) correlated to 3-year disease-free survival rates of 100%, 74%, and 21%, respectively [47]. It seems that a high PSA nadir provides an early warning sign of disease recurrence. If an adequate PSA nadir is

**Table 3.2** Efficacy of HIFU for the treatment of localized prostate cancer.

| Study | Device | N | D'amico risk categories (unless otherwise specified) | Hormones | Follow-up (months) (mean/median) | Biochemical control (PSA, ng/mL) | Positive biopsy |
|---|---|---|---|---|---|---|---|
| Ahmed et al [53,64] | S | 172 (1.0 sessions) | 28% (low) 38% (intermediate) 34% (high) | 29% | 12 | 92% No evidence of disease 61% (PSA <0.2) 83% (PSA <0.5) | 8% |
| Mearini et al [65] | S | 163 (1.17 sessions) | 49% (low) 29% (intermediate) 9% (high) | 0 | 24 | 78% (Phoenix) PSA nadir 0.15 70% (PSA <0.4) | 34% |
| Blana et al [13,37] | A | 163 (first 47 HIFU only; 116 pre-HIFU TURP) (1.2 sessions) | 52% (low) 49% (intermediate) | 37% | 58 | 75% (Phoenix) 86% (PSA <1.0) 64% (PSA <0.2) | 7% ("vital prostate cancer" |
| Misrai et al (2008) | A | 119 (71% pre-HIFU TURP) (1.4 sessions) | 55% (low) 42% (intermediate) 3% (high) | 0 | 47 | 56% (Phoenix) | 65% |
| Blana et al [13,37] | A | 140 (1.3 HIFU sessions) | 51% (low) 49% (intermediate) | 16% | 77 | 66% and 59% at 5 and 7 years (Phoenix ASTRO) 68.4% (PSA <0.5) | 14% |
| Poissonnier et al [45] | A | 227 (pre-HIFU TURP) (1.4 HIFU sessions) | | 34% | 27 | 84% (PSA<0.5) 66% disease-free survival at 5 years[b] | 14% |
| Uchida et al [31,44] | S | 63 (1.2 HIFU sessions) | 35% (low) 41% (intermediate) 24% (high) | 0 | 22 | 75% (old ASTRO criteria) | 13% |
| Ficarra et al (2006) | A | 30 (pre-HIFU TURP) | 100% (high)[a] | 100% (3 yrs) | 12 | 90% (PSA <0.3) 100% (PSA <1) | 23% |

(Continued)

**Table 3.2** (*Continued*)

| Study | Device | N | D'amico risk categories (unless otherwise specified) | Hormones | Follow-up (months) (mean/median) | Biochemical control (PSA, ng/mL) | Positive biopsy |
|---|---|---|---|---|---|---|---|
| Uchida et al [31,44] | S | 181 (1.2 HIFU sessions) | 29% (low) 45% (intermediate) 26% (high) | 52% | 18 | 78% (5 years) (old ASTRO) | – |
| Vallancien et al [24] | A | 30 (pre-HIFU TURP) | – | – | 20 | Mean 0.9 | 14% |
| Blana et al [56] | A | 146 (1.17 HIFU sessions) | – | 0 | 22 | 92% (PSA <1); 83% (PSA <0.5); 56% (PSA <0.1) | 7% |
| Thüroff et al [43] | A | 402 (1.5 HIFU sessions) | 28% (low) 48% (intermediate) 24% (high) | 0 | 11 | Median 0.6 Mean 1.8 | 13% |
| Chaussy and Thüroff [63] | A | 271 (96 HIFU only; 175 pre-HIFU TURP) | – | – | 19 | 80–84% (old ASTRO) | 29–34% |
| Gelet et al (2001) | A | 102 | – | – | 19 | 66% (3 consecutive increases in PSA + velocity >0.75/year or positive biopsy) 80–84% (old ASTRO) | 25% |

[a]Clinical stage of ≥T3 a or Gleason score 8–10, or total PSA >20 ng/mL.
[b]Any positive biopsy or a PSA >1 ng/mL with three consecutive rises

not reached within 3–4 months, additional HIFU therapy or an alternative therapy should be considered. Nevertheless, a major advantage of HIFU in this situation is that no bridges are burned and all forms of other curative therapy are still possible, albeit at a slightly higher complication rate [48,49]. Ahmed et al have used a definition of "no evidence of disease" combining histological and biochemical outcomes showing 92% were free of disease a median of just under 12 months follow-up. Although encouraging, this series suffered from short follow-up and lack of mandatory biopsies in all men undergoing HIFU [64]. Mearini et al showed 72% biochemical control by Phoenix criteria in 163 over a median follow-up of 24 months [65].

Longer term data is now starting to emerge from the more experienced centers. Uchida has recently updated his results on 517 patients over a maximum follow-up of 8 years showing an overall success rate of 72% using Phoenix ASTRO criteria with low-, intermediate-, and high-risk groups at 5 years showing 84%, 64%, and 45% success by this criteria, respectively ($P < 0.0001$) [66]. Blana et al reported on 8-year follow-up data showing a biochemical control rate of 75% at 5 years in 164 patients, who had undergone 4.8 +/– 1.2 years of follow-up [37]. Blana et al have also attempted to define the optimal definition of failure in men undergoing whole-gland HIFU. They have shown that PSA nadir plus 1.2 ng/mL seemed to best predict failure, although it remains to be validated in other cohorts [67].

An inherent problem of HIFU in treating prostate cancer is the limited penetration depth of the transducer. Curative treatment is limited to prostates with a volume below 40 mL. The decisive factor is the maximum anterior–posterior diameter, and with transducers of shorter focal depth this cannot exceed 25 mm [50]. To overcome this problem combining HIFU ablation with TURP in the same procedure has been recommended [32,50]. The reduction of prostate volume renders anterior parts of the prostate more accessible, especially when it is also flattened by compression with the transrectal balloon. With this approach, Poissonnier et al [45] reduced obstructive complications after HIFU from 31% to 6%, and Chaussy et al [50] reported a need for second HIFU procedures in only 5% of patients. Others have used short-term hormonal deprivation to cytoreduce prostate volume, although this carries systemic side effects (albeit reversible) and

impacts on PSA measures after treatment even if the half-life is short.

## Focal therapy

The rationale behind focal therapy is to minimize morbidity by treating only the cancer-bearing part of the prostate [68,69]. Early attempts were made by Madersbacher et al, who treated patients with one positive core in a unilateral palpable nodule and with an otherwise normal prostate on ultrasonography [8]. The lobe with the positive core and a surrounding "safety zone" were ablated by transrectal HIFU. The prostate was then removed by radical prostatectomy and examined by whole-mount histology. The tumor was always correctly targeted, but due to unexpected tumor distribution, only three out of ten patients showed complete tumor ablation. The authors concluded that because of the unpredictable tumor location the entire prostate had to be ablated. Since that time advances in imaging and biopsy techniques such as template transperineal mapping permit a more reliable detection of index cancers [51]. Phase II trials are currently ongoing and are expected to formally report soon, although early indications from conference proceedings is that genitourinary side effects are low (<5% erectile dysfunction, <5% pad-free incontinence, 90% cancer control at 1 year) [70]. The main problem currently lies in determining treatment failure. Since only part of the prostate is ablated, PSA fails as a surrogate marker, leaving only imaging techniques and repeat biopsy to detect recurrence.

## Recurrent prostate cancer

Salvage HIFU for locally recurrent prostate cancer after failure of curative surgery or radiotherapy seems appealing due to the ability to control lesion size and the good accessibility, but clinical experience is limited. In a retrospective analysis of 72 patients treated with HIFU for recurrent or residual tumor after external beam radiotherapy, negative biopsies were reported in 80% of patients at a mean follow-up of 39 months and with a median nadir PSA of 0.10 ng/mL [52]. Complications were significant, with 32% of patients developing grade II or III incontinence, 30% a urethral stricture or bladder neck stenosis, and a rectourethral fistula rate of 6% [48,52]. The UK group based in University College London reported on a smaller cohort of 31 men treated with whole-gland HIFU after external beam radiotherapy failure. They demonstrated a stricture or necrotic tissue retention of 36%, UTI/dysuria syndrome of 26%. Pad-free incontinence was low at 94%, although the rectourethral fistula rate was 3%. 71% had no evidence of disease but follow-up was short (median 9 months) [71]. For salvage HIFU after combined brachytherapy and external beam radiotherapy, even higher rates of rectourethral fistula formation have been reported, with as many as three out of five developing a rectourethral fistula [53]. Radiation therapy renders the anterior wall of the rectum considerably more vulnerable to injury, predisposing to rectourethral fistula. The use of transrectal biopsies to determine the presence of cancer in the radiotherapy treated prostate may also contribute to fistula formation. Thus, ablative treatments that utilize a perineal approach, such as cryoablation, may be more advantageous in this situation. This is not true for HIFU after failed radical prostatectomy. Chaussy et al performed HIFU 36 men who had undergone surgery and developed PSA progression with biopsy proven recurrent tumor [50]. With a mean follow-up of 59.7 weeks, 74% had negative biopsies and 65% reached a PSA nadir of <0.5 ng/mL. Complication rates were not reported, but these results suggest that salvage HIFU is a viable alternative to conventional therapies, particularly when the complication rates of other salvage options are considered.

## Renal tumors

In contrast to radiofrequency ablation and cryoablation, HIFU does not require puncturing the tumor, avoiding the high risk of hemorrhage or theoretical tumor spillage [54]. Ideally, this could be performed by an extracorporeal approach with a noninvasive approach [55].

Two HIFU systems operating in the 1–1.8-MHz range have been tested for extracorporeal HIFU of kidney tumors. A Storz HIFU prototype device (Storz Medical AG, Kreuzlingen, Switzerland) utilizes a 1-MHz piezoelectric element with a focal point at 100 mm using a parabolic reflector with a 10-cm aperture. The Chongqing HAIFU system (Chongqing Haifu Technology Co. Ltd., China) has exchangeable ellipsoidal therapeutic transducers of 12-cm or 15-cm diameter with frequencies of 0.5 MHz, 1.2 MHz, and

1.5 MHz. Both systems use a 3.5-MHz B-mode ultrasound transducer integrated in the device for in-line imaging of the targeted area.

Köhrmann et al reported partial remissions at radiological follow-up in 2 of 3 tumors treated with the Storz device. Marberger et al also observed tumor shrinkage with this technique and system at radiological follow-up in two patients, but residual tumor was detected at histological examination of the targeted tumor zone in all 14 patients in whom the tumor was removed after HIFU [26] (Figure 3.7). Häcker et al observed similarly insufficient results, with no correlation between energy administered and lesion achieved [27]. Experience with the Chongqing device was similar—radiological follow-up suggested some efficacy, but histological confirmation consistently documented insufficient ablation [25,56]. Possible explanations for the disappointing results are the respiratory movement of the kidney and complex acoustical interphases between transducer and target. Attempts to limit target movement by controlling ventilation during general anesthesia have proven unreliable [26]. Target mobility also renders MRI thermometry too unreliable with the present systems [57]. Theoretically, movement of the target can be corrected by using multichannel focused ultrasonic systems and multiprobe systems of small-aperture confocal HIFU transducers. These options are currently being studied experimentally, but have not reached clinical evaluation at this time [41].

The problems with target mobility and multiple acoustic interphases are avoided if the transducer is

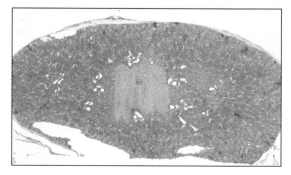

**Fig 3.7** HIFU lesion in normal parenchyma of a human kidney (kidney exposed surgically, 4-MHz, 3.5-cm transducer, site intensity 1650 cm$^2$, targeted lesion 10×10 mm). (Reproduced with permission from Department of Urology, Medical University Vienna)

brought directly to the target by laparoscopic HIFU (Figure 3.8). A laparoscopic HIFU probe (Sonatherm, Misonix Inc, Farmingdale, NY, USA) has recently undergone first clinical testing. It consists of a 4-MHz transducer with a 30 mm × 13 mm aperture and 35-mm focal length, which can be brought directly to the tumor through an 18-mm port. Real-time imaging of the target area in two planes is provided with an integrated single-element, 12-mm diameter imaging transducer aligned confocally with the therapy transducer. Insonication is performed in a continuous mode, with a maximum treatment depth of 3 cm.

Paterson et al evaluated a prototype in a porcine model [58]. Twelve of 13 kidneys showed homogeneous, complete coagulative necrosis throughout the entire target lesion with sharp demarcation to adjacent normal tissues [58]. Klingler et al tested the device in a phase I clinical trial [10]. In the first two patients, a defined target lesion was placed within the tumor prior to nephrectomy. Histological evaluation showed complete irreversible thermal damage within the tumor corresponding in position and size to the target. Subsequently, small renal masses with a mean diameter of 2.2 cm (range 1.1–4.0 cm) were completely ablated and then removed by laparoscopic partial nephrectomy. Histology showed complete destruction of the tumors in four patients. Two of the tumors showed a 1–3-mm rim of viable tumor at the surface of the tumor immediately adjacent to the transducer. Obviously, the transducer was too close to obtain sufficient site intensity at this location. By keeping the transducer >7 mm from the tumor, this problem was subsequently avoided. Only one tumor showed central areas of vital tissue (i.e., skip lesions), corresponding to about 20% of the tumor volume. No intra or postoperative complications or side effects were observed.

## Bladder tumors

HIFU therapy for the treatment of superficial bladder tumors has only been described by a single group, and data on this approach are limited. Vallencien et al used the Pyrotech system (EDAP Company, Croissy Beaubourg, France) with a 1-MHz generator and 16 piezoelectric elements with a fixed focus at 32 cm [59,60]. A phase II study included 20 patients with superficial bladder tumors (3 cm$^3$ mean treated tumor volume) [61]. The procedure was performed under general or spinal anesthesia. Overall, 15 patients (75%) had a normal urinary cytology and cystoscopy at 1 month. At 1 year, 33% of the patients had recurrent tumors. Of note, two patients sustained moderate skin toxicity, and one patient developed acute urinary retention after HIFU. The procedure took longer than standard TUR and still required anesthesia.

HIFU ablation may not prove to be a feasible option for the treatment of bladder tumors due to the multiple acoustic interphases between tumor tissue and urine as well as difficulty accessing the bladder with an ultrasound probe. In addition, ablating a hollow organ with HIFU has additional challenges of causing perforation that can necessitate a laparotomy.

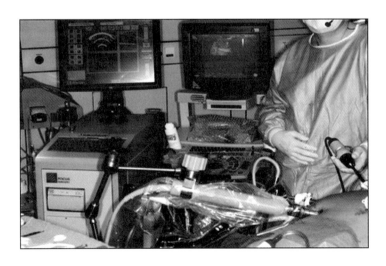

**Fig 3.8** Intraoperative setup with laparoscopic HIFU probe in place (center), HIFU treatment unit (left), and laparoscopic ultrasound probe (right). (Reproduced with permission from Department of Urology, Medical University Vienna)

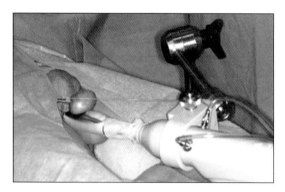

**Fig 3.9** Intraoperative setup with HIFU probe in place (right). The testis is held in place with a retractor (left).

## Testicular tumors

Testicular tumors are appealing for HIFU ablation because they can be perfectly visualized by ultrasonography, are easily accessed with few acoustic interphases, and lie within an organ of homogenous echogenicity. Clearly, HIFU ablation cannot be an alternative to orchidectomy in the presence of a normal contralateral testis, but it may be a useful alternative in patients with bilateral testis tumors or a tumor in a solitary testis. Organ-sparing surgical excision of tumors carries a considerable risk of irreversible loss of endocrine function and in this situation Madersbacher et al [12] first showed the efficacy of HIFU ablation. With the patient in the supine position, the treatment probe of the previous Sonablate 200 system was approximated to the scrotum, which was immersed in degassed water. Using a very similar approach as in transrectal HIFU of the prostate, the entire tumor with a safety margin of 5 mm was insonicated with a 4-second-on/12-second-off mode (Figure 3.9).

In a phase I trial, four patients with prostate cancer were subjected to transcutaneous HIFU therapy of the testis prior to scrotal orchiectomy. Homogeneous severe thermal damage consistent with complete coagulative necrosis was obtained within the entire target zone. Subsequently, four patients with a testicular tumor in a solitary testis were treated with transcutaneous HIFU with curative intent. All patients had lost the contralateral testis for cancer and were assumed to have carcinoma in situ in the remaining testis, and prophylactic irradiation of the testis with 18–20 Gy was performed 6 weeks following HIFU. No complications other than one superficial skin burn were observed, and no patient needed testosterone substitution. With a mean follow-up of 23.3 months, (range 16–31 months) only one patient who had refused post-HIFU irradiation developed a recurrent tumor. This was at a different site than the original tumor and clearly represented a de novo lesion. Kratzik et al added three more patients and reported long-term results with a mean follow-up of 42 months (range 3 to 93 months) (Figure 3.10). All six patients who had HIFU ablation of their tumor and prophylactic irradiation remained free of tumor recurrence, needed no testosterone substitution, and maintained normal sexual function and libido [62].

## Future directions

The most important factors for successful HIFU treatment are imaging and guidance. Current HIFU

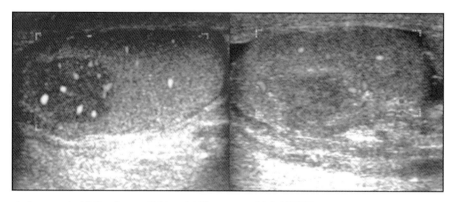

**Fig 3.10** Scrotal ultrasound with Duplex pre (left) and 48 hours post (right) HIFU treatment.

systems utilize ultrasonography and MRI for targeting and monitoring the success of therapy. Unfortunately, the ability to monitor temperature with ultrasonography is not yet possible. MRI is more expensive but has the distinct advantage of providing precise temperature monitoring at the focal point within seconds after HIFU exposure. New MRI and 3D-ultrasound systems represent the future of HIFU, and refinements in HIFU devices as well as improvements in imaging techniques are expected to improve cancer control while reducing side effects and complications. However, further studies and long-term data will be necessary before the widespread use of HIFU can be recommended.

## Conclusions

HIFU has been proposed as a noninvasive treatment for malignant tumors. Early reports including recent long-term studies suggest that this ablative technology provides appropriate oncological control with low morbidity. HIFU is based on ultrasound, and therefore, the same limitations apply. In particular, problems with acoustic shadowing, target movement, and monitoring for therapeutic failure remain challenging. Extracorporeal treatment of renal masses has shown unsatisfactory results because of the acoustic complexity of intervening structures and mobility of the kidney. For renal masses, the difficulties with respiratory movement and interphases have been avoided by using laparoscopic HIFU transducers.

With respect to homogeneous, nonmoving organs, HIFU achieves excellent tissue ablation with millimeter accuracy and minimal damage to intervening structures. Thus, prostate cancer and testicular cancer are optimal tumors for HIFU therapy. In patients with low-risk prostate cancer, primary HIFU treatment appears to be an alternative to active surveillance protocols as well as in men who are not candidates for surgery.

## References

1. Frey R (1950) Experimental investigations on the effect of ultrasonic therapy in Jensen-sarcoma of the rat. Langenbecks Arch Klin Chir Ver Dtsch Z Chir 264: 233–235.

2. Lochmann H (1950) Results of experimental and clinical ultrasonic treatment of malignant tumors. Langenbecks Arch Klin Chir Ver Dtsch Z Chir 264: 235–238.

3. Burov AK (1956) High-intensity ultrasonic vibrations for action on animal and human malignant tumors. Dokl Akad Nauk SSSR 106: 239–241.

4. Wang X, Sun J (2002) High-intensity focused ultrasound in patients with late-stage pancreatic carcinoma. Chin Med J (Engl) 115: 1332–1335.

5. Wu F et al (2003) A randomised clinical trial of high-intensity focused ultrasound ablation for the treatment of patients with localised breast cancer. Br J Cancer 89: 2227–2233.

6. Chapelon JY et al (1992) In vivo effects of high-intensity ultrasound on prostatic adenocarcinoma Dunning R3327. Cancer Res 52: 6353–6357.

7. Gelet A et al (1996) Treatment of prostate cancer with transrectal focused ultrasound: Early clinical experience. Eur Urol 29: 174–183.

8. Madersbacher S et al (1995) Effect of high-intensity focused ultrasound on human prostate cancer in vivo. Cancer Res 55: 3346–3351.

9. Gelet A et al (2004) Prostate cancer control with transrectal HIFU in 242 consecutive patients: 5-year results. Eur Urol Suppl. 3:214.

10. Klingler HC et al (2008) A novel approach to energy ablative therapy of small renal tumors: Laparoscopic high-intensity focused ultrasound. Eur Urol 53: 810–816

11. Vallancien G et al (1995) Destruction of superficial bladder tumors with focused extracorporeal pyrotherapy. In: M Marberger (ed.) *Application of Newer Forms of Therapeutic Energy in Urology*. Vol 10. Oxford: Isis Medical Media Ltd., pp. 99–106.

12. Madersbacher S et al (1998) Transcutaneous high-intensity focused ultrasound and irradiation: An organ-preserving treatment of cancer in a solitary testis. Eur Urol 33: 195–201.

13. Blana A et al (2008) First analysis of the long-term results with transrectal HIFU in patients with localised prostate cancer. Eur Urol 53: 1194–2001.

14. Madersbacher S, Marberger M (1995) Therapeutic applications of ultrasound in urology. In: M Marberger (ed.) *Application of Newer Forms of Therapeutic Energy in Urology*. Vol 12. Oxford: Isis Medical Media Ltd., pp. 115–136.

15. Ter Haar GR, Robertson G (1993) Tissue destruction with focused ultrasound in vivo. Eur Urol 23: 8–14.

16. Hill CR, Ter Haar GR (1995) High intensity focused ultrasound – potential for cancer treatment. Br J Radiol 68: 1296–1303.

17. Fry FJ et al (1970) Threshold ultrasonic dosages for structural changes in the mammalian brain. J Acoust Soc Am 48: 1413.

18. Dunn F, Lohnes JE, Fry FJ (1975) Frequency dependence of threshold ultrasonic dosages for irreversible structural changes in mammalian brain. J Acoust Soc Am 58: 512–514.

19. Roberts WW (2005) Focused ultrasound ablation of renal and prostate cancer: Current technology and future directions. Urol Oncol 23: 367–371.

20. Roberts WW et al (2006) Pulsed cavitational ultrasound: A noninvasive technology for controlled tissue ablation (histotripsy) in the rabbit kidney. J Urol 175: 734–738.

21. Lake AM et al (2008) Renal ablation by histotripsy–does it spare the collecting system? J Urol 179: 1150–1154.

22. Lake AM et al (2008) Histotripsy: Minimally invasive technology for prostatic tissue ablation in an in vivo canine model. Urology 72: 682–686.

23. Oosterhof GO et al (1997) Influence of high-intensity focused ultrasound on the development of metastases. Eur Urol 32: 91–95.

24. Vallancien G et al (2004) Transrectal focused ultrasound combined with transurethral resection of the prostate for the treatment of localized prostate cancer: Feasibility study. J Urol 171: 2265–2267.

25. Wu F et al (2003) Preliminary experience using high intensity focused ultrasound for the treatment of patients with advanced stage renal malignancy. J Urol 170: 2237–2240.

26. Marberger M et al (2005) Extracorporeal ablation of renal tumours with high-intensity focused ultrasound. BJU Int 95(suppl. 2): 52–55.

27. Häcker A et al (2006) Extracorporeally induced ablation of renal tissue by high-intensity focused ultrasound. BJU Int 97: 779–785.

28. Penna MA et al (2007) Modeling prostate anatomy from multiple view TRUS images for image-guided HIFU therapy. IEEE Trans Ultrason Ferroelectr Freq Control 54: 52–69.

29. Boyes A et al (2007) Prostate tissue analysis immediately following magnetic resonance imaging guided transurethral ultrasound thermal therapy. J Urol 178: 1080–1085.

30. Chopra R et al (2008) MRI-compatible transurethral ultrasound system for the treatment of localized prostate cancer using rotational control. Med Phys 35: 1346–1357.

31. Uchida T et al (2006) Treatment of localized prostate cancer using high-intensity focused ultrasound. BJU Int 97: 56–61.

32. Illing R, Emberton M (2006) Sonablate-500: Transrectal high-intensity focused ultrasound for the treatment of prostate cancer. Expert Rev Med Devices 3: 717–729.

33. Beerlage HP et al (1999) Transrectal high-intensity focused ultrasound using the Ablatherm device in the treatment of localized prostate carcinoma. Urology 54: 273–277.

34. Tsakiris P et al (2008) Transrectal high-intensity focused ultrasound devices: A critical appraisal of the available evidence. J Endourol 22: 221–229.

35. Ophir J et al (1991) Elastography: A quantitative method for imaging the elasticity of biological tissues. Ultrason Imaging 13: 111–134.

36. Souchon R et al (2003) Visualisation of HIFU lesions using elastography of the human prostate in vivo: Preliminary results. Ultrasound Med Biol 29: 1007–1015.

37. Blana A et al (2008) Eight years' experience with high-intensity focused ultrasonography for treatment of localized prostate cancer. Urology 72: 1329–1333.

38. Chen H, Li X, Wan M, Wang S (2009) High-speed observation of cavitation bubble clouds near a tissue boundary in high-intensity focused ultrasound fields. Ultrasonics 49: 289–292.

39. Illing RO et al (2006) Visually directed high-intensity focused ultrasound for organ-confined prostate cancer: A proposed standard for the conduct of therapy. BJU Int 98: 1187–1192.

40. Schatzl G, Waldert M, Marberger M Algorithm based HIFU of prostate cancer is more effective and safer than visually directed HIFU. Unpublished data..

41. Smith NB, Buchanan MT, Hynynen K (1999) Transrectal ultrasound applicator for prostate heating monitored using MRI thermometry. Int J Radiat Oncol Biol Phys 43: 217–225.

42. Canney MS et al (2008) Acoustic characterization of high intensity focused ultrasound fields: A combined measurement and modeling approach. J Acoust Soc Am 124: 2406–2420.

43. Thüroff S et al (2003) High-intensity focused ultrasound and localized prostate cancer efficacy results from the European multicentric study. J Endourol 17: 673–677.

44. Uchida T et al (2006) Five year experience of transrectal high-intensity focused ultrasound using the Sonablate device in the treatment of localized prostate cancer. Int J Urol 13: 228–233.

45. Poissonnier L et al (2007) Control of prostate cancer by transrectal HIFU in 227 patents. Eur Urol 51: 381–387.

46. Blana A et al (2006) Morbidity associated with repeated transrectal high intensity focused ultrasound treatment of localized prostate cancer. World J Urol 24: 585–590.

47. Ganzer R et al (2008) PSA nadir is a significant predictor of treatment failure after high-intensity focused ultrasound (HIFU) treatment of localised prostate cancer. Eur Urol 53: 547–553

48. Gelet A et al (2004) Local recurrence of prostate cancer after external beam radiotherapy: Early experience of salvage therapy using high intensity focused ultrasonography. Urology 63: 625–629.

49. Pasticier G et al (2008) Salvage radiotherapy after high-intensity focused ultrasound for localized prostate cancer: Early clinical results. Urology 72: 1305–1309.

50. Chaussy Y, Thüroff S, Bergsdorf T (2006) Local recurrence of prostate cancer after curative therapy. HIFU (Ablatherm) as a treatment option. Urologe A 45: 1271–1275.

51. Kirkham AP, Emberton M, Allen C (2006) How good is MRI at detecting and characterising cancer within the prostate? Eur Urol 50: 1163–1174.

52. Poissonnier L et al (2008) Locally recurrent prostatic adenocarcinoma after exclusive radiotherapy: Results of high intensity focused ultrasound. Prog Urol 18: 223–229.

53. Ahmed HU et al (2009) Rectal fistulae after salvage high-intensity focused ultrasound for recurrent prostate cancer after combined brachytherapy and external beam radiotherapy. BJU Int 103: 321–323.

54. Marberger M (2007) Ablation of renal tumours with extracorporeal high-intensity focused ultrasound. BJU Int 99: 1273–1276.

55. Klatte T, Marberger M (2009) High-intensity focused ultrasound for the treatment of renal masses: Current status and future potential. Curr Opin Urol 19(2): 188–191.

56. Blana A et al (2004) High intensity focused ultrasound for the treatment of localized prostate cancer. Urology 63: 297–300.

57. Illing RO et al (2005) The safety and feasibility of extracorporeal high intensity focused ultrasound (HIFU) for the treatment of liver and kidney tumours in a Western population. Br J Cancer 93: 890–895.

58. Damianou C et al (2004) High intensity focused ultrasound ablation of kidney guided by MRI. Ultrasound Med Biol 30: 397–404.

59. Peters NH, Bartels LW, Lalezari F (2006) Respiratory and cardiac motion-induced Bo fluctuations in the breast: Implications for PRFS-based temperature monitoring. In: GR Clement, NJ McDannold, K Hynynen (eds.) *Therapeutic Ultrasound: 5th ISTU Symposium, Boston, Massachusetts. AIP Proceedings 829,* New York: Melville, pp. 81–85.

60. Chartier-Kastler E, Chopin D, Vallancien G (1993) The effects of focused extracorporeal pyrotherapy on a human bladder tumor cell line (647 V). J Urol 149: 643–647.

61. Bataille N, Vallancien G, Chopin D (1996) Antitumoral local effect and metastatic risk of focused extracorporeal pyrotherapy on Dunning R-3327 tumors. Eur Urol 29: 72–77.

62. Vallancien G et al (1996) Ablation of superficial bladder tumors with focused extracorporeal pyrotherapy. Urology 47: 204–207.

63. Chaussy C, Thüroff S (2003) The status of high-intensity focused ultrasound in the treatment of localized prostate cancer and the impact of a combined resection. Curr Urol Rep 4: 248–252.

64. Ahmed HU et al (2009) High-intensity-focused ultrasound in the treatment of primary prostate cancer: The first UK series. Br J Cancer 101(1): 19–26.

65. Mearini L et al (2009) Visually directed transrectal high intensity focused ultrasound for the treatment of prostate cancer: A preliminary report on the Italian experience. J Urol 181(1): 105–111.

66. Uchida T et al (2009) Transrectal high-intensity focused ultrasound for the treatment of localized prostate cancer: Eight-year experience. Int J Urol 16(11): 881–886.

67. Blana A et al (2009) High-intensity focused ultrasound for prostate cancer: Comparative definitions of biochemical failure. BJU Int 104(8): 1058–1062.

68. Ahmed HU et al (2007) Will focal therapy become a standard of care for men with localized prostate cancer? Nat Clin Pract Oncol 4(11): 632–642.

69. Ahmed HU (2009) The index lesion and the origin of prostate cancer. N Engl J Med 361(17): 1704–1706.

70. Ahmed HU, Moore C, Emberton M (2009) Minimally-invasive technologies in uro-oncology: The role of cryotherapy, HIFU and photodynamic therapy in whole gland and focal therapy of localised prostate cancer. Surg Oncol 18(3): 219–232.

71. Zacharakis E et al (2008) The feasibility and safety of high-intensity focused ultrasound as salvage therapy for recurrent prostate cancer following external beam radiotherapy. BJU Int 102(7): 786–792.

72. Ficarra V, Antoniolli SZ, Novara G, Parisi A, Fracalanza S, Martignoni G, Artibani W (2006) Short-term outcome after high-intensity focused ultrasound in the treatment of patients with high-risk prostate cancer. BJU Int. 98: 1193–1198.

73. Misrai V, Roupret M, Chartier-Kastler E, Comperat E, Renard-Penna R, Haertig A, Bitker MO, Richard F, Conort P (2008) Oncologic control provided by HIFU therapy as single treatment in men with clinically localized prostate cancer. World J Urol. 26: 481–485.

74. Ficarra V, Antoniolli SZ, Novara G, Parisi A, Fracalanza S, Martignoni G, Artibani W (2006) Short-term outcome after high-intensity focused ultrasound in the treatment of patients with high-risk prostate cancer. BJU Int. 98: 1193–1198.

75. Gelet A, Chapelon JY, Bouvier R, Rouviere O, Lyonnet D, Dubernard JM (2001) Transrectal high intensity focused ultrasound for the treatment of localized prostate cancer: factors influencing the outcome. Eur Urol. 40: 124–129.

# 4 Prostate and renal cryotherapy

*Chad R. Ritch*[1], *Aaron E. Katz*[1], *Hashim U. Ahmed*[2], *and Manit Arya*[3]

[1]Department of Urology, Columbia University Medical Center, NY Presbyterian Hospital, New York, USA
[2]Division of Surgery and Interventional Science, University College London, University College London Hospitals NHS Foundation Trust, London, UK
[3]Laparoscopic and Minimally Invasive Surgery, King's College Hospital, London, UK

## Prostate cryotherapy

The origins of cryotherapy can be dated back to the 1840s when scientists first administered salt solutions with crushed ice to freeze tumors of the breast and cervix [1]. They found that it led to tumor shrinkage and reduced drainage while providing local pain control. Throughout the latter part of the nineteenth and early twentieth century, cryosurgery gradually evolved with more complex cooling agents being developed, specifically liquid nitrogen. With the emergence of this new technology, the first application of cryosurgery for the prostate was introduced in the mid 1960s [1]. Gonder et al developed a liquid nitrogen cooled transurethral probe that was used to administer cryotherapy for prostate cancer and benign prostatic hyperplasia [2] Several years later, in the 1970s Flocks et al described an open perineal approach to freezing the prostate [2,3]. These procedures were done using a finger in the rectum to guide the surgeon, and there was little control over the freezing process leading to high complication rates from rectourethral fistulas and incontinence. Prostate cryosurgery therefore fell out of favor until the early 1990s when transrectal ultrasound (TRUS) monitoring became available along with the use of a urethral warmer to protect the urethra from subzero temperatures.

With the use of TRUS monitoring, the size of the iceball could be estimated based on acoustic shadowing, and this improved control minimized exposure of the rectum and bladder to the extremely low temperatures

[4] Another technological advancement was the ability to place multiple cryoprobes under ultrasound guidance to allow maximal freezing of the prostate [4,5]. These so-called second-generation cryosystems with TRUS guidance, real-time monitoring of the freezing process, multiple cryoprobes, and use of a urethral warmer led to markedly decreased complication rates compared to the first-generation cryosystems and heralded in a resurgence of this therapeutic option.

In 1996 the American Urology Association recognized prostate cryotherapy as a therapeutic modality for the treatment of clinically localized prostate cancer. Shortly following this endorsement, a new era of technological advancement further improved prostate cryotherapy. The third-generation cryosystems featured a new method of cooling using Argon gas as opposed to liquid nitrogen. The scientific principle (known as the Joule-Thompson effect) is based on extreme temperature changes experienced by inert gases as they undergo rapid expansion from a pressurized to an unpressurized state. In the case of the third-generation systems, when pressurized Argon gas reaches the tip of the cryoprobe and becomes depressurized the temperature falls rapidly to approximately −200°C. The ability to defrost and also to better control the freezing process is provided by Helium gas, which, in contrast to Argon, heats up as it becomes depressurized on reaching the tip of the cryoprobe.

Prior generation devices utilized probes that were 2.4–3 mm in size, but the use of gas cooling allowed the cryoprobes to be much smaller for the

*Interventional Techniques in Uro-oncology*, First Edition. Edited by Hashim Uddin Ahmed, Manit Arya, Peter T. Scardino & Mark Emberton. © 2011 Blackwell Publishing Ltd. Published 2011 by Blackwell Publishing Ltd.

third-generation systems – on the order of 17 G or 1.5 mm [6]. These ultrathin probes can be placed percutaneously into the prostate using a perineal grid and TRUS guidance with little difficulty. Third-generation systems are also equipped with thermocouple probes that allow for real-time temperature monitoring. These are useful in controlling the temperature at the periphery of the iceball and to prevent freezing of the rectum, urethra, and bladder. Thermocouples also ensure that the maximum amount of freezing is occurring in the appropriate areas, with the lethal temperature for cancer cells being −40°C. Finally, the use of computer software has allowed surgeons to create isothermal maps that allow preoperative planning for the freezing process. The result is maximum exposure of the prostate to lethal low temperatures with minimal damage to the surrounding structures.

## Pathophysiology

The principles of cryobiology are based on the use of extreme low temperatures (-40°C) to cause cellular damage and apoptosis. The mechanism by which cellular damage and apoptosis occurs is multifactorial [7]. During the process of freezing, there is direct cellular damage caused by dehydration, ice crystal formation, and disruption of the cell membrane [8]. Another contributing factor is vascular injury and stasis of blood flow, which then leads to ischemia and necrosis [8,9]. The temperature and duration of freezing are directly proportional to the amount of cellular damage. Lower temperatures and longer duration of freezing (i.e., hold-time) are more lethal [10–12]. At the point of freezing, there are two compartments for ice formation: extracellular and intracellular. Extracellular ice forms first due to the protective effect of the cell membrane, which slows intracellular ice formation. Solute precipitation in the extracellular fluid leads to a change in the osmotic gradient and cellular dehydration, which initiates membrane rupture [8]. Continued exposure to freezing temperatures leads to intracellular ice formation wherein ice nucleates in the cell and DNA damage occurs. However, the complete mechanistic role of intracellular ice has not been completely elucidated. Controversy remains as to whether or not this is an actual lethal event or a result of cell death [7–9].

In addition to the direct lethal effects of ice formation on the target cancer cells, there is mechanical injury to the vascular endothelium that disrupts blood flow to cells. Injury to the microvasculature is believed to play an important role in the success of cryotherapy via both immediate and delayed effects [8]. Immediate effects of microvascular damage by cryotherapy result from direct effects on the endothelial cells followed by vessel wall leakage [13,14]. The compromised blood flow causes a lack of nutrient and oxygen supply to the tumor cells and ultimately, apoptosis. The delayed effects of vascular injury from cryotherapy are a result of necrosis following thawing and reperfusion [8]. Studies using the tissue engineered from AT-1 prostate cancer cells lines demonstrate that after cryotherapy, necrosis develops within 3 days [15]. Hyperperfusion that occurs upon thawing can enhance cellular damage due to the high oxygen delivery leading to the formation of harmful free radicals that are destructive to the cellular lipid membranes [7]. In addition to direct cellular injury and vascular stasis, theories have been proposed that suggest that an immune response to cryoinjury may cause cell death, although this is not completely understood [8].

The nadir temperature during cryotherapy is the main determinant of therapeutic efficacy. At temperatures of −15°C and below, cell death becomes progressive and at −30°C, the majority of cells are dead [9]. In vitro studies have demonstrated that at the critical freezing temperature of −40°C, LNCaP prostate cancer cells have significantly decreased viability and a diminished ability to regrow in culture after thawing [16]. Furthermore, these studies showed that a double freeze thaw cycle is much more effective than a single freeze thaw cycle. These experiments clearly demonstrate that lower temperatures, even beyond −40°C increase the degree of cell death. However, due to the proximity of the rectum and bladder, as well as the urethral margins, the clinically safe and efficacious thermal limit has remained at −40°C. Other technical parameters are varied during prostate cryotherapy in order to enhance the lethality of freezing. Specifically, the rate of freezing, the number of freeze thaw cycles, the rate of thawing, and the duration of freezing are all secondary parameters that have an effect on cell death and can easily be manipulated during the procedure to maximize ablation [9].

The histopathological changes that occur after prostate cryosurgery are mainly the result of coagulative necrosis from freezing, and this is confined to a radius of approximately 6 mm around the cryoprobe

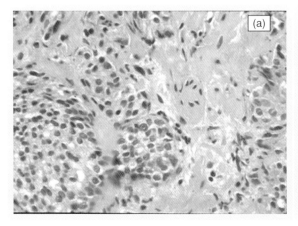
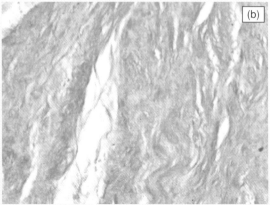

**Fig 4.1** Histopathological changes seen after prostate cryotherapy. (a) Gleason 6 (3+3) adenocarcinoma of the prostate and (b) postcryo coagulative necrosis.

[17]. (Figure 4.1) A thin peripheral zone around the primary cryogenic lesion, referred to as the freeze margin, is the border between dead tissue and viable cells. This region is slightly within the edge of the iceball that is seen on TRUS monitoring (Figure 4.2). The temperature in this zone just outside of the freeze margin can range from 0°C to −20°C and in this area, some cells may survive. Therefore, the ability to monitor the freezing process and advancement of the iceball in real time has been a critical factor for good oncological outcome.

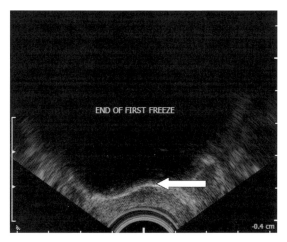

END OF FIRST FREEZE

-0.4 cm

**Fig 4.2** Edge of iceball (arrow: thin white line) and extent of freezing after first cycle.

## Operative technique

### Patient Selection

Suitable patients for primary prostate cryotherapy are those with organ-confined disease since this is a locally ablative treatment modality. A standard 12-core TRUS biopsy of the prostate is suitable for most cryotherapy candidates except those in whom focal therapy is being considered. For focal ablation, patients are considered candidates who have low volume disease on saturation biopsy and the cancer is confined to a single lobe of the prostate. The ideal patients are those with low-risk features (PSA <10 ng/mL, no Gleason pattern 4 or 5) and who are desirous of focal therapy [18]. In these cases, we routinely perform a saturation biopsy with at least 12 cores on the contralateral side of the cancer, although others recommend template transperineal mapping biopsies with a 5-mm sampling frame.

Prostate volume is an important factor to consider in patient selection for primary and salvage whole-gland therapy, as the ability to achieve uniform freezing of the entire gland is critical to oncological success. In patients with a large gland (>60 mL), we prefer to use neoadjuvant hormone therapy with an LHRH agonist such as leuprolide depot for 3 months to cytoreduce the prostate in order to achieve maximum therapeutic efficacy with cryotherapy. Recent data from the radiation oncology literature has revealed that long-term use of hormones is associated with an increased risk of cardiotoxicity and all-cause mortality, and therefore special consideration should be given to cryotherapy patients with preexisting cardiac conditions and large prostates volumes prior to initiating androgen deprivation therapy [19].

In general, there are few absolute contraindications to prostate cryotherapy. Patients who have a history of gastrointestinal fistulas (from inflammatory bowel disease), urethral stricture disease, or prior urethroplasty, and those with severe radiation proctitis and radiation-induced hemorrhagic cystitis, should not be considered for cryotherapy. These are at high risk of developing rectal pain, irritative voiding symptoms, recurrent fistulas, and strictures. Prior transurethral resection of the prostate (TURP) is a relative contraindication due to risk of urethral sloughing as well as the possibility of either retention or incontinence. When evaluating these patients is it important to perform a TRUS prior to performing the cryoablation to ensure there is enough tissue to ablate and that the TURP cavity is not too large. In addition, assessment of urethral length should be performed, as those patients with a prior TURP or laser resection of the prostate may have a shortened urethral length (<3 cm), which may increase the risk of the iceball extending into the urinary sphincter [20]. Patients with significant rectal pathology or abdominoperineal resection are unable to undergo real-time TRUS guided monitoring, and therefore are at a higher risk for poor outcomes and complications.

### Equipment

*Trus* Ultrasound monitoring is critical to the success of cryotherapy, and advances in this technology have provided excellent resolution for visualization of the iceball during the procedure. The standard TRUS probe (7.5 MHz) used for prostate biopsy is utilized during cryosurgery. The ability to switch between the sagittal and transverse planes is important for probe placement as well as monitoring. The edge of the iceball appears as a thin white line preceded by a hypoechoic area on the ultrasound monitor (Figure 4.2). This margin can be used to judge the extent of the freezing process and prevent damage to bladder, urethra, and rectum, which can also be seen on TRUS. However, this does not give any indication of the temperature in that region. Doppler ultrasound may be used to demonstrate vascular stasis during freezing and can help to delineate the neurovascular bundles (Plate 4.1).

*Brachytherapy grid* A brachytherapy template grid is used as a guide for needle insertion during the procedure. The letters on the grid allow for precise transperineal needle placement under ultrasound guidance (Figure 4.3). The use of the grid and the brachytherapy-style stepper has allowed the needles and thermocouples to be kept stable during the procedure.

*Needles, probes, and thermocouples* Currently, there are two commercially available systems in the United States that have Food and Drug Agency (FDA) approval for prostate cryosurgery. One employs the use of 17G cryoablation needles (Galil Medical Inc, Arden Hill, MN) (Figure 4.4) and the other uses 2.4 mm cryoprobes (Healthtronics, Austin TX). The Healthtronics system has the advantage of varying the length of the iceball along the cryoprobe by adjusting a knob on the handle. Both of these systems use argon gas to generate lethal ice, as well as helium for the thaw process. In addition to the freezing needles/probes, there are now commercially available thermocouples that measure temperature along the length of the needle (MTS[TM,] Galil Medical Inc, Arden Hill, MN) (Plate 4.2).

*Urethral warmer* After insertion and correct placement of the needles is confirmed, a urethral warmer (similar to a Foley catheter) is placed. This consists of a closed fluid circuit that cycles saline at 42°C through the catheter to maintain warm temperatures in the urethra during the procedure (Plate 4.2).

*Computer simulation* In order to help guide new cryotherapy users, there are commercially available systems that allow the surgeon to overlay the image of the prostate on ultrasound into a computer planning software (Figure 4.5). The software allows for patient specific freezing simulation and isotherm modeling prior to the actual procedure (Figure 4.6). The surgeon can monitor the temperature using the visual isotherm map in real-time to ensure adequate freezing of targeted areas. The two currently available cryosystems have similar features (Figure 4.5).

### Surgical Technique

After induction of general or spinal anesthesia, the patient is placed in the dorsal lithotomy position. This allows good exposure and access to the perineum while

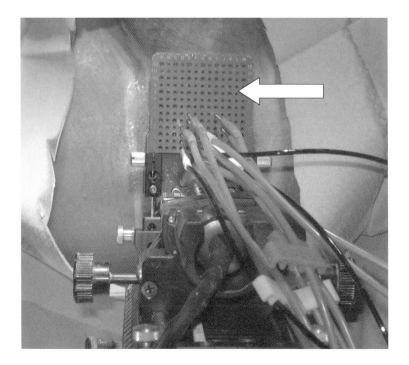

**Fig 4.3** Brachytherapy grid (arrow) placed in position against perineum for needle placement.

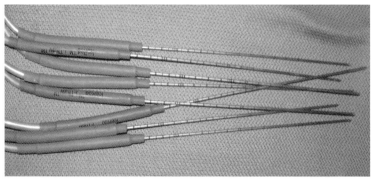

(a)

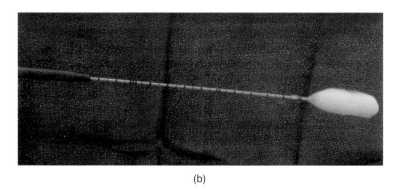

(b)

**Fig 4.4** (a) IceRod™ cryoneedles (Galil Medical Inc, Arden Hill, MN); (b) ice formation ex vivo on cryoneedle.

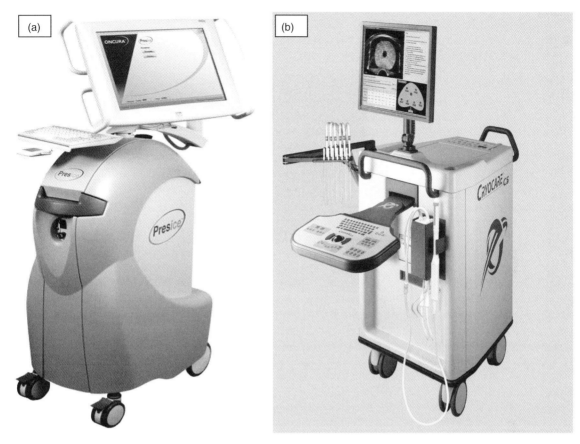

**Fig 4.5** Available cryoablation systems for operative planning and real-time monitoring of freezing process: (a) Precise™ Cryoablation system (Galil Medical Inc, Arden Hill, MN) and (b) Cryocare CS™ (Endocare/Healthtronics, Austin TX).

permitting placement of the thermocouples and cryoneedles. The 17G cryoablation needles are placed ≤20 mm apart (Figure 4.7). The needles are placed 10 mm away from the urethra and at least 10 mm from the posterior surface of the prostate capsule (Figure 4.7). For focal cryotherapy, since the NVB on the treated side will be intentionally ablated, the cryoneedles should be positioned within 10 mm from the lateral capsule.

Based on cryoneedle placement for conventional whole-gland therapy, a standard prostate measuring ≥3 cm in width and weighing approximately 45 mL typically requires eight cryoneedles for effective whole-gland ablation (Figure 4.7). For focal cryoablation, the standard needle configuration for unilateral nerve-sparing cryoablation will require four cryonee-

dles (i.e., for ablation of one side of the gland it will be the standard template for the 8 needle configuration placed in half the prostate) (Figure 4.8). An additional cryoprobe may be necessary for prostates of estimated TRUS volume between 45–60 mL. Similarly, for smaller prostates of estimated volume 20–30 mL, the operator may need to use fewer needles. These decisions are based on the necessity to maintain appropriate distances between adjacent cryoneedles and anatomic structures. The final dose can only be formulated based on the configuration of the prostate that is to be treated at the time of treatment.

The Precise™ Cryoablation System (Galil Medical, Arden Hills, MN) utilizes the multipoint thermal sensor (MTS™) that is capable of measuring 4 simultaneous temperatures, spaced 1 cm apart, along the

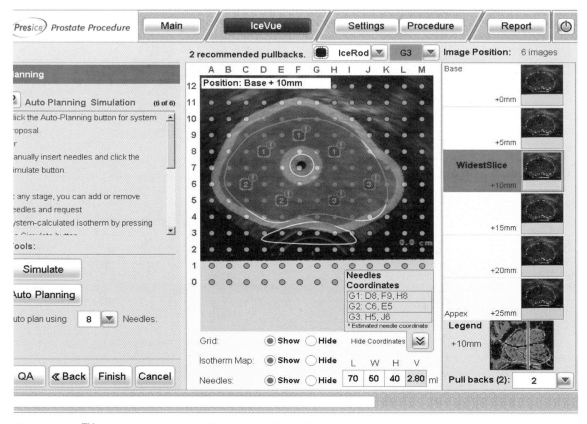

**Fig 4.6** Precise™ Cryoablation system (Galil Medical, Arden Hill, MN) user interface for preoperative simulation and isothermal mapping.

distal shaft of the thermocouple (Figure 4.9). MTS™ 1 is placed 2 cm into the prostate parallel to and 5–10 mm from the lateral edge of the urethra, thereby providing the following temperatures: mid-gland, apex, periprostatic capsule, and urinary sphincter (from needle tip to proximal shaft). During cryotherapy, all recorded temperatures are expected to be negative ($<0°C$) except the urinary sphincter, which should be targeted to remain $>0°C$. MTS™ 2 measures temperatures within Denonvillier's fascia (the posterior capsule is expected to reach at least $-20°C$). MTS™ 3 records the temperature of the NVB. It is positioned at the prostatic capsule or just exterior to it, posterolaterally where the NVB runs (this temperature is expected to reach $-20°C$). During focal cryotherapy, MTS™ 4 can be used to monitor the temperature of the untreated NVB. So as not to cause probe induced injury to the spared NVB during focal cryotherapy,

the placement of this thermocouple is made just inside the capsule, posterolaterally where it is expected that the temperature will be near normal as this side will be untreated.

Following placement of all cryoneedles and thermocouples, cystoscopy is performed to see if any needles need to be repositioned and to ensure that none of the needles have inadvertently entered the urethra or bladder. Following this, the urethral warming catheter is placed over a guidewire and water circulating at $42°C$ will continue for the duration of the procedure. Freezing proceeds from anterior to posterior because the ice completely absorbs ultrasound waves and it becomes technically difficult to visualize any structure behind the near margin of frozen tissue. In order to estimate the extent of freezing, the operator relies largely on the thermocouple readings, knowledge of the original cryoneedle placements, knowledge of ice generation,

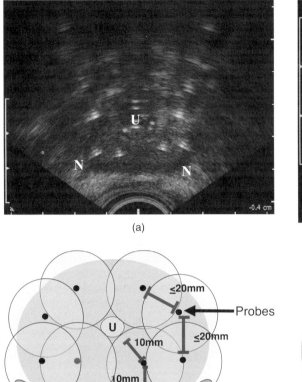

(a)

(b)

Fig 4.7 Ultrasound (a) and schematic diagram (b) demonstrating placement of cryoneedles for whole-gland cryotherapy: U, urethra; N, neurovascular bundle.

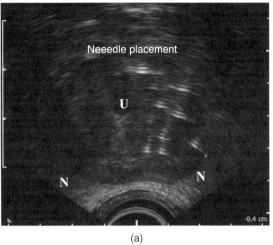

(a)

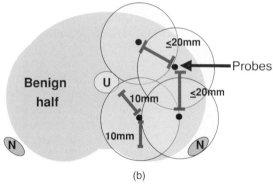

(b)

Fig 4.8 Ultrasound (a) and schematic diagram (b) demonstrating placement of cryoneedles for focal cryotherapy: U, urethra; N, neurovascular bundle.

and the location of the leading ice edge as visualized on ultrasound.

As the freezing continues, the iceballs from each of the cryoablation needles coalesce so that the targeted portion of the prostate and close periprostatic tissues are frozen. Sonographic and thermocouple temperature monitoring are performed continuously during the procedure to ensure that the prostate is adequately frozen. Two freeze-thaw cycles are always utilized. After the first freeze, passive thawing is usually employed for two minutes to augment cell death. Following this, active thawing can be carried out until no ice is visible on ultrasound. Only then will a second freeze be started. Following the second freeze, a brief active thaw (up to 5 minute) is used to loosen the needles before they are subsequently removed. Passive thaw-

ing completes the melting of ice. Ultrasound images are then recorded in the transverse and longitudinal planes showing the greatest extent of freeze. On the transverse view, the medial extent of the ice must encompass all treated tissue up to or slightly (≤5 mm) beyond the midline urethra. Lowest temperatures achieved per freeze cycle are recorded by the MTS™.

After the procedure is terminated and the cryoneedles are removed, direct digital pressure is held on the perineal puncture sites for 3–5 minutes. To protect the urethra from latent freezing by the remaining iceball, the urethral warmer will not be removed until at least 10 minutes following the completion of the second freeze. Following removal of all needles and the urethral warming catheter, a urethral Foley catheter or

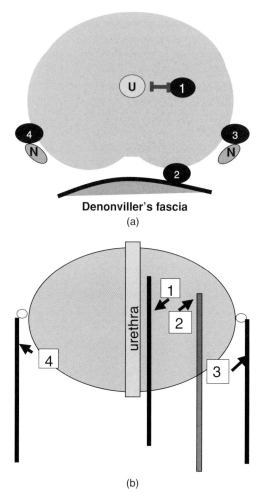

**Denonviller's fascia**

(a)

(b)

**Fig 4.9** Thermocouple placement for monitoring of temperature during freezing. (a) Schematic view of transverse section and (b) schematic view of coronal section. U, urethra; N, neurovascular bundle.

suprapubic catheter is placed for bladder drainage and a gauze pressure dressing is applied to the perineum.

*Postoperative Management*

Patients are given 5 days of a flouroquinolone antibiotic, as well as started on an alpha-blocker, for at least 3–4 weeks. In addition, all patients are discharged home the same day with a Foley catheter for 5–7 days after a complete gland ablation. In the case of a focal ablation, the catheter remains for only 3 days. Patients are seen up to a week after the procedure and then given an active trial of void in the office. Rarely, if

the residual volume on bladder scan following voiding is more than 200 mL the Foley can be reinserted for several additional days, or the patient can be taught self-intermittent catheterization. This is uncommon. PSA evaluation is performed 3 months after the initial procedure and then continued every 3 months for 2 years. For patients undergoing focal cryoablation, it is recommended that a repeat prostate biopsy be performed at 1 year or when there is evidence of a rising PSA to ensure that the side ablated has no residual cancer, and at the same time evaluate the contrateral, untreated side.

Primary cryotherapy

Prostate cryotherapy has been approved as a treatment by Medicare in both the primary and salvage settings. As a primary treatment, men who have low-risk disease (PSA <10 ng/mL, Stage ≤T2, Gleason ≤ 7) are considered ideal candidates for total gland ablation. One of the advantages of cryotherapy is that this procedure has not been associated with any blood loss or fluid shifts, and therefore patients with considerable comorbidities such as congestive heart failure or pulmonary disease that preclude major surgery generally fit into the category of patients who receive primary cryotherapy. Oncological success after cryotherapy varies depending on the definition of biochemical recurrence. Currently, there are two accepted definitions: the American Society of Therapeutic Radiation Oncology (ASTRO) criteria of 3 consecutive PSA rises 3 months apart after a nadir PSA and the ASTRO-Phoenix criteria that define failure as a rise in PSA of 2 points above the nadir value ("nadir plus 2").

Though long-term, randomized, controlled data are limited, published 10-year biochemical disease free survival (bDFS) rates of 56–62% have been reported based on various definitions of biochemical failure (ASTRO vs. Phoenix) [21]. As expected, low-risk patients have significantly higher bDFS rates (80.56%) compared with intermediate- and high-risk patients (74.16% and 45.54%, respectively) [21]. A retrospective analysis of 590 patients undergoing primary cryotherapy with 7 years of follow-up reported bDFS rates of 87%, 79%, and 71% using a PSA cut-off of <1.0 ng/mL for high-, medium-, and low-risk patients [22]. However, with the ASTRO definition, bDFS increased to 92%, 89%, and 89% for those same risk groups. With the advent of improved technology,

Table 4.1 Biochemical disease free survival (bDFS) rates for contemporary primary cryotherapy series.

| Reference | Number of patients | Follow-up (mos) | Median clinical stage | Pretreatment PSA (ng/mL) | Overall bDFS | Criteria |
|---|---|---|---|---|---|---|
| Jones et al [23] | 1198 | 24.4 | T2 a | 9.6 | 77% (5 year) | ASTRO |
| Cohen et al [21] | 204 | 144 | T2 | 9.3 | 56% (10 year) | ASTRO |
|  |  |  |  |  | 62% (10 year) | ASTRO-Phoenix |
| Long et al [24] | 975 | 24 | T2 | – | 63% (5 year) | threshold PSA <1.0 |
|  |  |  |  |  | 52% (5 year) | threshold PSA <0.5 |
| Bahn et al [22] | 590 | 68 | T2 | – | 89.5%(7 year) | ASTRO |
|  |  |  |  |  | 76%(7 year) | threshold PSA <1.0 |
| Hubosky et al [25][a] | 89 | 11 | T1 c | 11.8 | 94% (1 year) | ASTRO |
|  |  |  |  |  | 70% (1 year) | threshold PSA ≤0.4 |
| Polascik et al [26][a] | 50 | 18 | T1 c | 5.1 | 90% (at last follow-up) | threshold PSA ≤0.5 |
| Cresswell et al [27][a] | 15 | 9 | T2 |  | 60%(1 year) | threshold PSA ≤0.5 |
| Han et al [28][a] | 110 | 12 | T2 | – | 73%(1 year) | threshold PSA ≤0.4 |

[a]Third-generation cryosystems only.

results of primary cryotherapy are expected to improve. The majority of published studies report outcomes from a combination of new and older generation cryotherapy systems, but results from only third-generation systems with longer follow-up will be available within the coming years. Emerging bDFS data from the contemporary series show modest results in terms of efficacy despite short-term (≤10 year) follow-up [21–28] (Table 4.1).

Direct comparison to other primary treatment modalities, namely radical prostatectomy and radiotherapy is difficult due to the heterogeneity in the definition of biochemical failure between these therapies. While, the presence of a detectable PSA post-prostatectomy indicates disease recurrence, neither an optimal post-treatment nadir nor surveillance cut-off level has been established for cryotherapy [6]. Both the ASTRO and ASTRO-Phoenix definitions of biochemical failure can miss cancer recurrence after cryotherapy.

In an attempt to compare two therapeutic modalities, Chin et al conducted a randomized trial of cryoablation to EBRT for locally advanced (T2C–T3B) prostate cancer [29]. The authors concluded that bDFS was less favorable for cryotherapy, but that there was no difference in disease specific or overall survival [29]. They also made note of the fact that the study and conclusions were limited by poor accrual ($N = 64$: 31 radiation therapy vs. 33 cryotherapy patients) and short mean follow-up of only 37 months. In a larger study of cryotherapy versus external beam radiation therapy (EBRT), Donnelly et al randomized 244 patients to either modality (122 cryotherapy and 122 EBRT) with a median follow-up of 100 months. The primary endpoint was failure at 36 months postrandomization [30]. Failure was defined as a trifecta of (1) biochemical failure, (2) radiological evidence of disease recurrence, and (3) the initiation of further prostate cancer treatment. Biochemical failure was analyzed in two ways: (1) nadir + 2 ng/mL and (2) two consecutive rises above nadir PSA with failure occurring when a value >1.0 ng/mL was achieved. There was no significant difference in failure at 36 months using the nadir + two definitions of biochemical recurrence (17.1% cryotherapy vs. 13.2% EBRT) and, similarly there was no difference using the second definition of biochemical recurrence as defined above (23.9% cryotherapy vs. 23.7% EBRT). Interestingly, there was a significantly higher positive biopsy rate at 36 months for EBRT patients compared with cryotherapy patients (28.9% vs. 7.7%). However, there was no difference in 5-year overall and disease-specific survival between the two groups.

The cryo-online database (COLD) registry is a multicenter database that was developed to standardize recording and improve outcome data for prostate cryotherapy. The registry incorporates information from 4 academic medical centers and 34 community urologists [23]. A total of 1198 patients who underwent primary whole-gland cryoablation have been registered [23]. Median pretreatment PSA was 9.6 ng/mL, GS 7, and stage was T2 [23)]. Of these patients, 49.5% received neoadjuvant hormonal ablation. The 5-year bDFS for the entire group was 77.1% using the ASTRO criteria and 72.9% using the ASTRO-Phoenix criteria [23]. When risk stratified as low-, medium-, and high-risk, the 5-year bDFS was 84.7%, 73.4%, and 75.3% (ASTRO) and 91.1%, 78.5%, and 62.2% (ASTRO-Phoenix). While these data represent the largest combined experience for primary prostate cryotherapy, results should be interpreted with the understanding that they represent multiple different surgeons' practices using both second- and third-generation cryosystems.

### Salvage cryotherapy

Primary radiation therapy (RT) for localized prostate cancer has had similar results in comparison to radical prostatectomy with respect to long-term bDFS [31]. However, management of recurrence after radiation therapy usually requires ablative therapy or salvage surgery as this typically occurs within the gland, as demonstrated by positive post-treatment biopsy rates for prostate cancer ranging from 21% to 51% [32,33]. Salvage prostatectomy, even in experienced hands, is technically difficult and carries significant morbidity including: rectal injury (2%), urinary incontinence (23%), and anastomotic stricture (30%) [34]. In contrast, salvage cryotherapy is less invasive and morbid and therefore may be a more acceptable alternative for patients who fail RT. This is demonstrated by studies that report a lower incidence of complications in comparison to salvage prostatectomy, specifically incontinence rates of 3% and urethrorectal fistula rates of 2% [35]. In addition, survival for salvage cryotherapy is excellent with 97% of patients alive at 5 year(s) and biochemical failure rates ranging from 44% to 59% [35,36].

The COLD registry for salvage cryotherapy reported on 5-year bDFS for 279 patients, which was 59% using ASTRO criteria and 54.5% using Phoenix criteria [36]. Ismail et al reported their 5-year salvage therapy bDFS rates of 73%, 45%, and 11% for low-, medium-, and high-risk groups [37]. Given the locally ablative nature of cryotherapy, it is accepted that there may be viable tumor cells in the prostate after treatment particularly in the periurethral region where the urethral warmer protects the tissue from achieving the necessary lethal low temperatures. As a result, positive postsalvage cryotherapy biopsy rates range from 14.2% to 23% and may necessitate repeat salvage cryotherapy procedures [37–39]. The bDFS of the larger, more recent salvage cryosurgery series are shown in Table 4.2 [36,37,40,41].

As patients who recur after RT represent a high-risk population the use of androgen deprivation therapy (ADT) is widespread in this group. It is therefore not surprising that the use of ADT in salvage cryotherapy series ranges from 8.2% to 32%, which will inevitably affect posttreatment biopsy rates as

Table 4.2 Biochemical disease free survival (bDFS) rates for contemporary salvage cryotherapy series.

| Reference | Number of patients | Follow-up (mos) | Median clinical stage | Pretreatment PSA (ng/mL) | Overall bDFS | Criteria |
|---|---|---|---|---|---|---|
| Pisters et al [36] | 279 | 21.6 | – | 7.6 | 59% (5 year) | ASTRO |
| | | | – | | 55% (5 year) | ASTRO-Phoenix |
| Ng et al [40] | 187 | 39 | T2 | 4.9 | 97% (5 year) | ASTRO-Phoenix |
| | | | | | 92% (8 year) | ASTRO-Phoenix |
| Ismail et al [37] | 100 | 33.5 | T2 | 5.4 | 55% (5 year) | ASTRO |
| Katz et al [41] | 187 | 37 | T2 | 5 | 73.3% (5 year) | ASTRO |
| Izawa et al [42] | 131 | 57 | T2 | – | 40% (5 year) | ASTRO-Phoenix |

well as bDFS [36,40]. ADT in this setting is typically used to treat possible micrometastases as most patients treated in the salvage setting have relatively small size glands, which do not need to be downsized to adequately freeze the prostate [43]. Depending on the timing and duration of ADT, it may make biochemical surveillance difficult especially in conjunction with the confounding effects of prior radiation and cryotherapy-induced injury. Further studies are therefore needed to standardize duration and dose of ADT and surveillance criteria of patients undergoing salvage cryotherapy.

## Focal cryotherapy

Further attempts to decrease morbidity with cryotherapy have led to the development of focal targeted cryoablation with the hope that intervention on only one half of the prostate may improve the side effect profile, particularly with regard to ED. Whole-gland cryotherapy is associated with a relatively high rate of ED compared to nerve-sparing radical prostatectomy; therefore focal targeted cryotherapy may be more desirable than whole-gland ablation in select patients [44]. Understandably, with bilateral, multifocal disease the neurovascular bundle is adversely impacted as the iceball's "kill zone" must extend just down to or beyond the prostatic capsule. However, given that certain patients may demonstrate unilateral or unifocal disease on prostate biopsy, whole-gland ablation may be unnecessary [45]. With current TRUS techniques and biopsy sampling patterns, the surgeon's ability to predict unilateral, unifocal cancer with just nine or more tissue cores may be sufficiently good. Therefore, in carefully selected low-risk (PSA<10, GS<7, stage T1 c) patients with unifocal, unilateral disease, focal cryoablation may have a role in treatment while preserving erectile function.

Recent preliminary experience with focal cryotherapy has shown promising short-term efficacy with bDFS of 84% at 3 years of follow-up with over half of these patients potent posttreatment [46]. Onik et al reported that 94% of patients who underwent primary focal cryoablation had a stable PSA at 2 years and 90% maintained potency [47]. Of the 48 patients, 24 underwent routine biopsy at 1 year, all of which were negative [47]. In the largest published focal cryotherapy series to date ($N = 60$), Ellis et al reported slightly lower rates of potency and bDFS of 80.4% and 70.6%

after 15.4 months of follow-up, respectively [48]. After treatment, 35 patients underwent prostate biopsy of which 14 (40%) showed demonstrable disease, which resulted in a 23.3% overall positive biopsy rate [48]. These results indicate that further studies are needed to evaluate focal cryotherapy prior to its use as a standard treatment option.

Biochemical surveillance following focal cryotherapy proposes a unique challenge because only one half of the gland is ablated. In our experience, we incorporate the factor of hemiablation by assume that PSA production after treatment should fall by a similar percentage of the gland that is ablated. Therefore, if the PSA after focal cryotherapy is reduced by more than 50% of the preoperative PSA and remains below this threshold, then it is reasonable to assume that BCR has not occurred.

## Complications

The major benefit to cryotherapy is the minimally invasive nature of the procedure. Initially, when cryotechnology was introduced, there were significant concerns due to the high rates of rectourethral fistulas, incontinence, urethral sloughing, and erectile dysfunction. However, with the technological advancements mentioned in the previous section there have been major improvements.

### Primary Cryotherapy

Incontinence rates during the early era of cryotherapy, were noted to be as high as 83% [49]. In contrast, using third-generation technology, Han et al reported good outcomes in a series of 106 patients who underwent primary cryotherapy with only 3% incontinence [50]. Other notable side effects in this series were: 5% urethral sloughing, 5% urge incontinence requiring no pads, 3.3% transient urinary retention, and 2.6% rectal pain [50]. None of these patients experienced rectourethral fistulas demonstrating marked improvement over historic series [50]. Even lower rates of urethral sloughing (2%) and incontinence (2%) have been reported in single institution experiences by using only third-generation technology [25]. When compared to brachytherapy patients, cryosurgery patients had better urinary function after 18 months of follow-up and this difference was maintained up to two years after therapy [25]. The COLD database reported

Table 4.3 Complication rates for primary cryotherapy series using third-generation cryosystems only.

| Reference | Total no. of patients | Follow-up (mos) | Erectile dysfunction | Incontinence | Fistula | Retention/ Obstruction | Urethral sloughing | Urethral stricture | Perineal pain |
|---|---|---|---|---|---|---|---|---|---|
| Han et al [50] | 106 | 12 | 87 | 3 | 0 | – | 5 | 0 | 6 |
| Hubosky et al [25] | 89 | 11 | – | 2 | 1 | 4 | 2 | – | 6 |
| Polascik et al [26] | 50 | 18 | 88 | 3.7 | 0 | 0 | 0 | 0 | 0 |

incontinence rates of 4.8% for any leakage, and 2.9% for leakage requiring pad usage [23].

While it is possible to achieve good extension of the iceball into the prostatic capsule to allow maximal oncologic efficacy, it is not possible to prevent damage to the neurovascular bundle. It is therefore not surprising that even with current technology the rates of erectile dysfunction after primary whole-gland cryotherapy are high and range from 49% to 93% [6]. Hubosky et al reported that sexual function was diminished after cryosurgery, and the entire cohort only achieved 20% return to baseline sexual function at 1 year follow-up [25]. In a prospective study of a small cohort of patients undergoing third-generation cryotherapy, Cresswell et al reported that 13/29 (45%) patients had ED after primary cryoablation despite having normal erectile function prior to the procedure [27]. Table 4.3 shows complication rates noted among the most recent studies using third-generation cryotherapy systems for primary therapy [25,26,28].

Rectourethral fistula formation after primary cryotherapy is rare and rates of 0–2.4% have been reported [6]. With improvement in technology, more recent series have demonstrated fistula rates of only 0–1% [25,51]. Urethral sloughing is another feared complication and occurs when the prostatic urethra is exposed to freezing temperatures for prolonged periods and then undergoes necrosis and ulceration. Patients typically present with urinary retention and may eventually need to undergo transurethral resection of the necrotic tissue. In the recent COLD series, 2.1% of patients had to undergo resection of necrotic tissue for urinary retention caused by sloughing [23]. Data from older studies have demonstrated urethral sloughing rates after primary cryotherapy as high as 23% [52]. The key to avoiding both fistula formation and urethral sloughing is the use of thermocouple

monitoring and the urethral warmer. These instruments enable controlled freezing and minimal damage to vital anatomy, and have permitted us to achieve no incidences of either complications even in our earlier experience [53].

*Salvage Cryotherapy*

Given the prior exposure to RT and the ensuing poor tissue viability and healing within the field of radiation, salvage cryotherapy has higher complication rates than primary therapy. While there may be a slightly increased risk of urinary tract infections, intraprostatic abscesses, urethral sloughing, and urinary retention compared to primary cryotherapy, the major complications after salvage cryotherapy are still fistula formation, incontinence, and ED. The incidence of rectourethral fistulas is significant for salvage patients and has been shown to be as high as 3.3% [54]. Data from the COLD database demonstrate fistula rates of 1.2%, but it should be noted that some of the patients in this series underwent treatment with older generation technology [36].

Incontinence rates after salvage cryotherapy appear to be similar to primary therapy and for third-generation technology these rates are generally in the region of 4.7–17.5% [36]. Older salvage cryotherapy series had high incontinence rates from 73% to 95% [55]. In a more recent experience, Ng et al have reported improvement in incontinence after salvage cryotherapy with published rates as low as 3% [40].

Postsalvage cryotherapy rates of ED are high despite the shift in technology, but this is due to the combined damage to the NVB from exposure to radiation therapy followed by cryoablation, and typically affects up to 90% of patients [56]. Another contributing factor to the high rates of ED is the use of hormone therapy along with radiation. However, the COLD registry

Table 4.4 Complication rates for modern salvage cryotherapy series.

| Reference | Total no. of patients | Follow-up (mos) | Erectile dysfunction | Incontinence | Fistula | Retention/ Obstruction | Urethral sloughing | Urethral stricture | Perineal pain |
|---|---|---|---|---|---|---|---|---|---|
| Pisters et al [36] | 279 | 21.6 | 69.2 | 4.7 | 1.2 | – | – | – | – |
| Ng et al [40] | 187 | 39 | – | 3* | 2 | 21 | – | – | 14 |
| Ismail et al [37] | 100 | 33.5 | 86 | 13 | 1 | 2 | – | – | 4 |
| Katz et al [41] | 187 | 37 | – | 9.7 | 0 | 1.9 | – | – | 12.8 |

has published lower rates of impotence (69.2%) indicating better outcomes that are likely related to increased use of current technology that provides less exposure of the NVB to low temperatures [36]. Salvage cryotherapy in a series of 100 patients demonstrated ED rates of 86% overall indicating that while technology is improving, ED remains a significant side effect and patients should be counseled regarding the impact of sexual dysfunction on their quality of life [37]. A comparison of salvage cryotherapy morbidity among modern series of patients is shown in Table 4.4 [36,37,40,41].

*Focal Cryotherapy*

Studies assessing the complications of focal cryotherapy are limited due to the relatively recent practice of this technique. This approach in theory spares the contralateral NVB and can potentially preserve erectile function. Early data demonstrate that after focal ablation in 40 preoperatively potent patients, 36 (90%) maintained potency after a single focal cryotherapy treatment [47]. In addition, no patients experienced incontinence and only 1 patient had urethral sloughing requiring TURP [47]. Similarly, in a smaller group of patients with slightly more than 2 years follow-up from the Columbia University cryosurgery database, 71% of patients were potent postoperatively out of a total 24 patients who reported preoperative potency [57]. Only 1 patient had retention, which resolved weeks postoperatively, and there were no occurrences of fistulas, incontinence, or pain [57]. While these data are encouraging with respect to the low morbidity of focal cryotherapy, larger series with longer follow-up are necessary to better evaluate this treatment as standard therapy in unifocal, unilateral prostate cancer.

Recurrence following cryotherapy

One of the future challenges for cryotherapy is defining an accurate method of assessing bDFS. The 1997 ASTRO and 2006 ASTRO-Phoenix criteria have been used in RT to determine successful endpoints and define recurrence. However, cryogenically induced necrosis of the prostate may be different from that of radiation induced injury, and a more standard PSA endpoint based on cryotherapy should be developed. It is the variation in definition of biochemical failure in several cryotherapy studies that makes direct comparison of results difficult. In our experience, we have typically considered a postoperative nadir PSA <50% of the initial PSA to indicate a successful cryoablation. However, different groups vary on their definition of an acceptable PSA nadir after cryotherapy.

Levy et al performed a review of the COLD registry to determine a suitable nadir PSA that correlates with biochemical failure (ASTRO-Phoenix in this case) after prostate cryotherapy [58]. They found that a nadir PSA of 0.6 ng/mL or more was associated with a 29.5% biochemical failure rate regardless of risk stratification. As a result, the authors concluded that a nadir PSA $\leq 0.5$ is associated with more favorable bDFS [58]. While posttreatment PSA values can help with surveillance, the presence of cancer on posttreatment prostate biopsy remains the definitive method for diagnosing recurrence. Izawa et al have shown that up to 1 year after salvage cryotherapy, positive biopsy rates are as high as 17% [39]. Chin et al have shown even higher positive biopsy rates of 26% in their series of salvage cryotherapy patients [38]. Therefore, a biopsy should be considered in all patients suspected of having a recurrence based on acceptable PSA criteria.

## Renal cryotherapy

Renal tissue requires exposure temperatures at or below $-19.4°C$ for cell death, although clinical practice tends to be cautious and freeze to temperatures at $-40°C$. If the collecting system is not directly punctured with the probe, there is usually healing without urinary fistulas--which may be an advantage over radiofrequency ablation (RFA), where there is a greater risk of urinary leakage.

Four cryoablation manufacturers are existent at present with the Endocare (Irvine, California, USA), Galil Medical (Yokneam, Israel), Oncura (Arlington Heights, Illinois, USA), and Cryomedical Sciences (Rockville, Maryland, USA) systems. The first three use argon gas to cause rapid freezing at the probe tip, which is based on the Joule–Thomson effect. The Cryomedical Sciences device uses nitrogen and is used for prostate, and liver applications, and ot renal tumors. The recent development of third-generation cryotechnology using argon/helium gas circulation and ultrathin 17-gauge needles has made the procedure somewhat less traumatic as it penetrates the renal capsule. This has also facilitated precision insertion of the cryoprobes into the tumor under intraoperative ultrasound guidance with multiple small probes placed into the tumor. This seems to minimize blood loss when the probes are removed compared to larger probes.

Renal cryoablation can be performed laparoscopically or percutaneously. Surgeon preference and experience determine the optimal approach since each route has advantages and limitations. Laparoscopic renal cryoablation offers the advantage of precise cryoprobe positioning and monitoring of the iceball under real-time ultrasound as well as direct vision. As in the prostate, ultrasound demonstrates the iceball as a hyperechoic advancing area with a posterior acoustic shadow. Anterior or medial tumors can be difficult to target through a percutaneous route so are best approached via the laparoscopic route. Percutaneous renal cryoablation is commonly performed with the use of CT guidance, but open gantry magnetic resonance imaging guidance is also possible.

A meta-analysis conducted in 2008 evaluated forty-seven studies (1375 kidney lesions in total) treated by cryoablation or RFA [59]. Cryoablation was on the main performed laparoscopically (65%), whereas the vast majority (94%) of lesions treated with RFA were carried out via the percutaneous route. The meta-analysis found no differences between ablation modalities with regard to mean patient age, tumor size, or duration of follow-up. However, pretreatment biopsy was performed significantly more often for cryoablated lesions (82.3%) compared to RFA (62.2%; $p < 0.0001$). Unknown pathology occurred at a significantly higher rate for small renal masses that underwent RFA (40.4%) as opposed to cryoablation (24.5%; $p < 0.0001$). Repeat ablative intervention was required more often after RFA (8.5% vs. 1.3%; $p < 0.0001$), and the rates of local tumor progression were significantly higher with RFA compared with cryotherapy (12.9% vs. 5.2%; $p < 0.0001$). Metastasis was reported less frequently for cryoablation (1.0% vs. 2.5%; $p = 0.06$). Although this did not reach statistical significance there may be some clinical significance in the difference. It was not surprising therefore that the meta-analysis concluded that cryoablation was better than RFA with respect to short-term parameters, such as tumor ablation, retreatment, and local tumor progression. However, development of metastases and long-term survival are yet to be shown to be superior, and this area requires a large prospective multicenter randomized controlled trial that should also incorporate partial nephrectomy.

## Future directions

Further investigation into the role of targeted focal cryoablation is of much interest with respect to innovations in the field. The ability to spare nerves while targeting only cancerous tissue has great potential for oncological control with minimal morbidity, and will be of great benefit to patients. Imaging modalities, such as MRI and 3D ultrasound are already under investigation [60]. Studies of MRI-guided cryoablation have been performed in canine models and may potentially be used to follow the cryolesion over time after therapy [61].

While cryotechnology advances have paved the way in recent times, future scientific breakthroughs in immunology and oncology may have promising roles for adjuvant therapy. In vivo studies combining 5-fluorouracil and cisplatin with cryotherapy on human prostate cancer cell lines have demonstrated enhancement in chemo-induced apoptosis with freezing

[62]. Immuno-cryotherapy incorporates the cellular response to cryotherapy with the release of tumor antigens and inflammatory signals in order to enhance dendritic cell maturation thereby making the tumor more sensitive to immunotherapy after freezing [63]. Using a tumor necrosis factor related apoptosis inducing ligand (TRAIL) in combination with cryotherapy, Ismail et al has shown that prostate cancer cells exhibit increased sensitivity to freezing and complete loss of viability at $-10°C$ and $-20°C$ [64]. Further studies investigating the use of immunotherapeutic agents, chemotherapy, and novel targeted molecular therapies in combination with cryotherapy could have promising roles for future treatment.

## Conclusions

With the advent of PSA screening and the subsequent stage migration in prostate cancer, there are more men being identified with low-risk disease, but who are not interested in watchful waiting or active surveillance. These men are not necessarily candidates for radical treatment or wish to avoid the morbidity of surgery and radiation therapy. These men may instead be better served by minimally invasive ablative therapies such as cryotherapy. Medium and emerging long-term data have shown this ablative technology to be safe and effective with low urinary morbidity. Further improvements in erectile function outcomes may be achieved by applying the ablative target to only one lobe or areas of cancer alone in focal therapy. Further research into the therapeutic efficacy of cryotherapy is therefore essential in order to serve our patients better and offer them maximal benefit with minimal complication.

Renal tumors have also increased in incidence due to imaging for other diseases. Many of these tumors are small and a significant minority is benign. The ability of preoperative diagnostic tests to differentiate between benign and malignant lesions is yet to be accurate enough to rely on, and the morbidity of nephrectomy is high. Therefore, the need for minimally invasive interventions such as cryotherapy is paramount. It seems from retrospective studies that cryotherapy may have advantages over radiofrequency ablation, but this has yet to be proven in comparative prospective trials.

## References

1. Gage AA (1998) History of cryosurgery. Semin Surg Oncol 14(2): 99–109.
2. Gonder MJ, Soanes WA, Smith V (1964) Experimental prostate cryosurgery. Invest Urol 1: 610–619.
3. Flocks RH, Nelson CM, Boatman DL (1972) Perineal cryosurgery for prostatic carcinoma. J Urol 108(6): 933–935.
4. Onik GM et al (1993) Transrectal ultrasound-guided percutaneous radical cryosurgical ablation of the prostate. Cancer 72(4): 1291–1299.
5. Chang Z et al (1994) Development of a high-performance multiprobe cryosurgical device. Biomed Instrum Technol 28(5): 383–390.
6. Babaian RJ et al (2008) Best practice statement on cryosurgery for the treatment of localized prostate cancer. J Urol 180(5): 1993–2004.
7. Gage AA, Baust J (1998) Mechanisms of tissue injury in cryosurgery. Cryobiology 37(3): 171–186.
8. Hoffmann NE, Bischof JC (2002) The cryobiology of cryosurgical injury. Urology 60(2 suppl. 1): 40–49.
9. Baust JG et al (2009) The pathophysiology of thermoablation: optimizing cryoablation. Curr Opin Urol 19(2): 127–132.
10. Daum PS et al (1987) Vascular casts demonstrate microcirculatory insufficiency in acute frostbite. Cryobiology 24(1): 65–73.
11. Tatsutani K et al (1996) Effect of thermal variables on frozen human primary prostatic adenocarcinoma cells. Urology 48(3): 441–447.
12. Bischof J et al (2001) A parametric study of freezing injury in ELT-3 uterine leiomyoma tumour cells. Hum Reprod 16(2): 340–348.
13. Adams-Ray J, Bellman S (1956) Vascular reactions after experimental cold injury; a microangiographic study of rabbit ears. Angiology 7(4): 339–367.
14. Pollock GA, Pegg DE, Hardie IR (1986) An isolated perfused rat mesentery model for direct observation of the vasculature during cryopreservation. Cryobiology 23(6): 500–511.
15. Hoffmann NE, Bischof JC (2001) Cryosurgery of normal and tumor tissue in the dorsal skin flap chamber: Part I–thermal response. J Biomech Eng 123(4): 301–309.
16. Klossner DP et al (2008) Cryoablative response of prostate cancer cells is influenced by androgen receptor expression. BJU Int 101(10): 1310–1316.
17. Larson BT et al (2003) Histological changes of minimally invasive procedures for the treatment of benign prostatic hyperplasia and prostate cancer: clinical implications. J Urol 170(1): 12–19.

18. Jayram G, Eggener SE (2009) Patient selection for focal therapy of localized prostate cancer. Curr Opin Urol 19(3): 268–273.

19. Nanda A et al (2009) Hormonal therapy use for prostate cancer and mortality in men with coronary artery disease-induced congestive heart failure or myocardial infarction. JAMA 302(8): 866–873.

20. Talcott JA et al (2001) Long-term treatment related complications of brachytherapy for early prostate cancer: a survey of patients previously treated. J Urol 166(2): 494–499.

21. Cohen JK et al (2008) Ten-year biochemical disease control for patients with prostate cancer treated with cryosurgery as primary therapy. Urology 71(3): 515–518.

22. Bahn DK et al (2002) Targeted cryoablation of the prostate: 7-year outcomes in the primary treatment of prostate cancer. Urology 60(2 suppl. 1): 3–11.

23. Jones JS et al (2008) Whole gland primary prostate cryoablation: initial results from the cryo on-line data registry. J Urol 180(2): 554–558.

24. Long JP et al (2001) Five-year retrospective, multi-institutional pooled analysis of cancer-related outcomes after cryosurgical ablation of the prostate. Urology 57(3): 518–523.

25. Hubosky SG et al (2007) Single center experience with third-generation cryosurgery for management of organ-confined prostate cancer: critical evaluation of short-term outcomes, complications, and patient quality of life. J Endourol 21(12): 1521–1531.

26. Polascik TJ et al (2007) Short-term cancer control after primary cryosurgical ablation for clinically localized prostate cancer using third-generation cryotechnology. Urology 70(1): 117–121.

27. Cresswell J et al (2006) Third-generation cryotherapy for prostate cancer in the UK: a prospective study of the early outcomes in primary and recurrent disease. BJU Int 97(5): 969–974.

28. Han KR et al (2003) Treatment of organ confined prostate cancer with third generation cryosurgery: preliminary multicenter experience. J Urol 170(4 Pt 1): 1126–1130.

29. Chin JL et al (2008) Randomized trial comparing cryoablation and external beam radiotherapy for T2 C-T3B prostate cancer. Prostate Cancer Prostatic Dis 11(1): 40–45.

30. Donnelly BJ et al (2010) A randomized trial of external beam radiotherapy versus cryoablation in patients with localized prostate cancer. Cancer 116(2): 323–330.

31. Sylvester JE et al (2007) 15-Year biochemical relapse free survival in clinical Stage T1-T3 prostate cancer following combined external beam radiotherapy and brachyther-apy; Seattle experience. Int J Radiat Oncol Biol Phys 67(1): 57–64.

32. Zapatero A et al (2009) Post-treatment prostate biopsies in the era of three-dimensional conformal radiotherapy: what can they teach us? Eur Urol 55(4): 902–909.

33. De Meerleer G et al (2007) Intensity-modulated radiation therapy for prostate cancer: late morbidity and results on biochemical control. Radiother Oncol 82(2): 160–166.

34. Stephenson AJ et al (2004) Morbidity and functional outcomes of salvage radical prostatectomy for locally recurrent prostate cancer after radiation therapy. J Urol 172(6 Pt 1): 2239–2243.

35. Izawa JI et al (2001) Local tumor control with salvage cryotherapy for locally recurrent prostate cancer after external beam radiotherapy. J Urol 165(3): 867–870.

36. Pisters LL et al (2008) Salvage prostate cryoablation: initial results from the cryo on-line data registry. J Urol 180(2): 559–563; discussion 563–564.

37. Ismail M et al (2007) Salvage cryotherapy for recurrent prostate cancer after radiation failure: a prospective case series of the first 100 patients. BJU Int 100(4): 760–764.

38. Chin JL et al (2003) Serial histopathology results of salvage cryoablation for prostate cancer after radiation failure. J Urol 170(4 Pt 1): 1199–1202.

39. Izawa JI et al (2006) Histological changes in prostate biopsies after salvage cryotherapy: effect of chronology and the method of biopsy. BJU Int 98(3): 554–558.

40. Ng CK et al (2007) Salvage cryoablation of the prostate: follow-up and analysis of predictive factors for outcome. J Urol 178(4 Pt 1): 1253–1257.

41. Katz AE et al (2005) Salvage cryosurgical ablation of the prostate (TCAP) for patients failing radiation: 10-year experience. American Urology Association Annual Meeting Program [Abstracts, #1662]. J Urol 173: 450–451.

42. Izawa JI et al (2002) Salvage cryotherapy for recurrent prostate cancer after radiotherapy: variables affecting patient outcome. J Clin Oncol 20(11): 2664–2671.

43. Ghafar MA et al (2001) Salvage cryotherapy using an argon based system for locally recurrent prostate cancer after radiation therapy: the Columbia experience. J Urol 166(4): 1333–1337; discussion 1337–1338.

44. Asterling S, Greene DR (2009) Prospective evaluation of sexual function in patients receiving cryosurgery as a primary radical treatment for localized prostate cancer. BJU Int 103(6): 788–792.

45. Iczkowski KA et al (2008) Preoperative prediction of unifocal, unilateral, margin-negative, and small volume prostate cancer. Urology 71(6): 1166–1171.

46. Katz AE, Kacker R (2008) Focal treatment for low-risk prostate cancer. BJU Int 102(2): 158–159.

47. Onik G et al (2008) The "male lumpectomy": focal therapy for prostate cancer using cryoablation results in 48 patients with at least 2-year follow-up. Urol Oncol 26(5): 500–505.

48. Ellis DS, Manny TB Jr, Rewcastle JC (2007) Focal cryosurgery followed by penile rehabilitation as primary treatment for localized prostate cancer: initial results. Urology 70(6 suppl.): 9–15.

49. Long JP et al (1998) Preliminary outcomes following cryosurgical ablation of the prostate in patients with clinically localized prostate carcinoma. J Urol 159(2): 477–484.

50. Han KR, Belldegrun AS (2004) Third-generation cryosurgery for primary and recurrent prostate cancer. BJU Int 93(1): 14–18.

51. Donnelly BJ et al (2002) Prospective trial of cryosurgical ablation of the prostate: five-year results. Urology 60(4): 645–649.

52. Shinohara K et al (1996)) Cryosurgical treatment of localized prostate cancer (stages T1 to T4): preliminary results. J Urol 156(1): 115–120.

53. De La Taille A et al (2000) Cryoablation for clinically localized prostate cancer using an argon-based system: complication rates and biochemical recurrence. BJU Int 85(3): 281–286.

54. Chin JL et al (2001) Results of salvage cryoablation of the prostate after radiation: identifying predictors of treatment failure and complications. J Urol 165(6 Pt 1): 1937–1941

55. Bales GT et al (1995) Short-term outcomes after cryosurgical ablation of the prostate in men with recurrent prostate carcinoma following radiation therapy. Urology 46(5): 676–680.

56. Anastasiadis AG et al (2003) Comparison of health-related quality of life and prostate-associated symptoms after primary and salvage cryotherapy for prostate cancer. J Cancer Res Clin Oncol 129(12): 676–682.

57. Lambert EH et al (2007) Focal cryosurgery: encouraging health outcomes for unifocal prostate cancer. Urology 69(6): 1117–1120.

58. Levy DA, Pisters LL, Jones JS (2009) Primary cryoablation nadir prostate specific antigen and biochemical failure. J Urol 182(3): 931–937.

59. Kunkle DA, Egleston BL, Uzzo RG (2008) Excise, ablate or observe: the small renal mass dilemma–a meta-analysis and review. J Urol 179(4): 1227–1233

60. Hou AH, Sullivan KF, Crawford ED (2009) Targeted focal therapy for prostate cancer: a review. Curr Opin Urol 19(3): 283–289.

61. Josan S et al (2009) MRI-guided cryoablation: in vivo assessment of focal canine prostate cryolesions. J Magn Reson Imaging 30(1): 169–176.

62. Baust JG et al (2004) Cryosurgery–a putative approach to molecular-based optimization. Cryobiology 48(2): 190–204.

63. Machlenkin A et al (2005) Combined dendritic cell cryotherapy of tumor induces systemic antimetastatic immunity. Clin Cancer Res 11(13): 4955–4961.

64. Ismail M et al (2009) Enhancing prostate cancer cryotherapy using tumour necrosis factor related apoptosis-inducing ligand (TRAIL) sensitisation in an in vitro cryotherapy model. Cryobiology 59(2): 207–213.

# 5 Radiofrequency ablation

Adam S. Feldman[1], Peter R. Mueller[2], and W. Scott McDougal[1]
[1]Department of Urology, Massachusetts General Hospital, Harvard Medical School, Boston, MA, USA
[2]Department of Radiology, Massachusetts General Hospital, Harvard Medical School, Boston, MA, USA

## Introduction

Thermal ablation techniques have gained considerable attention in the field of urologic oncology. Methods such as cryoablation, high-intensity focused ultrasound (HIFU), interstitial laser therapy, and microwave ablation are all being investigated for their potential use as forms of minimally invasive treatments for genitourinary malignancies. Over the past several years the utilization of radiofrequency ablation (RFA) has increased and gained considerable clinical acceptance in localized treatment of primary and metastatic tumors. Initial experiences in RFA were in the intraoperative ablation of colon cancer metastases in the liver. However, as understanding and experience with this technology developed, RFA was employed percutaneously. Considerable work has been done in the evaluation of RFA in the liver for the treatment of hepatocellular carcinoma [1–3]. With increased technical experience in RFA, interventionalists broadened the application of this treatment modality to other sites, including the kidney for the treatment of renal cell carcinoma (RCC).

The accepted and expected management of small renal masses has significantly changed over the past several years. With the widespread use of abdominal imaging, a majority of renal masses are now discovered incidentally. These otherwise asymptomatic incidental renal masses tend to be smaller in size and of lower grade than those that are diagnosed as a result of symptomatic presentation [4,5]. With a shift in the size of renal masses at presentation, treatment goals include the preservation of renal function via nephron-sparing techniques, as this approach may provide long-term benefits to the patient [6]. Partial nephrectomy (PN) in appropriately selected patients has been demonstrated to be as effective as radical nephrectomy in oncologic control [7,8]. Partial nephrectomy, however, may carry with it elevated operative risk in older patients with greater comorbidity. In an effort to expand the realm of nephron-sparing techniques, RFA has provided an alternative minimally invasive treatment option. Since the initial case report of RFA in RCC in 1999 [9], this technique has become more widely accepted as a viable treatment modality for small renal masses. This chapter explores the science, technique, and efficacy of this relatively new technology and explores its comparison with the traditional surgical approach for the management of RCC. In addition, RFA has been briefly explored in other genitourinary malignancies, and this experience will be discussed.

## Scientific basis for radiofrequency ablation

### Mechanism of effect

RFA produces its effect by the transmission of radiofrequency energy into tissues. This method combines physics with biology to transform an alternating current into heat, resulting in coagulation necrosis of

*Interventional Techniques in Uro-oncology*, First Edition. Edited by Hashim Uddin Ahmed, Manit Arya, Peter T. Scardino & Mark Emberton. © 2011 Blackwell Publishing Ltd. Published 2011 by Blackwell Publishing Ltd.

tumor. A generator supplying 60 W to 250 W of radiofrequency energy is the source of this current. RFA applicator electrodes are inserted into the tumor. Current flows through the applicator electrode from the generator into the targeted tissue, and then through the patient into a grounding pad that is connected back to the generator to complete the electrical circuit. The RFA generator produces an alternating current, which causes agitation of the ions in the surrounding cells and tissue. This ionic agitation produces friction and thus heat, resulting in an elevation of local tissue temperatures. Target tissue temperatures of 60–100°C result in instantaneous irreversible cellular damage resulting in coagulation necrosis [10]. Lower tissue temperatures between 50–60°C also results in coagulation necrosis, however, this occurs within minutes. Temperatures below 46°C appear to produce tissue hyperthermia, which however, is repairable by the native tissue. Target tissue temperatures above 100°C are avoided as this will result in tissue vaporization, leading to boiling and gas formation, as well as significant tissue charring on the electrode. (Table 5.1) The formation of gas and tissue charring both act as significant insulators that prevent diffusion of heat into the surrounding tissues and effectively decrease the size of the thermal zone of tissue ablation.

One method devised to avoid tissue vaporization and charring is the use of energy pulsing. This technique utilizes a rapid alternation of high and low energy deposition into the target tissue. This method allows the tissue immediately adjacent to the electrode to cool momentarily, while the more distant tissue maintains its temperature [11]. Repeated cycles of pulsed heating and transient cooling prevents the temperature in the tissue nearest to the electrode from reaching elevated temperatures that would otherwise result in vaporization and charring.

## Applicator electrode

The earliest and simplest form of applicator electrode is a monopolar single straight needle with an insulated shaft and an uninsulated metal tip through which the current flows into the tissue. Since the inception of RFA, variations on the monopolar electrode have been developed, including straight cluster electrodes with multiple adjacent tips and multitined expandable electrodes. These electrodes allow for an increase in size of a single ablation zone from the applicator electrode.

The single-tip monopolar electrode (Figure 5.1) delivers the alternating electrical current directly to the target tissue in a manner such that the current delivered to the adjacent tissue is inversely proportional to the square of the distance from the electrode [12].

Table 5.1 Biological tissue effects of thermal ablation.

| Tissue temperature | Tissue effect |
| --- | --- |
| 42–46°C | Tissue hyperthermia with reversible cellular injury |
| 46–48°C | Irreversible cellular injury that occurs at 45 minutes of ablation |
| 50–55°C | Irreversible coagulation tissue necrosis that occurs at 4 to 6 minutes of ablation |
| 60–100°C | Irreversible coagulation tissue necrosis that occurs instantaneously |
| >110°C | Immediate tissue vaporization and tissue charring, which can decrease transmission of current and decrease RFA efficacy |

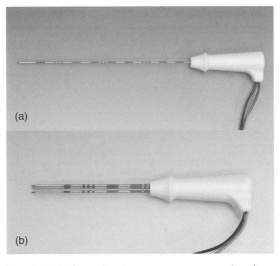

Fig 5.1 RFA Electrodes. Demonstrates two examples of RFA electrodes. The single-tip monopolar electrode is seen in (a) and the cluster electrode, designed with three evenly spaced 17-gauge electrodes in a triangular configuration is seen in (b).

These properties of the rapid diffusion of the electrical current and energy result in a decrease in the area of coagulation necrosis achievable with the single electrode. The maximum diameter ablation zone achievable with such a single monopolar electrode appears to be 1.6 cm in an in vivo model [13].

One method devised to increase the zone of ablation with a single monopolar electrode is through the use of an internally cooled electrode in which chilled saline is perfused into and then out of the applicator tip. This perfusion mechanism effectively reduces the temperature at the tip of the applicator electrode, reducing the risk of gas formation and charring and allowing for an environment that can produce a larger zone of ablation.

Another advance in electrode design was in the development of a cluster electrode (Figure 5.1). This applicator electrode is designed with three evenly spaced 17-gauge electrodes in a triangular configuration and held together as a single unit (Valley Lab, Boulder, CO). This array of three adjacent electrodes effectively increases the diameter of the ablation zone. This model is also designed with an internally cooled tip to avoid insulating vaporization and charring and effectively improving the size of the ablation zone.

A third physical design with the intent of increasing the size of the ablation zone is a multi-tined expandable electrode. This electrode is configured in such a way that the applicator needle is placed and then an umbrella-style hooked array expands within the tissue. This expandable electrode significantly increases the size of the ablation zone, such that early devices could result in treatment zones up to 4 cm and more recent systems allowing ablation zones up to 5 or 6 cm [11,12].

More recently, a bipolar applicator electrode has been designed for use of thermal tumor ablation. As opposed to a monopolar electrode, which delivers current through the target tissue and then completes the circuit by traveling through the patient to a separate grounding pad electrode, the bipolar electrode works by passing the current through the target tissue between two adjacent electrodes. This technology allows for destruction of target tissue between the two electrodes, however, limits the adjacent collateral damage to other tissues. A surgical bipolar RFA device (Boston Scientific) is available in the United States, and a percutaneous bipolar device is undergoing investigational trials in Europe [14,15].

# Radiofrequency ablation in renal cell carcinoma

## Rationale

In 2009 there was expected to be 57,760 new cases of kidney cancers in the United States [16]. With the prevalent use of abdominal imaging, there is a much greater proportion of RCCs that are discovered as incidental renal masses. These masses, when discovered incidentally, tend to be smaller and of lower grade than those that are diagnosed due to symptomatic presentation [4,5] Concordant with this shift in tumor size and stage of presentation has been a paradigm shift in our algorithm for treating these small renal masses. Attention has now focused on preservation of functional renal tissue, which has resulted in a move toward performing PN in appropriately selected patients. Justification for this interest in nephron-sparing surgery has recently been supported with evidence that PN results in long-term preservation of renal function and perhaps overall survival [6,17] Furthermore, follow-up data has demonstrated that in the appropriately selected patients, PN results in equivalent oncologic control as total nephrectomy [7,8]. A nephron-sparing approach is especially attractive in patients with a genetic predisposition to the development of multiple RCCs, such as in patients with Von Hippel-Lindau (VHL) disease. This approach is essential in patients with a solitary kidney to avoid the need for dialysis.

Given the demonstrated oncologic efficacy of partial nephrectomy, improvements in technology have moved the field toward the development of minimally invasive methods for a nephron sparing approach. Developments in laparascopic techniques and skill have made laparoscopic PN an attractive minimally invasive alternative to the standard open partial nephrectomy. Even less invasive, percutaneous techniques, including RFA and cryoablation have now also become available and more commonly accepted alternatives.

## Early experience and short-term outcomes

The use of RFA in RCC developed in the late 1990s with reports of animal studies demonstrating the feasibility of using this technology in the kidney [18,19]. Zlotta, et al [20] reported on two renal tumors that were ablated and then resected, demonstrating the efficacy of renal tissue ablation with this technique. In

1999 McGovern, et al [9] from Massachusetts General Hospital (MGH) reported on the first percutaneous in vivo treatment of RCC with RFA. This report demonstrated the ability of this technology to ablate a 3 cm tumor, with no resulting tumor enhancement on follow-up contrast-enhanced computed tomography (CT).

In 2000 the group at MGH reported on their experience with RFA in 9 tumors in 8 patients [21]. This was the first series reported with imaging follow-up in RFA in RCC. Gervais and colleagues prospectively studied their experience, with the indications for RFA being a life expectancy shorter than 10 years, substantial coexistent medical comorbidities that would make a surgical approach very risky, and/or a solitary kidney. Patients who had metastatic disease or were considerable surgical candidates were excluded. All tumors were biopsy proven to be RCC and ranged in size from 1.2 to 5.0 cm, with a mean diameter of 3.3 cm.

Electrodes were placed percutaneously by either ultrasound or CT guidance and placed under intravenous conscious sedation. Cooled-tip electrodes were used with a pulsed current to avoid tissue vaporization and charring. Post-RFA imaging protocol was to evaluate with contrast-enhanced CT scans at 1, 3, and 6 months. One patient with a serum creatinine (Cr) above 2 mg/dL was evaluated with gadolinium-enhanced magnetic resonance imaging (MRI). Any lesion enhancement of greater than 10 hounsfield units (HU) on CT was considered to be untreated or residual tumor. Similarly, an increase in signal intensity on MRI was also considered to be untreated tumor.

Five tumors were completely treated in one ablation session, and four required additional visits. Three of these four patients completed treatment in two sessions and one patient required four sessions.

With a mean follow-up time of 10.3 months (range 3–21), seven of the nine tumors were completely treated. No patients developed metastatic disease during the course of the study and their serum Cr all remained stable during treatment. Two complications were noted in the study. One was a complication of intravenous sedation in which the patient developed a 5- to 10-minute dystonic reaction to fentanyl. The other complication was in a large central lesion in a solitary kindey, in which the patient developed gross hematuria and a perinephric hematoma within one hour after RFA. Clot within the collecting system resulted in anuric obstruction and the patient required a cystoscopic placement of a ureteral stent and blood transfusion. This patient recovered from this complication within several days and he ultimately proceeded with additional RFA of residual tumor.

To better analyze the results by tumor location within the kidney, this study classified each tumor as either exophytic, central, or mixed. Figure 5.2 demonstrates these categories. Exophytic tumors are those in which 25% or more of the tumor diameter is in contact with the perinephric fact. Central tumors are defined as a tumor that extends into the renal sinus, but not beyond the renal capsule. Mixed tumors are those with components in both the renal sinus fat and perinephric fat. In reviewing the results, it was clear that the small exophytic tumors are those that are most readily treated by RFA. In fact, the two tumors that were not completely treated in this series were central tumors greater than 4 cm in size.

Tumor location was one of the major predictors of treatment success that was identified in this study. It was clear that the exophytic tumors were more readily treated than the central tumors. Central tumors, which are embedded in highly vascular renal parenchyma as well as the surrounding high-flow vessels of the hilar

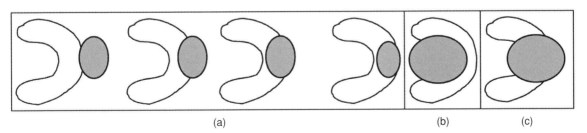

**Fig 5.2** CT images of exophytic, central, and mixed tumors. Demonstrates examples of exophytic (a), central (b), and mixed (c) tumors.

area, are more challenging to maintain at the elevated temperatures necessary for coagulation necrosis. The surrounding vasculature and highly vascular tissue has a cooling or "heat sink" effect as the heated blood is carried away and replaced with the cooler blood at body temperature. This difficulty is in contrast to an exophytic tumor, which is surrounded by perinephric fat. The fat around these tumors acts as an insulator of heat and therefore results in an ideal environment to heat and maintain required temperatures in the target tissue.

Gervais and colleagues updated their experience in 2005, reporting on 100 tumors ablated [22]. This report confirmed the challenges of treating larger tumors and centrally located tumors. Of the 100 tumors, 90 demonstrated complete necrosis by imaging criteria. These completely treated tumors ranged in size from 1.1 to 5.5 cm, with a mean diameter of 2.9 cm. The remaining incompletely treated tumors ranged in size from 4.0 to 8.9 cm. In fact, no tumors over 5.5 cm in size were completely ablated. In multivariate analysis, both smaller tumor size and noncentral location were the strongest predictors of successful treatment.

Pavlovich, et al [23] reported on the early experience of the group at the National Cancer Institute with RFA for 24 RCC tumors in 21 patients with hereditary renal tumors from VHL and hereditary papillary RCC. All tumors were 3 cm or less in diameter and solid, with no cystic components. Treatment was performed with ultrasound or CT guidance and follow-up imaging protocol consisted of contrast-enhanced CT scan at 3, 6, and 12 months postablation. All ablations were performed with the multi-tined hooked array expandable electrodes (RITA Medical Systems, Inc. Mountain View, CA). All tumors were treated once. Treatments were considered satisfactory when tissue temperatures greater than 70°C were maintained throughout the ablation. Five of the 24 tumors did not maintain temperature and thus were considered poor or unsatisfactory treatments.

Follow-up imaging consisted of a contrast-enhanced CT scan at two months postablation. Five of the tumors ablated demonstrated persistent enhancement at 2 month imaging, with four of these being those tumors that were also considered poor or unsatisfactory treatments at the time of ablation. Patients experienced mild pain and some postprocedural nausea, likely related to the sedatives used during ablation. There were no major complications during or after

the ablations. Minor complications included transient gross hematuria in one patient, transient pain on hip flexion in two patients, and cutaneous flank numbness that was persistent at 2 months in two patients. A 1.5 cm postprocedure perinephric hematoma was visualized in one patient and this was resolved at 2 month imaging.

The group at University of Texas Southwestern reported on their early experience with RFA in RCC [24]. This series included 13 tumors treated percutaneously in 12 patients. All tumors were less than 4 cm in diameter (mean 2.4 ± 0.6 cm). All ablations were performed with the multi-tined hooked array expandable electrodes (RITA Medical Systems, Inc. Mountain View, CA) and follow-up imaging protocol included contrast-enhanced CT scans at 6 weeks, 3, 6, and 12 months, and every 6 months thereafter. Of all 13 tumors, one demonstrated a rim of persistent enhancement on follow-up CT. This tumor was reablated at 6 months and did not demonstrate any enhancement on the subsequent 6-week scan. The remaining 12 tumors did not demonstrate any recurrent tumor enhancement on any follow-up imaging. No major complications occurred and one patient developed a small nonclinically significant perinephric hematoma postablation.

Based on their series, Cadeddu and colleagues at UT Southwestern reflected on the importance of deploying the electrode tines 0.5 to 1 cm beyond the visible edge of the tumor, such that the outer tumor margin is adequately treated. Furthermore, they recommended that multiple electrode placements or ablations may be necessary during a treatment session in order to cover the entirety of tumor area. This measure is necessary in larger tumors with inhomogeneous shape such that one deployment of the electrode will not adequately cover the entirety of the targeted tumor.

Several other institutions, including Johns Hopkins [25], Mayo Clinic [26], and Wake Forest [27] have reported their early experiences with RFA in RCC. The group at Hopkins [25] reported on 35 tumors less than 4 cm in size in 29 patients. All but two patients were treated under IV sedation and 85% of the patients were treated on an outpatient basis. Over a mean follow-up period of 9 months (range 0–23 months), 2 patients required a second ablation for small areas of residual enhancement. These both were treated successfully with no further enhancement on repeated imaging.

The early series from the Mayo Clinic [28] included 35 tumors in 20 patients. Twenty-seven of these tumors were treated percutaneously, while two patients with eight tumors were treated with intraoperative RFA due to the risk of injury to adjacent organs including the bowel or gallbladder. Of those who were treated percutaneously, all but one were treated as outpatients. At a mean follow-up time of 9 months (range 1–23 months), no tumors demonstrated residual or recurrent enhancement by either contrast-enhanced CT or MRI.

Zagoria, et al [27] reported a retrospective analysis of the Wake Forest experience with RFA in RCC. Twenty-four renal tumors were ablated in 22 patients, seventeen of which were proven to have RCC by percutaneous biopsy. All ablations were carried out under CT guidance and were performed using cooled-tip electrodes of either the single-tip or cluster-array type. Follow-up ranged from 1 to 35 months, with a mean of 7 months.

On the initial follow-up imaging at 1–3 months, residual tumor was demonstrated in 4/24 tumors. The mean tumor size in these four patients with residual tumor was 4.4 cm (range 3.1–5 cm). Two of these patients underwent additional ablation sessions with follow-up imaging showing no residual tumor. Two of the remaining four patients with residual tumor chose observation due to severe medical comorbidities. No metastases were detected in any of the patients during this limited time of follow-up.

The group at Wake Forest updated their experience in 2007, reporting on a total of 125 tumors in 104 patients [29]. This analysis reiterated their earlier results, demonstrating that larger tumor size correlated with a greater risk of residual tumor on follow-up after the initial RFA treatment. In fact, no recurrent disease was demonstrated in any tumor less than 3.7 cm in diameter. Despite the findings of residual disease in 16 of 30 larger tumors, 7 were successfully retreated with no further evidence of recurrent disease on follow-up imaging. However, three patients who opted for additional ablative treatments ultimately developed evidence of viable recurrent tumor. The remainder of the 16 patients with recurrent disease either declined treatment, were lost to follow-up, or underwent salvage nephrectomy. Of the entire series, 2 patients demonstrated evidence of metastatic disease on follow-up. One patient in retrospect, likely had metastatic disease at the time of RFA given that he had small pulmonary nodules on pre-RFA CT, which eventually became evident to be metastatic disease. The second patient developed pulmonary nodules on CT one year after RFA, indicating that he also may have had otherwise undetectable metastatic disease at the time of RFA.

These initial short-term results from multiple separate institutions have been extremely encouraging in evaluating the safety and efficacy of RFA for RCC. Nevertheless, long-term data is critical in truly evaluating the oncologic control of RCC with RFA. A few groups with early experience have presented their more recent longer term data in an attempt to address this concern.

## Results with extended follow-up

Paramount in the evaluation of any emerging treatment modality is long-term efficacy in comparison to the gold standard. McDougal et al [30] reported on 16 patients undergoing RFA for biopsy proven RCC with a minimum of 4 years since the procedure. Three of these patients had multiple tumors for a total of 20 tumors treated, ranging in size from 1.1 to 7.1 cm (mean $3.2 \pm 1.4$ cm). Patients were followed with contrast- enhanced CT or gadolinium-enhanced MRI at 1 month, 3 months, 6 months, and then 6 month to yearly intervals thereafter. The presence of recurrent or untreated tumor was based on contrast enhancement. No lesions were rebiopsied.

Of the 16 patients, 5 died of unrelated causes before 4 years, leaving 11 patients with a mean follow-up time of $4.6 \pm 0.8$ years. All exophytic and central tumors were treated successfully without recurrence or metastasis. Of the 2 mixed tumors, 1 was successfully treated, but the other progressively enlarged after the initial treatment and was thus considered unsuccessful. No patients developed metastatic disease during this follow-up period.

More recently, Levinson et al [31] reported on the long-term follow-up of RFA in RCC at Johns Hopkins. Although only 18 tumors were pathologically confirmed RCC, 31 patients with solitary tumors were followed for a mean time of 5.1 years (range 41–80 months) after treatment for renal masses ranging in size from 1.1 to 4.0 cm (mean 2.1 cm).Imaging was performed at 3, 6, and 12 months, and then 6 to 9 month intervals thereafter. One of the total 31 patients demonstrated inadequate ablation, as evidenced by

Derby Hospitals NHS Foundation Trust Library and Knowledge Service initial postablation imaging. This patient underwent repeat RFA and was recurrence-free after 76 months.

Local tumor recurrence was identified in 3 of 31 patients, as evidenced by contrast enhancement on follow-up imaging. These occurred at 7, 13, and 31 months post-RFA. These patients underwent salvage treatment with repeat RFA, cryoablation, and laparoscopic radical nephrectomy. Two of the recurrences were confirmed pathologically, however, the third revealed only postablation scar on biopsy prior to re-ablation. None of the patients developed metastatic disease and there was no disease specific mortality.

These reports suggest that with a modest follow-up period RFA appears to be efficacious in treating small renal tumors. However, before we can truly accept the oncologic efficacy of this technique as comparable to the gold standard, we must first have longer term follow-up data in larger cohorts spanning at least 5 years, and preferably 10 years.

## Oncologic efficacy – controversies

One of the difficulties in assessing an ablative technique as opposed to an extirpative method of tumor treatment is the question of how to measure success in treating the malignancy. These questions have been raised over the past several years as RFA has been investigated. CT scan enhanced with intravenous contrast has largely been the preferred method for following lesions after ablation. Any persistent or new enhancement is considered to be persistent or recurrent disease, respectively. The accuracy of this method for detecting persistent or recurrent disease has been questioned, however. Furthermore, the ability of RFA to achieve total tumor cell destruction has also been questioned.

The group at Lahey clinic questioned the ability of RFA to achieve total tumor destruction [32]. They performed open tumor RFA in a total of 20 tumors (15 patients) just prior to open resection by partial nephrectomy. Tumors were then analyzed by standard histologic hematoxylin and eosin (H&E) staining, as well as staining for nicotinamide adenine dinucleotide (NADH) diaphorase for enzymatic activity. In all tumors, they reported that there were histologically viable tumor cells within the regions of tumor destruction by coagulative necrosis. In 5 of the tumors, they also performed NADH diaphorase staining and demonstrated enzymatic activity in 4 of the

5 specimens. These findings certainly raised questions as to the efficacy of complete tumor destruction by RFA. However, it must be noted that ablations were only single needle placements and tissue temperatures reached up to 110 °C, which as discussed previously can result in tissue charring on the electrode and thus ineffective energy transfer. Furthermore, it appears that the histologic effects of RFA on renal tissue mature over time [33] and therefore the immediate microscopic evaluation in this study may not represent the true long-term effect.

Rendon et al [34] evaluated four patients who underwent partial or radical nephrectomy immediately after RFA and six patients who underwent partial or radical nephrectomy one week after RFA. In the group with immediate nephrectomy, their analysis demonstrated the difficulty in determining cell viability at this time point, thus questioning the findings of the Michaels et al [32] study discussed above. The group with surgical excision delayed by one week had a contrast-enhanced CT scan on day 7 prior to resection. Three patients demonstrated what appeared to be viable tumor in 5–10% of the original tumor volume. Two of these patients had no evidence of contrast enhancement on CT scan prior to resection. These findings again questioned the ability of RFA to effectively achieve tumor cell death, however, also questioned the ability of contrast-enhanced CT to adequately assess for tumor recurrence. It must be noted, however, that the tissues obtained were only analyzed by H&E staining, which may be inadequate for assessing tumor viability in this setting. In addition, CT scans were obtained at only one week post-RFA, which as discussed above, may not represent the actual long-term effect.

Cadeddu's group [35] reported on three patients who underwent surgical excision at 11, 18, and 24 months after RFA. These resections were performed for what appeared to be new enhancement on CT at the periphery of the ablation zone margin in two patients and an unrepairable UPJ obstruction in the third patient. All three patients had no evidence of any viable tumor in the entire specimen. The area of contrast enhancement seen on CT scan appeared to be as a result of a granulomatous giant cell reaction in the area of the ablation margin. Although this reports on only a few patients, it does demonstrate a long-term effectiveness of tumor cell killing by RFA. It also, however, raises the critical features of post-RFA imaging by contrast-enhanced CT scan. Whereas new enhancement within the ablation zone should absolutely be considered a tumor recurrence, a so-called "halo" of enhancement around the periablation zone may be an atypical finding that does not truly represent a recurrence. Of course, the authors admit that we can only begin to truly define what are benign and what are malignant imaging findings with increased experience, however, this report begins to shed light on what these imaging findings may truly represent.

This same group also evaluated 17 biopsy proven RCC tumors treated by RFA with a post-RFA tumor biopsy all being done at least one year after the ablation (mean 26.9 months) [36]. In all of these patients, standard follow-up imaging was negative for any evidence of recurrence. All biopsied tumor beds demonstrated no evidence of viable tumor and histopathologic findings varied from extensive coagulation necrosis to complete tissue necrosis and inflammatory reaction. These findings suggest that RFA does result in effective long-term tumor cell death within the ablation zone. These longer term histopathologic results correlate more closely with the clinically observed success rates discussed previously. It is clear that the true histologic evolution within a tumor following RFA is not entirely defined and evalution at early time points may be misleading in determining cellular viability.

## Technical considerations

Optimal treatment of renal tumors with RFA has been found to be dependent on multiple factors and over time with increased experience, various measures for achieving success have been identified. It is clear that exophytic tumors at the periphery of the renal parenchyma and polar regions are more easily treated than those lesions that are central or intraparenchymal. The exophytic tumors are typically surrounded by fat, which insulates the treatment area, both serving to maximize thermal coagulation effect in the target tissue and also protecting surrounding structures from collateral injury. Central tumors have been demonstrated to be more of a challenge to treat. These tumors are surrounded by multiple or large vessels, which serve as a heat sink dissipating the effective energy and potentially reducing the effectiveness of the treatment. Treatment of these central and intraparenchymal tumors also pose a relative risk of injury to the hilar structures and collecting system. These techni-

cal considerations identified by the MGH group [37] have been confirmed by others. Veltri et al [38] described that an exophytic nature of the tumor served as a significant predictor of complete ablation success in a single treatment session as compared with parenchymal or central tumors. Exophytic tumor extension also appeared to be significantly predictive of a reduced risk of complication compared with a central tumor extension and mid-kidney location. Central tumor extension was a negative predictor of treatment success of the tumor during both the first and second treatment sessions. In addition to the heat sink effect in the hilar area, it is likely that this relative difficulty of treatment of central tumors is also in part due to technical limitation of an inability to place the electrode needle tip beyond the deep margin of the tumor that is adjacent to large vessels and renal sinus and hilar structures. Treatment of an extended margin in this deep area would certainly pose a significant risk of injury to these hilar structures resulting in major complications.

In addition to the location of the tumor within the renal unit, the location of the tumor in relation to surrounding structures also plays a significant role in effective treatment of RCC with RFA. Adjacent structures in relation to the left kidney include the large and small bowel, the spleen, the pancreas, and the adrenal gland. On the right side, structures at risk include the liver, the duodenum, the large bowel, and the adrenal gland. Of course, with both kidneys, the hilar structures, renal pelvis, and proximal ureter are always at risk. In an effort to successfully treat tumors in spite of at risk adjacent organs, innovative methods have been employed to protect or move these innocent bystanders. Rendon et al [39] described a method of hydrodissection in a large animal model in which they used normal saline hydrodissection and carbon dioxide ($CO_2$) dissection to manipulate and move the tissues under ultrasound guidance. This method effectively created a thermal barrier between the target tumor and adjacent organ, thus protecting that organ from risk of collateral injury. There were no differences noted between the effectiveness of thermal protection from either method, however, it was noted that $CO_2$ was technically easier to confine within the created perirenal space, whereas saline more easily dissipated throughout the surrounding tissues. In addition, the group did not identify any increase in impedance of energy by having the electrode wires partially submerged in saline. One difference noted, however, was that the $CO_2$ did interfere with ultrasound visualization, whereas saline did not. It was clear from this analysis that this method of tissue manipulation for the protection of adjacent organs was easy to perform and did not result in any significant morbidity in this pig model.

Gervais et al [37] discussed using this method of hydrodissection in humans in order to displace the colon during treatment. This method used the instillation of 50–200 mL of sterile water to displace the colon from the tumor that was originally 0.1–0.4 cm from the tumor. Figure 5.3 demonstrates this method of hydrodissection. This method allowed the treatment of these tumors by displacing the at-risk organ and creating a protective thermal cushion between it and the target. The authors noted, however, that the displacement was transient and that due to dissipation of the water, repeat instillations needed to be performed at multiple time points during the treatment. Prior to using this technique, the authors would never place the electrode tip within 2–3 mm of the bowel perpendicularly or the shaft of the electrode no closer than 5–7 mm when parallel to the bowel. There were no complications with bowel perforation or inflammation in this group's experience.

Other groups have demonstrated the effective use of this technique of hydrodissection or $CO_2$ displacement. Chen et al [40] demonstrated the effective use of a 5% Dextrose solution (D5 W) to displace and protect the colon during RFA of a renal tumor. Farrell et al [41] utilized sterile water instillation and Liddell and Solomon [42] injected air to displace the bowel from the adjacent tumors. Kariya et al [43] successfully performed two cases of RFA after percutaneous instillation of $CO_2$ around the target tissue to displace the adjacent spleen, splenic vessels, and pancreas, which were at risk of collateral injury. The authors noted the attractiveness of $CO_2$ as an agent for this method given its properties of poor heat conduction and thus high heat insulation. Furthermore, its safety of use intra-abdominally has been proven by a long experience of use in laparoscopic surgery.

Due to the length of bowel normally adjacent to the kidneys on both sides, the colon is the most common structure to be adjacent to a renal tumor and at risk of secondary injury. Interestingly, however, in the MGH series the colon was also the most common structure that notably moved positions from prior diagnostic imaging to ablation and during ablation [37]. The authors also noted that at times the placement of the electrode needle itself pushed the kidney safely away from the bowel, and in another treatment, the colon spontaneously moved away from the tumor even without repositioning of the patient. This group commented that they were able to safely ablate 21 tumors that

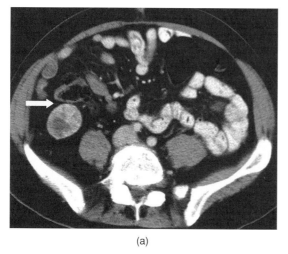

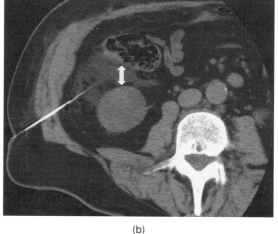

| (a) | (b) |

**Fig 5.3** CT images of the technique of hydrodissection. (a) Preoperative CT image in which the arrow points to the proximity of the tumor to the overlying colon. (b) CT image demonstrating hydrodissection being used to create a barrier between the tumor and the adjacent organ. This technique can be used to protect an adjacent organ from collateral injury by the RFA electrode.

were within 1 cm of the bowel by using cautious electrode positioning and no additional displacement techniques. There were no bowel complications within this series.

In addition to adjacent other organs, the ureter and collecting system are at risk of injury in the treatment of nearby tumors. Retrograde pyeloperfusion was for thermal protection of the collecting system during RFA was initially described by Schultze et al [44] who perfused cold saline into the collecting system of the kidney during a RFA of a renal pelvis transitional cell carcinoma. Wah et al then reported on retrograde pyeloperfusion of cold D5 W into the collecting system during RFA of a central RCC. This technique is employed by cystoscopically placing an open-ended ureteral catheter into the ureter and renal collecting system and infusing cold D5 W into the collecting system at a perfusion pressure of 80 cm $H_2O$. One-liter bags of D5 W were stored in refrigeration at 2–6°C prior to infusion. Figure 5.4 demonstrates the ureteral catheter in place for pyeloperfusion while the RFA probe is in place in the adjacent tumor.

Cantwell et al [45] reported on a two-institution retrospective analysis of 17 patients treated with this technique. The indication for this method of protection with pyeloperfusion was that the tumor was

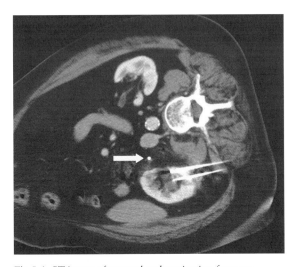

**Fig 5.4** CT image of ureteral catheterization for retrograde pyeloperfusion. The arrow points to the radio-opaque ureteral catheter which can be seen within the ureter as it is infusing cooled D5 W in a retrograde fashion into the renal collecting system and proximal ureter. The RFA electrode is seen within the tumor in the same image.

within 1.5 cm of the ureter. Pyeloperfusion was achieved as described above and the ureteral catheter was removed immediately upon termination of the RFA procedure. No complications occurred in any of the treated patients. There were no findings of hydronephrosis or ureteral strictures. Three patients demonstrated residual tumor at one month follow-up imaging and underwent a second RFA session with complete effectiveness. This report suggests that retrograde cold fluid pyeloperfusion is safe and may be effective in preventing ureteral injury or stricture during RFA of adjacent tumors. It does, however, raise the question of whether this method may make the RFA slightly less effective at tumor cell killing by producing a heat sink similar to that seen at the large hilar vessels. The choice to use this method must therefore be made with cautious judgement based on the architecture of the kidney and relative tumor location.

## Management of residual or recurrent disease

Following ablative therapy of RCC, residual disease is defined as persistent enhancement demonstrated on contrast-enhanced CT scan within three months of surveillance imaging. Recurrent disease is declared when initial follow-up images demonstrate no area of contrast enhancement, and enhancement then becomes evident on any subsequent scan after three months. Gervais et al [37] demonstrated that out of 100 tumors treated, 23 demonstrated some degree of residual disease. When residual disease occurs, the multi-tined hooked array systems are more associated with a residual pattern of multiple peripheral nodules. The straight needle systems tend to leave areas of enhancement, which are crescent-shaped edges; however, they may also leave small masses or residual nodules. These areas of residual disease after treatment are most often amenable to repeat ablation of the enhancing region(s).

Matin et al [46] reported on a multi-institutional retrospective analysis of residual and recurrent disease. Of the seven participating centers and a total of 410 RFA treated tumors, there were 55 (13.4%) residual or recurrent tumors. This study also included 8 cases of recurrence after cryoablation. A total of 69.8% of the cases were detected within 3 months of initial treatment and were thus labeled as residual disease. The majority of the remaining cases of residual and remaining cases were detected within the first

12 months, however, there were also a few cases detected after one year. Of the total 63 patients with residual/recurrent disease after ablative therapy, 46 received a salvage energy ablative technique. Thirty-seven of these patients demonstrated no further evidence of disease on follow-up, thus resulting in an overall rate of residual or recurrence disease of 4.2% after salvage ablation. Six patients underwent salvage nephrectomy, and in all of these cases residual RCC was detected in the specimen.

These reports demonstrate that residual disease within the first three months may occur and can be safely and successfully managed with repeat ablation to the areas of persistent disease. Later recurrences can also be managed with repeat or salvage ablation with apparent success. Another alternative is salvage nephrectomy or PN in select cases [47].

## Complications

As experience with RFA has increased, so has an understanding of its potential complications. In 2006 the Technology Assessment Committee of the Society of Interventional Radiology published reporting standards for percutaneous thermal ablation of renal tumors [48]. This group presented a list of known complications and classified them into various groups or classes (Table 5.2). Potential complications ranged from infectious, including abcess and sepsis, to vascular, including hematoma, pulmonary embolism, and renal infarct, to general non-vascular, including hematuria, collecting system/ureteral injury or stricture, perforation of hollow viscus, and respiratory, including pleural effusion and pneumothorax. This group also recognized that complications should be graded and reported according to the defined boundaries of minor and major complications as outlined by the Society of Interventional Radiology [49]. As shown in Table 5.3, major complications include those that require therapy with a minor hospitalization less than 48 hours, require major therapy with a prolonged hospitalization, result in permanent adverse sequelae or death. Minor complications require no or minimal therapy, resulting in no clinical consequence to the patient and may include an overnight admission for observation only.

Gervais et al [22,37] discussed that in 100 cases, their most common complication was hemorrhage, including hematoma formation or hematuria. Three

**Table 5.2** Classification of complications of RFA in RCC [48].

| Classification | Complication |
| --- | --- |
| General nonvascular | Hematuria |
| | Renal failure |
| | Stricture |
| | Collecting system |
| | Ureteral |
| | Tumor seeding |
| | Urinary fistula |
| | Unintended perforation of hollow viscus |
| Respiratory-pulmonary | Pleural effusion |
| | Pneumothorax |
| Cardiac | Angina/Coronary ischemia |
| | Myocardial infarction |
| | Hypotension |
| | Vagal reaction |
| Vascular | Hematoma bleeding |
| | Perirenal |
| | Subcapsular |
| | Retroperitoneal |
| | Puncture site |
| | Renal infarct |
| | Pulmonary embolism |
| Neurologic | Lumbar radiculopathy |
| | Stroke |
| Infectious/Inflammatory | Abcess |
| | Sepsis |
| Medication-related | Idiosyncratic reaction |
| Contrast agent-related | Allergic/Anaphylactoid reaction |
| Device-related | Skin burn |
| Death | Death related to procedure |
| | Death unrelated to procedure (30 day mortality) |

patients experienced minor hemorrhage that did not require transfusion, however, two of these patients had gross hematuria with clots resulting in bladder outlet obstruction and the need for bladder catheterization and irrigation. The third patient with minor hemorrhage had transient ureteral obstruction from clot, which was managed conservatively. One patient with a solitary kidney developed major hemorrhage

**Table 5.3** Grading of complications as defined by the Society of Interventional Radiology [49].

| | |
|---|---|
| Major complications | Requires therapy and/or minor hospitalization (<48 hours) |
| | Requires major therapy, an unplanned increase in level of care, and/or a prolonged hospitalization (>48 hours) |
| | Results in permanent adverse sequelae |
| | Results in death |
| Minor complications | No therapy required, no consequences |
| | Requires nominal therapy, but with no consequences. May include overnight admission for observation only. |

resulting in gross hematuria, which required a ureteral stent for ureteral clot obstruction and anuria. One other patient with major hemorrhage in the form of a subcapsular hematoma required blood transfusion.

After hemorrhage, the second most common clinically relevant complication was ureteral stricture. One patient with a solitary kidney developed a ureteral stricture and anuria within hours after RFA and required nephrostomy drainage and ureteral stenting. This tumor was located 2 mm away from the proximal ureter. Two clinically insignificant and asymptomatic ureteral strictures and one mild nonsignificant ureteropelvic junction obstruction were detected on follow-up imaging and required no intervention. These ureteral injuries occurred prior to the initiation of cold D5 W pyeloperfusion as described above for ureteral and collecting system protection and served as the impetus for the utilization of this technique.

Of the 100 cases reported, there were three urine leaks, however, only one that became clinically significant and required intervention. Two nonsignificant leaks were very small volume extravasation seen on post-RFA imaging and never resulted in any urinoma formation. The one patient who did develop a clinically significant leak was managed with drainage of the urinoma and placement of a nephroureteral catheter. This significant leak may have resulted from

a ureteral injury during treatment of an adjacent lower pole tumor. No bowel injuries or complications occurred in this series.

Veltri et al [38] reported complications in their series, confirming that hemorrhage, often in the form of a small insignificant hematoma was the most common complication. Of 44 total tumors treated, there were a total of 8 complications. The five minor complications included three asymptomatic perinephric hematomas, one case of pain at the procedure site, and one case of transient gross hematuria. Three major complications included one area of psoas necrosis, which subsequently resulted in the development of a posas abcess after 9 months. There was also a massive peri/pararenal bleed treated with arterial embolization. The authors commented that an exophytic location seemed to be a protective factor against complication, such that more central tumors demonstrated a higher rate of complication than noncentral tumors. This report also raises the issue that there may have been a tumor seeding of the tract through which the needle was passed. It is not clear, however, that this reported area of tumor seeding was ever truly evaluated pathologically.

In the MGH series [22] follow-up imaging demonstrated an anterior abdominal wall mass with inflammatory changes, which was initially thought to represent a tract seeding or recurrence. However, this mass was excised surgically and was found to only be an area of acute and chronic inflammation with histiocytes on pathologic anaylsis but no evidence of malignancy. Although we cannot definitively say that there is no risk, it appears that the risk of tract seeding, if present, is exceedingly low.

## Comparisons of RFA with other nephron-sparing techniques

Very little has been written directly comparing RFA with other nephron-sparing techniques, including cryoablation, laparoscopic PN, and open PN. Kunkle et al [50] published a meta-analysis comparing the published literature on the results of RFA, cryoablation, PN, and active surveillance. Across a total of 99 studies, the mean ages of the patients undergoing the various treatments were 60.1 years for PN, 67.2 years for RFA, 65.7 years for cryoablation, and 68.7 years for active surveillance. Mean tumor size for PN was 3.4 cm, 2.69 for RFA, 2.56 for cryoablation, and 3.04

for active surveillance. From a utilization perspective, these data indicate that older patients are undergoing the less invasive approaches of RFA and cryoablation, however, patients with slightly larger tumors are being selected for PN.

The authors of this study conclude that the rates of local recurrence in RFA and cryoablation are greater than for PN. They report that across the 99 studies, the rates of recurrence are 2.6% after PN, 4.6% after cyroablation, and 11.7% after RFA. However, the authors define recurrence as any lesion with evidence of local disease persistence at any time point after ablation. As Raman and Caddedu [51] point out in a letter to the editor of the Journal of Urology in review of this article, this definition does not account for the potential finding of residual disease on the initial one month CT scan after RFA. In assessing RFA, many authors differentiate the findings of residual disease from recurrent disease. The grouping of residual and recurrent disease, as done in this meta-analysis will severely overinflate the actual recurrence rate in the reviewed studies.

This notion of residual disease raises an interesting point. With percutaneous ablative techniques, any residual disease can be reablated during a separate visit without a significant increase in technical difficulty or patient morbidity. In fact, with some larger tumors the RFA treatment may be planned in a staged manner such that a repeat RFA is peformed within weeks of the initial treatment. This certainly is a novel approach to oncologic control, however, there is no evidence that there is a resultant increase in the development of metastatic disease. In fact, Kunkle's meta-analysis did not demonstrate any difference in the risk of developing metastatic disease between RFA, cryoablation, and PN.

Stern et al [52] compared the outcomes of patients undergoing laparoscopic PN, open PN, laparoscopic RFA, and percutaneous RFA for cT1 a tumors (≤4 cm). In a total of 37 patients with PN and 40 with RFA, there were three treatment failures in the RFA group and two recurrences in the PN group. The treatment failures in the RFA group included one incomplete ablation, which was reablated and remained recurrence-free at 42 months and two recurrences, one of which was successfully reablated and the other who underwent nephrectomy. The two recurrences in the PN group were a tumor in the contralateral kidney and an enhancing lesion adjacent to the previous tumor bed. In those tumors that were pathologically confirmed as RCC, the 3 year recurrence-free survival was 91.4% for RFA and 95.2% for PN. These rates were not statistically significant and demonstrate that RFA may have a similar rate of successful disease control in small renal masses as compared with PN, which must be taken as the gold standard for any nephron-sparing approach.

An additional aspect of comparison of any new method of treatment, is cost. It appears to be not only intuitive but also in actuality that the less invasive approach of RFA that is largely performed on an outpatient basis under conscious sedation is significantly less costly than PN. Lotan and Cadeddu [53] performed a cost comparison between RFA and PN, assessing acute care costs between the two procedures. RFA demonstrated a significant reduction in cost as compared with laparoscopic and open PN. This cost savings was in excess of $2500 and was largely accounted for by the difference in length of stay (LOS). RFA had a LOS of 0.5 days, which was significantly lower than that for laparoscopic PN (1.86 days) and open PN (4.94 days). Interestingly, there was no significant difference in costs between laparoscopic and open PN. It appears that the difference in LOS is offset by the greater operative costs of laparoscopic PN.

Pandharipande et al [54] performed a cost-effectiveness analysis comparing RFA and PN for small renal masses using a decision-analytic Markov model that was developed to assess life expectancy and lifetime costs for a 65-year-old man with a small renal mass. The life expectancy gained from PN vs. RFA in this analysis was only 2.5 days. The cost savings, however, was significant. Compared with RFA ablation, the incremental cost-effectiveness ratio of PN relative to RFA was $1,152,529 per quality-adjusted life-year (QALY). This striking amount certainly exceeds the assumed societal willingness to pay of $75,000 per QALY and demonstrates that from a cost-effectiveness perspective, RFA may be advantageous PN.

These two cost-analyses demonstrate the advantages of RFA from a financial standpoint. However, it must be reiterated that until true comparative long-term recurrence and survival data are available, surgical resection of the tumor must be held as the standard of care and should remain as such in a young, healthy surgical candidate with a small renal mass.

## Present status and potential future of a combined therapeutic approach

It would be attractive if the combination of RFA with some other therapeutic modality could improve tumor response and hence outcomes. Such investigations have been largely done thus far in experimental animal models. Ahmed et al [55] compared the effects of RFA alone and RFA in combination with intravenous liposomal doxorubicin, administered 30 minutes after RFA in rabbit kidneys. Induced coagulative necrosis in the target tissues were compared between the experimental groups. The authors found a significant increase in the zone of coagulation necrosis in the RFA group, which had been followed by the liposomal doxorubicin.

Hines-Peralta et al [56] investigated the effect of the combination of RFA and preoperative intraperitoneal arsenic trioxide administration in a human RCC model in nude mice. Mean tumor blood flow and resultant coagulation necrosis were assessed. Treatment with arsenic trioxide resulted in a significant decrease in RCC tumor blood flow. Although there was also a decrease in normal renal blood flow, the decrease in tumor flow was significantly greater. Treatment with arsenic trioxide resulted in a greater degree of coagulation necrosis in tumors as compared with that in controls. Furthermore, there was a positive dose-dependent relationship in coagulation necrosis seen in treated animals. This dose-dependent increase in coagulation necrosis correlated with the dose-related changes in tumor blood flow that were also observed. The most intense effect of combined treatment was observed when the arsenic trioxide was delivered 1 hour before RFA. At 6 hours, this combined effect began to diminish and after 24 hours the effect became negligible. These results certainly raise an interesting question about the potential benefits of combination therapy of RFA with arsenic trioxide or another agent that affects tumor blood flow.

Hakimé et al [57] further investigated this notion of combination therapy. This study randomly assigned three groups of six nude mice to receive 80 mg of sorafenib, 20 mg of sorafenib, or placebo. Sorafenib, a Raf kinase inhibitor and inhibitor of the vascular endothelial growth factor (VEGF) receptor is a known antiangiogenesis inhibitor used in the treatment of RCC [58]. The authors demonstrated that there was a significantly greater degree of tumor coagulation necrosis after RFA in the groups treated with sorafenib as compared with controls. Similar to that seen with arsenic trioxide as described above, this increase in coagulation necrosis occurred in a dose-dependent relationship. By histologic analysis, the authors also demonstrated a significant reduction in tumor microvascular density in the sorafenib treated animals and further revealed that this reduction also occurred in a dose-dependent fashion. These findings again suggest that combined therapy of RFA with an angiogenesis inhibitor or an agent that reduces tumor blood flow may improve the effectiveness and efficiency of tumor coagulation. This notion may hold practical implications for the treatment of larger tumors, such that these may be treated more safely and/or more efficiently with fewer treatment zones. Of course, these preliminary findings in animal models can only suggest the potential clinical applications and must be properly investigated in human trials.

## Radiofrequency ablation of localized prostate adenocarcinoma

The vast majority of the experience of RFA in genitourinary oncology has been in the treatment of RCC. However, there have been a few investigative reports into the potential application of RFA in the management of localized prostate cancer. Djavan et al [59]. reported on the use of transperineal RFA of localized prostate cancer under transrectal ultrasound (TRUS) guidance. Ten men scheduled for radical prostatectomy underwent transperineal RFA, followed by radical prostatectomy 1–7 days later. All patients had a zone of treatment in each lateral lobe. One patient had a third zone of treatment. No immediate complications were reported and all were performed under spinal anesthesia. Endorectal coil MRI was performed prior to radical prostatectomy and histological examination.

On MRI, the RFA lesions were clearly visible on T1-weighted images with gadolinium enhancement and no abnormalities were noted in the rectum, neurovascular bundle, or external sphincter on any patient. Histologic examination revealed that in 7/10 patients the region of cancer was totally or partially within the zone of ablation, however, the goal of this study was not to localize the actual area of tumor but to demonstrate feasibility of the technique and the postoperative imaging by MRI. Pathologic analysis did demonstrate that the area of ablation was accurately identified by MRI.

This same group reported on 14 patients treated with transperineal RFA to the prostate prior to radical prostatectomy [60]. One additional patient only underwent RFA and no additional treatment for his prostate cancer. No technical problems occurred during ablation and no complications were reported from treatment. During treatment, it was evident that the RFA energy interfered with the TRUS images, thus impeding the optimal visualization of the prostate. Furthermore, pathologic analysis revealed that the ultrasound images during treatment did not accurately correlate with the true zone of ablation. These findings question the ability of ultrasound to accurately guide RFA of the prostate.

Shariat et al [61]. reported on the treatment of 11 patients with localized prostate cancer using TRUS-guided RFA to the prostate. Eight patients had local recurrence of disease after prior failed external beam radiation (XRT) and 3 patients were not considered to be candidates for primary curative therapy. Patients were followed prospectively for a median follow-up of 20 months (3–38 months range). They underwent serial PSA testing and DRE, and were assessed for voiding symptoms, uroflow and postvoid residual. Repeat 12-core biopsies were performed at 6 and 12 months postablation.

In two patients the procedure was aborted due to increasing rectal temperatures. No major complications were reported, however, two patients experienced gross hematuria, one patient had bladder spasms, and one patient had dysuria. Ninety percent of patients demonstrated a decrease in PSA of over 50% and treated areas demonstrated extensive coagulation necrosis on repeat biopsy. Six out of eleven patients overall demonstrated no cancer in repeat biopsies at 6 months, and 5/9 patients had no cancer on repeated biopsy at 12 months postablation. There were no significant changes on any aspects of the validated questionnaires used to assess lower urinary tract symptoms (LUTS).

Unlike RFA in RCC, RFA in prostate cancer is only starting to be investigated. Although no major short-term complications occurred in these limited studies, it is not clear as to what longer term or short-term complications may occur in a larger cohort with a more prolonged follow-up time. It is also concerning that even in the small series discussed above there were a significant number of patients who had residual cancer on repeat biopsies. This questions the ability of this technique to effectively treat the whole gland and thus the entirety of tumor present. As a potential localized therapy for treating only the tumor within the gland, one of the major barriers to RFA for prostate cancer is that our ability to effectively and accurately image foci of prostate cancer within the gland is inadequate at this point in time. Only until we can accurately demonstrate where cancer lies within the gland by imaging, can we then consider such a localized therapy adequate treatment for adenocarcinoma of the prostate.

## Conclusion

RFA is a relatively new but promising technique for localized treatment of tumors and certainly does and will continue to play a significant role in the treatment of genitourinary malignancy. In RCC, this method appears to be safe and effective in appropriately selected renal masses that are amenable to a nephron-sparing technique. Although surgical resection still remains the standard of care in good surgical candidates, it appears from the literature that RFA can achieve similar oncologic outcomes at least by intermediate to early long-term follow-up. The use of RFA in other genitourinary cancers remains very much investigational and will need further development in the future if it is to become clinically applicable.

## References

1. Iannitti DA, Dupuy DE, Mayo-Smith WW, Murphy B (2002) Hepatic radiofrequency ablation. Arch.Surg 137(4): 422–426; discussion 427.

2. Jiao LR, Hansen PD, Havlik R, Mitry RR, Pignatelli M, Habib N (1999) Clinical short-term results of radiofrequency ablation in primary and secondary liver tumors. Am. J.Surg 177(4): 303–306.

3. Sutherland LM, Williams JA, Padbury RT, Gotley DC, Stokes B, Maddern GJ (2006) Radiofrequency ablation of liver tumors: A systematic review. Arch.Surg 141(2): 181–190.

4. Pantuck AJ, Zisman A, Rauch MK, Belldegrun A (2000) Incidental renal tumors. Urology 56(2): 190–196.

5. Luciani LG, Cestari R, Tallarigo C (2000) Incidental renal cell carcinoma-age and stage characterization

and clinical implications: Study of 1092 patients (1982–1997). Urology 56(1): 58–62.

6. Huang WC et al (2006) Chronic kidney disease after nephrectomy in patients with renal cortical tumours: A retrospective cohort study. Lancet Oncol 7(9): 735–740.

7. Herr HW (1999) Partial nephrectomy for unilateral renal carcinoma and a normal contralateral kidney: 10-year followup. J Urol 161(1): 33–34; discussion 34–35.

8. Licht MR, Novick AC (1993) Nephron sparing surgery for renal cell carcinoma. J Urol 149(1): 1–7.

9. McGovern FJ, Wood BJ, Goldberg SN, Mueller PR (1999) Radio frequency ablation of renal cell carcinoma via image guided needle electrodes. J Urol 161(2): 599–600.

10. Wood BJ, Ramkaransingh JR, Fojo T, Walther MM, Libutti SK (2002) Percutaneous tumor ablation with radiofrequency. Cancer 94(2): 443–451.

11. Goldberg SN, Gazelle GS, Mueller PR (2000) Thermal ablation therapy for focal malignancy: a unified approach to underlying principles, techniques, and diagnostic imaging guidance. AJR Am J Roentgenol 174(2): 323–331.

12. Beland M, Mueller PR, Gervais DA (2007) Thermal ablation in interventional oncology. Semin Roentgenol 42(3): 175–190.

13. Goldberg SN, Gazelle GS, Dawson SL, Rittman WJ, Mueller PR, Rosenthal DI (1995) Tissue ablation with radiofrequency: effect of probe size, gauge, duration, and temperature on lesion volume. Acad Radiol 2(5): 399–404.

14. Ritz JP et al (2006) Bipolar radiofrequency ablation of liver metastases during laparotomy. First clinical experiences with a new multipolar ablation concept. Int J Colorectal Dis 21(1): 25–32.

15. Ritz JP et al (2006) In-vivo evaluation of a novel bipolar radiofrequency device for interstitial thermotherapy of liver tumors during normal and interrupted hepatic perfusion. J Surg Res 133(2): 176–184.

16. Jemal A, Siegel R, Ward E, Hao Y, Xu J, Thun MJ (2009) Cancer statistics, 2009. CA Cancer. J Clin 59(4): 225–249.

17. Thompson RH et al (2008) Radical nephrectomy for pT1a renal masses may be associated with decreased overall survival compared with partial nephrectomy. J.Urol 179(2): 468–471; discussion 472–473.

18. Polascik TJ et al (1999) Ablation of renal tumors in a rabbit model with interstitial saline-augmented radiofrequency energy: preliminary report of a new technology. Urology 199953(3): 465–472; discussion 470–472.

19. Merkle EM, Shonk JR, Duerk JL, Jacobs GH, Lewin JS (1999) MR-guided RF thermal ablation of the kidney in a porcine model. AJR Am. J.Roentgenol 173(3): 645–651.

20. Zlotta AR et al (1997) Radiofrequency interstitial tumor ablation (RITA) is a possible new modality for treatment of renal cancer: ex vivo and in vivo experience. J.Endourol 11(4): 251–258.

21. Gervais DA, McGovern FJ, Wood BJ, Goldberg SN, McDougal WS, Mueller PR (2000) Radio-frequency ablation of renal cell carcinoma: early clinical experience. Radiology 217(3): 665–672.

22. Gervais DA, McGovern FJ, Arellano RS, McDougal WS, Mueller PR (2005) Radiofrequency ablation of renal cell carcinoma: part 1, Indications, results, and role in patient management over a 6-year period and ablation of 100 tumors. AJR Am J Roentgenol 185(1): 64–71.

23. Pavlovich CP et al (2002) Percutaneous radio frequency ablation of small renal tumors: initial results. J Urol 167(1): 10–15.

24. Ogan K et al (2002) Percutaneous radiofrequency ablation of renal tumors: technique, limitations, and morbidity. Urology 60(6): 954–958.

25. Su LM, Jarrett TW, Chan DY, Kavoussi LR, Solomon SB (2003) Percutaneous computed tomography-guided radiofrequency ablation of renal masses in high surgical risk patients: preliminary results. Urology 61(4 suppl. 1): 26–33.

26. Farrell MA et al (2003) Imaging-guided radiofrequency ablation of solid renal tumors. AJR Am J Roentgenol 180(6): 1509–1513.

27. Zagoria RJ et al (2004) Percutaneous CT-guided radiofrequency ablation of renal neoplasms: factors influencing success. AJR Am J Roentgenol 183(1): 201–207.

28. Farrell MA et al (2003) Imaging-guided radiofrequency ablation of solid renal tumors. AJR Am. J Roentgenol 180(6): 1509–1513.

29. Zagoria RJ, Traver MA, Werle DM, Perini M, Hayasaka S, Clark PE (2007) Oncologic efficacy of CT-guided percutaneous radiofrequency ablation of renal cell carcinomas. AJR Am J Roentgenol 189(2): 429–436.

30. McDougal WS, Gervais DA, McGovern FJ, Mueller PR (2005) Long-term followup of patients with renal cell carcinoma treated with radio frequency ablation with curative intent. J Urol 174(1): 61–63.

31. Levinson AW et al (2008) Long-term oncological and overall outcomes of percutaneous radio frequency ablation in high risk surgical patients with a solitary small renal mass. J Urol 180(2): 499–504; discussion 504.

32. Michaels MJ, Rhee HK, Mourtzinos AP, Summerhayes IC, Silverman ML, Libertino JA (2002) Incomplete renal tumor destruction using radio frequency interstitial

ablation. J Urol 168(6): 2406–2409; discussion 2409–2410.

33. Hsu TH, Fidler ME, Gill IS (2000) Radiofrequency ablation of the kidney: acute and chronic histology in porcine model. Urology 56(5): 872–875.

34. Rendon RA et al (2002) The uncertainty of radio frequency treatment of renal cell carcinoma: findings at immediate and delayed nephrectomy. J Urol 167(4): 1587–1592.

35. Park S, Strup SE, Saboorian H, Cadeddu JA (2006) No evidence of disease after radiofrequency ablation in delayed nephrectomy specimens. Urology 68(5): 964–967.

36. Raman JD, Stern JM, Zeltser I, Kabbani W, Cadeddu JA (2008) Absence of viable renal carcinoma in biopsies performed more than 1 year following radio frequency ablation confirms reliability of axial imaging. J Urol 179(6): 2142–2145.

37. Gervais DA, Arellano RS, McGovern FJ, McDougal WS, Mueller PR (2005) Radiofrequency ablation of renal cell carcinoma: part 2, lessons learned with ablation of 100 tumors. AJR Am J Roentgenol 185(1): 72–80.

38. Veltri A et al (2006) Experiences in US-guided percutaneous radiofrequency ablation of 44 renal tumors in 31 patients: analysis of predictors for complications and technical success. Cardiovasc Intervent Radiol 29(5): 811–818.

39. Rendon RA et al (2001) Development of a radiofrequency based thermal therapy technique in an in vivo porcine model for the treatment of small renal masses. J Urol 166(1): 292–298.

40. Chen EA, Neeman Z, Lee FT, Kam A, Wood B (2006) Thermal protection with 5% dextrose solution blanket during radiofrequency ablation. Cardiovasc Intervent Radiol 29(6): 1093–1096.

41. Farrell MA, Charboneau JW, Callstrom MR, Reading CC, Engen DE, Blute ML (2003) Paranephric water instillation: a technique to prevent bowel injury during percutaneous renal radiofrequency ablation. AJR Am. J.Roentgenol 181(5): 1315–1317.

42. Liddell RP, Solomon SB (2004) Thermal protection during radiofrequency ablation. AJR Am. J Roentgenol 182(6): 1459–1461.

43. Kariya S et al (2005) Radiofrequency ablation combined with CO2 injection for treatment of retroperitoneal tumor: protecting surrounding organs against thermal injury. AJR Am J Roentgenol 185(4): 890–893.

44. Schultze D, Morris CS, Bhave AD, Worgan BA, Najarian KE (2003) Radiofrequency ablation of renal transitional cell carcinoma with protective cold saline infusion. J Vasc Interv Radiol 14(4): 489–492.

45. Cantwell CP et al (2008) Protecting the ureter during radiofrequency ablation of renal cell cancer: a pilot study of retrograde pyeloperfusion with cooled dextrose 5% in water. J Vasc Interv Radiol 19(7): 1034–1040.

46. Matin SF et al (2006) Residual and recurrent disease following renal energy ablative therapy: a multi-institutional study. J Urol 176(5): 1973–1977.

47. Nguyen CT et al (2008) Surgical salvage of renal cell carcinoma recurrence after thermal ablative therapy. J Urol 180(1): 104–109; discussion 109.

48. Clark TW et al (2006) Reporting standards for percutaneous thermal ablation of renal cell carcinoma. J Vasc Interv Radiol 17(10): 1563–1570.

49. Burke DR et al (2003) Quality improvement guidelines for percutaneous transhepatic cholangiography and biliary drainage. J Vasc.Interv.Radiol 14(9 Pt 2): S243–S246.

50. Kunkle DA, Egleston BL, Uzzo RG (2008) Excise, ablate or observe: the small renal mass dilemma–a meta-analysis and review. J Urol 179(4): 1227–1233; discussion 1233–1234.

51. Raman JD, Cadeddu JA (2008) Re: excise, ablate or observe: the small renal mass dilemma–a meta-analysis and review. D.A. Kunkle, B.L. Egleston, and R. G. Uzzo J Urol 179;1227–1234. J Urol 180(4): 1567–1568; author reply 1568.

52. Stern JM et al (2007) Intermediate comparison of partial nephrectomy and radiofrequency ablation for clinical T1 a renal tumours. BJU Int 100(2): 287–290.

53. Lotan Y, Cadeddu JA (2005) A cost comparison of nephron-sparing surgical techniques for renal tumour. BJU Int 95(7): 1039–1042.

54. Pandharipande PV, Gervais DA, Mueller PR, Hur C, Gazelle GS (2008) Radiofrequency ablation versus nephron-sparing surgery for small unilateral renal cell carcinoma: cost-effectiveness analysis. Radiology 248(1): 169–178.

55. Ahmed M et al (2005) Combination radiofrequency ablation with intratumoral liposomal doxorubicin: effect on drug accumulation and coagulation in multiple tissues and tumor types in animals. Radiology 235(2): 469–477.

56. Hines-Peralta A, Sukhatme V, Regan M, Signoretti S, Liu ZJ, Goldberg SN (2006) Improved tumor destruction with arsenic trioxide and radiofrequency ablation in three animal models. Radiology 240(1): 82–89.

57. Hakime A et al (2007) Combination of radiofrequency ablation with antiangiogenic therapy for tumor ablation efficacy: study in mice. Radiology 244(2): 464–470.

58. Escudier B et al (2007) Sorafenib in advanced clear-cell renal-cell carcinoma. N.Engl. J Med. 356(2): 125–134.

59. Djavan B et al (1997) Transperineal radiofrequency interstitial tumor ablation of the prostate: correlation of magnetic resonance imaging with histopathologic examination. Urology 50(6): 986–992; discussion 992–993.

60. Zlotta AR et al (1998) Percutaneous transperineal radiofrequency ablation of prostate tumour: safety, feasibility and pathological effects on human prostate cancer. Br J Urol 81(2): 265–275.

61. Shariat SF, Raptidis G, Masatoschi M, Bergamaschi F, Slawin KM (2005) Pilot study of radiofrequency interstitial tumor ablation (RITA) for the treatment of radio-recurrent prostate cancer. Prostate 65(3): 260–267.

# 6

# Photodynamic therapy

*Caroline M. Moore[1], Stephen G. Bown[2], John Trachtenberg[3], and Mark Emberton[4]*

[1]University College London and University College London Hospitals Trust, London, UK
[2]National Medical Laser Center, University College London, London, UK
[3]Department of Surgery, University of Toronto, Princess Margaret Hospital, Toronto, Canada
[4]Division of Surgery and Interventional Science, University College London, London, UK

## Introduction

Photodynamic applications in urology use the interaction of light with a photosensitizing agent to produce an effect that can be used for diagnosis or treatment of different conditions, including cancer.

Photodynamic therapy (PDT) uses directed light of a specific wavelength to activate a photosensitizing drug. The activated drug reacts with molecular oxygen to produce reactive oxygen species, which are directly responsible for tissue damage. There is a delay between drug administration and light delivery (the drug light interval), which varies from minutes to days depending upon the photosensitizer used and the tissue to be treated. The photosensitizing drug can be given topically for superficial treatment, e.g., for skin cancers or intravesically for bladder cancer, or systemically in the treatment of solid organ tumors such as prostate or renal cancer. The light is often produced by a laser and directed using optical fibers, which, for interstitial treatment, are commonly positioned with the aid of real-time imaging. The light dose used to activate the drug is much less than when lasers are used to destroy tissue by heating.

For a photodynamic effect to occur, the photosensitizer, light, and oxygen must be present in the tissue in sufficient amounts [1]. For systemically administered photosensitizer, distribution throughout the body occurs, with different concentrations in different organs over time. This can be exploited therapeutically by choosing the time of light delivery when maximal differentiation of photosensitiser concentration between the tissue to be treated and other tissues occurs. Some photosensitizers may show selectivity between tumor tissue and normal tissue of the same organ. A side effect of systemic administration is that the photosensitizer may accumulate in the skin or eyes where it can be activated by sunlight or indoor lighting, causing a "sunburn" type reaction. Precautions against this must be taken, in the form of protective clothing and customized glasses, which, for some photosensitizers, are required for a few weeks. However, there are now photosensitizers in development that show rapid clearance from the body (minutes to hours), which make such precautions unnecessary.

Photodynamic diagnosis involves the differential accumulation of a fluorescent agent in tumor tissue, compared to surrounding normal tissue. Many fluorescent agents used for diagnosis are also photosensitizers suitable for photodynamic therapy. Fluorescent agents can either be endogenous or exogenous, and are usually best visualized by light of a specific wavelength, e.g., the blue light (380–450 nm) used to see accumulation of PpIX following administration of hexaminolevulinic acid in bladder cancer.

*Interventional Techniques in Uro-oncology*, First Edition. Edited by Hashim Uddin Ahmed, Manit Arya, Peter T. Scardino & Mark Emberton. © 2011 Blackwell Publishing Ltd. Published 2011 by Blackwell Publishing Ltd.

## Definitions

It is helpful to begin with some definitions of different aspects of photodynamics:

### Photosensitizer

A compound that is excited by light of a specific wavelength, in the presence of oxygen, to give a photodynamic effect.

### Drug light interval

The length of time between drug administration, and light activation. This can vary from minutes to days, depending on whether the photosensitizer is activated in the vasculature, or whether it has had time to accumulate preferentially in the target tissue.

### Light source

The source of low power light used to activate a photosensitizer. This is often a laser (single wavelength light), but could be as simple as a desk lamp.

### Laser (light amplification by stimulated emission of radiation)

Light of single wavelength (monochromatic), which is in phase, and can remain collimated (focused) over travel for long distances. It can be carried by optical fibers to allow illumination of solid organs, more easily and efficiently than nonlaser light.

### Optical fibers

These are used to deliver the light source from a laser to the treatment volumes. They can be classified as bare ended fibers, where the light is emitted from the end of the fiber, like a torchlight; or cylindrical diffusers, where the light is emitted along a defined distance, e.g., 3 cm, at the end of the fiber, like a strip light.

### Phototoxicity

This refers to unwanted photodynamic effects of a photosensitizer, and is usually taken to mean the unintended activation of a photosensitizer in the skin, leading to a sunburn like reaction.

## History

Phototherapy is the use of light in the treatment of disease, and it encompasses photochemotherapy (the use of light in combination with a drug) and photodynamic therapy (which requires a drug to be activated by light in the presence of oxygen). The beneficial effect of light has been known for centuries. Hippocrates formalized the use of phototherapy or heliotherapy, using sunbaths to build up wasted muscles, using a blanket as a protective head covering. A common contemporary use of phototherapy is in the treatment of neonatal hyperbilirubinemia, where light is used in two ways—for photosolubilization (the conversion of bilirubin to more soluble isomers) and photofragmentation (photo-oxidation of bilirubin to colorless soluble products).

In ancient India, an early form of photochemotherapy was used as a treatment for vitiligo. The leaves of the plant Psoralea coryfolia were eaten, and the patient then sat in the sunlight. It is now known that this plant contains furocoumarins, which are currently used as photochemotherapeutic agents in the treatment of psoriasis, when they are activated by ultraviolet light. Furocoumarins work by intercalating into DNA and then, when excited by ultraviolet light, react with DNA bases, which prevent the proliferation of the rapidly dividing cells that give rise to psoriatic plaques.

Photodynamic therapy is a form of photochemotherapy that requires oxygen. In 1903, Niels Ryberg Finsen, was awarded the Nobel prize for his work using photodynamic therapy in the treatment of lupus vulgaris, a tubercular skin condition common in Nordic countries.

The first modern scientific experiment with photodynamic therapy was performed by Oscar Raab, a medical student, and his supervisor Hermann Von Tappeiner in 1897 [2]. They observed that paramecia given the biological dye acridine survived ten times longer during a heavy thunderstorm than during an identical experiment at a different time. They concluded that the prolonged survival was due to the reduced light exposure during the storm. Further work revealed that oxygen was also necessary for a photodynamic effect to work [1].

In 1902, Von Tappeiner and Jesionek reported experiments in which tumors were treated with topical eosin and visible light. Von Tappeiner went on to publish a book of papers on PDT, including the use of topical photosensitizer to treat patients with basal cell carcinoma, and other skin diseases [3].

There were no further clinical reports of PDT until the early 1960s when Lipson showed that hematoporphyrin accumulated preferentially in tumors, and emitted a red fluorescence. The treatment of a recurrent breast tumor was then mentioned in a meeting abstract "Hematoporphyrin derivative for the detection and management of cancer," but later, the paper of the same title only discussed the use of hematoporphyrin derivative (HpD) in diagnosis [4,5].

In 1978, Dougherty and colleagues published a paper documenting the first clinical case series of PDT for cancer [6]. Using HpD they treated 25 patients with a range of subcutaneous or cutaneous metastatic tumors, including breast, colon, prostate, and skin, and declared that "no type has been found to be unresponsive."

The first approved use for PDT was in 1993 when hematoporphyrin derivative, under the trade name Photofrin, was approved for the treatment of recurrent superficial bladder cancer in Canada. Since then a variety of different compounds have been approved for use in a number of cancers, both localized and advanced, in different countries. These include most skin cancers (although not malignant melanoma), dysplasia and cancer of the esophagus, airways, and mouth. PDT is also used in a number of other diseases, which range from arterial stenosis and endometrial hyperplasia to psoriasis and other skin conditions. PDT using Visudyne (a benzoporphyrin derivative monoacid ring A – BPD-MA) has been approved worldwide for use in some types of age related macular degeneration. To date, this is the most successful commercial application of PDT [7].

## Basic science

The mechanism of action of PDT is complex, and differs between different photosensitizers and different treatment schedules. There are two types of reaction that contribute to the PDT effect. These are shown schematically in Plate 6.1.

The photosensitizer is administered in a stable form (ground state). It is then promoted to a higher energy state by light of a specific wavelength. The excited photosensitizer (singlet state) is then unstable and can release energy in one of 3 ways—emission of heat, emission of light (fluorescence), or conversion to an intermediate energy state (triplet state), before returning to stable ground state. In triplet state, the photosensitizer can either undergo photodegradation, or undergo either a type 1 or type 2 reaction. In a type 1 reaction, the photosensitizer reacts with the tissue to produce hydroxyl or superoxide radicals. In a type 2 reaction, the photosensitizer reacts with molecular oxygen to produce highly reactive singlet oxygen. The singlet oxygen, in turn, reacts with proteins, lipids, and nucleic acids in cells causing functional and structural damage that leads to cell death. Hydroxyl and superoxide radicals are also directly responsible for cell death, although it is thought likely that type 2 reactions are more important for many of the photosensitizers [8].

The above reactions can be demonstrated in *in vitro* cell culture experiments. However, tumor models in animal studies have demonstrated that there are three main mechanisms by which cells are killed. First, direct cell damage by free radical oxygen, as discussed above. Second, damage to vasculature causing disruption of blood supply (Figure 6.1). Third, by indirect responses or responses to the initial PDT injury. This includes the release of cytokines and other inflammatory mediators that initiate an inflammatory response [9]. It is thought that an immune response to PDT may also contribute to its effect. This has been well described by Korbelik and colleagues [10].

## Photosensitizing drugs

There are a number of different photosensitizing drugs available, belonging to different classes of photosensitizer. These vary in their drug light interval, mechanism of action, route, and timing of clearance from the body.

### Hematoporphyrin and hematoporphyrin derivative

Hematoporphyrin was one of the first photosensitizers. It is made by treating powdered blood with sulfuric acid. However, it is difficult to make it in a chemically pure form, and so hematoporphyrin derivative (HpD) was developed, which is a mixture of compounds derived from hematoporphyrin. These compounds are characterized by the presence of the porphyrin tetrapyrrole structure. HpD absorbs light at

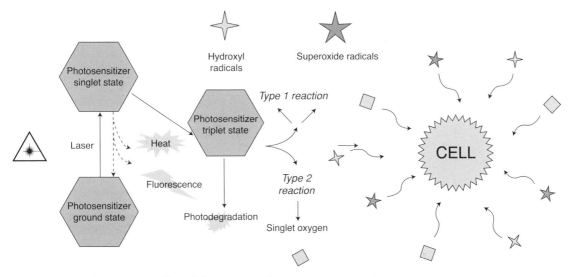

**Fig 6.1** Schematic diagram of the effect of photodynamic therapy on tumor vasculature.

both 400 nm and 630 nm. The longer wavelength of light (630 nm, which is in the red region of the visible spectrum) is used to activate it, as the longer wavelength is able to penetrate tissue more deeply. HpD causes skin photosensitivity that can persist for several weeks. Fraction D of HpD is the most biologically active fraction; this is marketed as Photofrin and Photosan. In the 1980s the search began for alternative photosensitizers, which could be manufactured in a pure form, with less skin photosensitivity.

## Chlorins

Chlorins have a porphyrin skeleton with one reduced double bond. They are stronger absorbers of red light than the hematoporphyrins, and so can produce a greater photodynamic effect for a given light dose. Meta-tetrahydroxyphenyl chlorin (mTHPC) (temoporfin, marketed as Foscan) has been used in photodynamic therapy for prostate cancer. Its maximal absorption occurs at 652 nm, which penetrates tissue more deeply than the 630 nm light used to activate HpD. The major disadvantage of temoporfin is the prolonged skin photosensitivity.

## 5-amino levulinic acid

Amino levulinic acid (5-ALA) is a prodrug that can be given either topically or systemically. 5-ALA is part of the endogenous haem synthesis pathway. When exogenous 5-ALA is administered, this causes excess production of a photoactive intermediate substance, protoporphyrin IX (PpIX). PpIX is the last substance in the chemical chain prior to the formation of haem. Although haem biosynthesis takes place in all nucleated cells, the amount of PpIX accumulated in different cell types following 5-ALA administration varies greatly. High quantities are found in epithelial lining tissues (urothelium, endothelium, mucosa of the GI tract), making 5-ALA a suitable photosensitizer for treatment of superficial lesions, e.g., Barrett esophagus, superficial bladder cancer, and skin tumors. PpIX is rapidly cleared from the body, so cutaneous photosensitivity lasts for less than 48 hours. PpIX levels reach their peak 3–6 hours after administration of 5-ALA, so this is the best time for light activation. The activating wavelength is 635 nm.

## Phthalocyanines

Aluminium disulfonated phthalocyanine (AlS2 Pc) is a purified phthalocyanine photosensitizer that is water soluble, with good fluorescence properties, excellent absorption at 675 nm, and little cutaneous photosensitivity [11]]. Photosens is a sulfonated aluminium phthalocyanine that has been used clinically in skin and lung cancers [12]. It has also been used for head and neck cancers [13,14].

## Hypericin

Hypericin is a phenanthroperylenquinone derivative that is extracted from *Hypericum* plants, of which St John's wort (*Hypericum perforatum*) is the commonest example [15]. Hypericum is activated by light from 450 to 605 nm, with absorption peaks at 548 and 590 nm. It is one of the photosensitizers that can accumulate preferentially in tumor tissue. Along with its fluorescent properties, it is suitable for photodynamic tumor detection, as well as PDT.

## Tin ethyl etiopurpurin (SnET2)

This is also known as rostaporfin and Sn (IV) etiopurpurin. It is one of the purpurin photosensitizers, and was initially used in dog prostate PDT by Selman and colleagues [16]. Since the approval of PDT for age related macular degeneration, it is being evaluated (under the name of rostaporfin) for this use [17]. It is activated by light of 664 nm. It is thought to selectively bind to plasma lipoproteins. The drug light interval used for ophthalmic work is 24 hours, although different drug light intervals have been evaluated in the canine prostate work.

## Bacteriochlorophyll derivatives

The palladium bacteriopheophorbides (WST-09, Tookad and WST-11, Tookad Soluble) are palladium substituted bacteriopheophorbides. WST-09 is lipophilic, with maximum absorption at 763 nm, and a high extinction coefficient of 105 in chloroform [18]. WST-09 is activated while in the vascular distribution stage. It is thought that this damages tumor vasculature and causes subsequent necrosis. Due to the lipophilic nature of WST-09, it needs to be given with Cremophor, a carrier, which has been associated with cardiovascular side effects. WST-11 is a water soluble bactereriopheophorbide, which does not require Cremophor, and is now replacing WST-09 in urological clinical studies. Since the palladium bactereophephorbides are activated while in the vascular phase, both drug and light are given in a single session. This could allow treatment to be carried out in an ambulatory setting in one visit. As they are cleared rapidly from the blood, they have little cutaneous sensitivity after 3 hours [19].

## The ideal photosensitizer

The ideal photosensitizer would have no toxicity in the dark, have a short drug light interval (to allow near simultaneous drug and light administration, within a single patient visit), be cheap to manufacture to high levels of chemical stability, and be simple to administer. It would also be highly efficient, requiring low light, and drug doses to produce necrosis, and would absorb light most strongly at a long wavelength, e.g., in the near infrared range (700 to 850 nm), as longer wavelengths of light are able to penetrate tissue more deeply. Other desirable characteristics would be simple pharmacokinetics, fluorescence that could be used to monitor drug levels, and rapid clearance from the skin. In addition, a photosensitizer that preferentially accumulated in the tissue to be treated, in comparison to surrounding normal tissue, would be highly advantageous. One way to increase this tumor selectivity would be to use monoclonal antibodies to deliver the photosensitizer. Such delivery systems are currently under development.

## Light sources

The light sources used for PDT and photodynamic diagnosis depend on the site to be treated or assessed. For superficial applications, e.g., genital warts, a simple lamp- based light source can be used. When the light delivery fiber is not touching the target tissue, the light dose is expressed in Joules per square cm of the illuminated surface.

For intravesical photodynamic diagnosis, it is necessary to use a light source with an adapted cystoscope, so that the urologist can alternate between white light for standard cystoscopy, and the wavelength of light required to detect fluorescence, e.g., blue light for heaminolaevulinic acid. For intravesical treatment, light delivery systems have been developed using a variety of balloon devices to distribute light evenly throughout the bladder.

For interstitial treatments, optical fibers are used. These allow the transmission of laser light deep within a tissue, such as the prostate or kidney. Thin needles are inserted into the target tissue using image guidance (e.g., with ultrasound, CT, or MRI), and the laser fibers inserted through the needles. When a bare ended fiber is used, the light dose is given in Joules per square centimeter; when a cylindrical diffuser is used, the light dose is given in Joules per centimeter.

## Bladder cancer

### Photodynamic diagnosis

Bladder cancer is the fifth most common malignancy in Europe, and the fourth most common malignancy in the USA. The majority (95%) of bladder cancers are transitional cell carcinoma, which can be classified into muscle-invasive and nonmuscle-invasive disease. Muscle-invasive disease (T2 and greater) requires radical treatment, with either surgery, or radiotherapy, with or without neoadjuvant chemotherapy. Nonmuscle-invasive disease (T1, Ta, and carcinoma in situ (CIS)) can be treated with transurethral resection and intravesical therapies, such as mitomycin-C and BCG. The two problems with nonmuscle-invasive bladder cancer are: (1) recurrence, which can occur in 70% when no additional treatment is given post resection; (2) progression, which is a particular risk with CIS.

It is known that white light cystoscopy can miss small papillary tumors and flat urothelial tumors, including CIS. The timely treatment of such lesions, particularly carcinoma in situ, is important in reducing progression and recurrence of nonmuscle-invasive bladder cancer. Photodynamic diagnosis of lesions that are difficult to detect with white light cystoscopy alone is of interest in increasing the sensitivity of cystoscopy for such lesions.

Photodynamic detection of bladder tumors, using PpIX formed from the precursor 5–5-ALA, or its derivative hexaminolevulinic acid, is recognized as a method to reveal areas suspicious for CIS, by the European Association of Urology. Hexaminolevulinic acid is the commonest agent used for fluorescence diagnosis in the bladder. It has a number of advantages over 5-ALA, such as a deeper penetration into the urothelium and a higher PpIX concentration at significantly lower prodrug concentrations [20]. Other drugs that have been investigated for fluorescence diagnosis of urothelial tumors are hematoporhyrin derivatives (HpD) and hypericin [21].

To date, there have been three randomized prospective multicenter studies published that compare fluorescence diagnosis with white light cystoscopy [22–24], as well as a large number of studies of other designs. A number of studies in different centers have shown that the sensitivity of fluorescence-guided cystoscopy is superior to white-light cystoscopy, with a mean sensitivity of 93% (range 82–97%) for fluorescence-guided cystoscopy, compared to a mean sensitivity of 73% (range 62–84%) for white light cystoscopy [21]. It has been shown that there is a significant reduction in the number of tumors seen at second look cystoscopy, following fluorescence-guided cystoscopy and resection when compared to white light alone [22,25–27]. Three studies have shown a reduction in recurrence rates at 24 months with fluorescence-guided resection compared to white light resection, with recurrence free survival of 40–88% vs. 28–64%, respectively [28–30]. Two studies did not show any difference in recurrence rates [22,31]. One study that reported the long-term outcome of initial T1 high-grade bladder cancer showed an improvement in recurrence free survival for fluorescence-guided resection versus white light resection, with rates of 91% and 69% at 4 years, and 80% and 52% at 8 years, respectively. However, there was no significant difference in the number of patients in each group who progressed to muscle-invasive disease [32].

### Photodynamic therapy

PDT has been investigated as a treatment for nonmuscle-invasive bladder cancer, in an attempt to reduce both recurrence and progression. It can be used in bladder cancer in a number of ways. First, as a treatment for papillary lesions, using light directed at visible lesions only. Second, as a whole-bladder treatment, where it is known that CIS is present. Third, in combination with other treatments, such as the use of photosensitizing drugs that act as radiosensitizing agents prior to whole-bladder radiotherapy. Last, PDT can be used in combination with well- established treatments, such as intravesial chemotherapy or immunotherapy.

This was a report of a single patient given hematoporphyrin derivative (HpD), activated with a mercury vapor lamp, and necrosis was noted, by Kelly in 1975 [33]. As with other uses of PDT in urology, there have been advances in both photosensitizer and light delivery systems. In terms of photosensitizers, the first to be used were the Hematoporphyrin derivatives. These penetrate into bladder muscle as well as mucosa and have therefore been associated with bladder fibrosis and contracture. HpD can be activated by 630 nm light, which has tissue penetration of up to 1 cm. Alternatively, due to another absorption peak, it can be activated by 514 nm light, which has less tissue penetration (3–5 mm); so that at least theoretically this may lead to a lower incidence of bladder contracture.

More recent work has been done with 5-ALA that has significant advantages over HpD (Table 6.1). The PpIX that is generated by exogenous 5-ALA is preferentially accumulated in mucosa, and is not seen in significant concentrations in bladder muscle. PpIX is also found in significantly higher concentrations in tumor compared to benign tissue and can be given topically by intravesical instillation. Further, it is not associated with skin photosensitivity when given intravesically. It can be given orally, although this is associated with cardiovascular side effects (tachycardia and hypotension) in some patients. Clinical work has been carried out to assess different concentrations of 5-ALA to be used as an intravesical instillation. An instillation time of 4 hours provides good selectivity of PpIX concentration in malignant versus benign mucosa.

Light delivery in the bladder poses a particular challenge. For treatment of an individual lesion, a single fiber can be passed along a cystoscope and positioned at a suitable distance from the bladder wall, either under direct vision or with the aid of ultrasound guidance. For whole-bladder PDT, different systems using an optical fiber within either a single- or double-layered bladder balloon, mounted on a catheter, have been developed. Some groups have tried using intralipid within the inner balloon, which acts to scatter light. This has the effect of a larger and more spherical intravesical light source, which should give a more consistent light dose to the whole- bladder wall. One group has looked at delivering 5-ALA PDT using a flexible cystoscope under local anesthetic [37]. They found that the procedure was associated with bladder spasm and pain, which was in direct proportion to the 5-ALA concentration. At an 5-ALA concentration of 3%, this pain could be alleviated by passive diffusion of local anesthetic into the bladder; at the higher concentration of 6%, electro motive diffusion (EMDA) was needed to give the required anesthetic effect to allow the procedure to take place without regional or general anesthesia This group found that, due to short term irritative bladder symptoms, the procedure could not be performed as a day case.

In bladder PDT studies there are a number of parameters that can be modified to alter the treatment effect: the photosensitizer and its mode of administration, including the concentration and dwell time of intravesical instillations; the wavelength, delivery device, and total energy dose of the light source; the drug light interval, and importantly, the patient group studied. This makes comparison of different studies difficult. However, it seems that the lowest response rates for HpD PDT were for non-resected papillary tumors, with a response of 54%, with a response rate for CIS of 66–77% at 3 months, albeit with a 5-year recurrence rate estimated at 70% [40]. Most patients experienced post-PDT irritative symptoms and hematuria, which could last for weeks. Overall rates for bladder contracture were 16% with reflux occurring in 24%. Around one in five patients experienced skin phototoxicity [41].

5-ALA PDT has undergone clinical trials in Germany, Belgium, Austria, and England [34–39]. Study protocols differ significantly, with inclusion criteria ranging from CIS alone to G1pTa disease, to a combination of CIS and T1 lesions. Most studies use red light (630 nm) to activate 5-ALA, although some use green light (514 nm), with light doses ranging from 15 to 100 J/cm². Three month complete response rates vary from 33% to 100% with recurrence free rates also varying between studies. Similar to HpD PDT, patients experience irritative symptoms in the initial posttreatment period. Again, CIS seems to have a better response rate than papillary tumors [40]. As photodynamic detection of bladder tumors, particularly CIS is now a well-established procedure in the urological community, it may be that larger studies of therapeutic 5-ALA PDT may be undertaken.

## Prostate cancer

### Photodynamic therapy

The first clinical report of PDT for prostate cancer was in 1990 by Windahl et al [42]. Two cases of the use of hematoporphyrin derivative and porfimer sodium were described; each patient had prostate cancer diagnosed following transurethral resection of the prostate, and subsequently underwent a second resection to remove as much tissue as possible, prior to PDT. The photosensitizer was given intravenously, and activated with a bare-tipped fiber inserted transurethrally. Post-PDT biopsy did not show any evidence of recurrent or residual cancer; one

**Table 6.1** Summary of clinical studies of ALA photodynamic therapy for bladder cancer

| Author [reference] | 5-ALA dose and retention time | Light dose | Patient group (number) | Three month complete response rate (%) | Duration of disease free recurrence |
|---|---|---|---|---|---|
| Kriegmar 1997 [34] | 5 g<br>Mean 5.1 h | 635 nm; 15–30 J/cm$^2$ (2 pts)<br>514 nm 40 J/cm$^2$ and<br>635 nm 20 J/cm$^2$ (8 pts) | pTA G2–G3 +CIS [4]<br>pTa G1–G3 [6] | 2/4 (50)<br>2/6 (33) | 9 and 27 months<br>6 months |
| D'Hallewin 1997 [35]<br>Waidelich 2001 [36] | 1.5 g; 3–4 h<br>40 mg/kg orally<br>4–6 h drug light interval | 630 nm 75 J/cm$^2$<br>514 nm 40 J/cm$^2$ and<br>635 nm 20 J/cm$^2$ | CIS [6]<br>CIS [5]<br>pTa G1–2 [9]<br>pTa G1–G2 + CIS [2]<br>pT1 G1–G3 [4]<br>pT1 G1–G3 + CIS [4] | 2/6 (33)<br>5/5 (100)<br>7/9 (78)<br>1/2 (50)<br>3/4 (75)<br>3/4 (75) | 3 at 36 months<br>2 at 33 months<br>0 at 33 months<br>1 at 23 months<br>1 at 37 months |
| Shackley 2002 [37] | 1.5 g for 10 pts<br>3 g for 9 pts<br>4 h | 633 nm 25–50 J/cm$^2$ | CIS [2]<br>pTa G1 [7]<br>pTa G2 [10] | ? | |
| Berger 2003 [39] | 1.5 g<br>"as long as possible" | 633 nm 30 J/cm$^2$ (28 pts)<br>633 nm 50 J/cm$^2$ (3 pts) | CIS [1]<br>pTa [6]<br>pTa + CIS [6]<br>pT1 [15]<br>pT1 +CIS [3] | [CIS5/6 (83)] | 1 at 26 months<br>3 at 43 months<br>3 at 18 months<br>7 at 15 months<br>2 at 33 months |
| Waidelich 2003 [38] | 5 g<br>2–4.5 h (mean 3.6 h) | White light<br>100 J/cm$^2$ | CIS [7]<br>pTa G1–G2 [2]<br>pTa G1–G3 + CIS [3] | 4/7 (57)<br>2/2 (100)<br>1/2 (50) | 3 at 6, 16 and 23 months<br>1 at 22 months<br>1 at 6 months |

patient died from an undiagnosed lung tumor at 6 months post-PDT; postmortem examination of the prostate did not show any evidence of prostate cancer.

A number of groups then investigated PDT for prostate cancer using a benign canine prostate model. Chang and colleagues at University College London, UK assessed 5-ALA, AlS2 Pc, and mTHPC in the canine model [43,44]; and concluded that mTHPC was the most promising of these photosensitizers for clinical work. Selman and colleagues in Philadelphia have carried out extensive work using SnET2 in the canine model, resulting in some of the more advanced software planning systems for prostate PDT [16,45,46]. However, this has not yet been carried into the clinical setting with this particular photosensitizer. Other photosensitizers assessed in the canine model include Porfimer sodium [47,48], WST-09 [49], and motexafin lutetium [50].

The next clinical report of prostate PDT to follow Windahls' work was a study of mTHPC in recurrent prostate cancer following radiotherapy [51]. The dose of mTHPC was constant at 0.15 mg/kg, while the light dose varied between patients. An initial low light dose of 20 J/cm$^2$ was used in 5 patients. Small areas of devascularization were noted on contrast-enhanced CT scan a few days later, although no reduction in PSA was seen. The light dose was then increased to 50 J/cm$^2$, and 13 patients were given this higher dose, including four of the original five. The procedures were carried out using either ultrasound or open access MRI guidance, with a freehand transperineal approach. A combination of bare fibers were used, with a pullback technique, along with cylindrical diffusers. It was intended to treat selected areas of the prostate, based on biopsy and pretreatment imaging. Contrast-enhanced imaging showed a marked inflammatory response at 2 to 5 days. Necrosis, as shown by areas of devascularisation, was patchy, but involved up to 49% of the prostate for a single lobe treatment, and up to 91% for a bilateral treatment. PSA decreased in nine out of fourteen patients, to undetectable levels in two patients. All patients underwent flexible sigmoidoscopy to assess the rectal mucosa; in one patient a biopsy of a red patch was performed, and, following the biopsy a rectourethral fistula developed that required a defunctioning colostomy until the fistula had healed. Preclinical experiments had shown that the mechanical integrity of the rectum was maintained by the submucosal collagen, which is not affected by PDT, even when there was rectal mucosal damage. As this patient did not have any evidence of fistula in the first month post-PDT, it seems that it was the inclusion of submucosal collagen in the biopsy, along with a red patch of mucosa, which led to fistula formation. Temporary stress urinary incontinence was seen in two patients with acute urinary retention in three patients.

The same group at University College London also carried out a pilot study using mTHPC in previously untreated men with prostate cancer [52]. This study, of ten treatments in six patients, used the same drug dose (0.15 mg/kg) with a drug light interval that varied from 3 to 5 days. Again, a combination of bare tip and cylindrical diffusers were used, with a light dose of up to 1800 J per lobe. Each treatment was confined to a single lobe only. Volumes of necrosis of up to 51 cubic cm were seen. Side effects were less serious in this group, with two treatments associated with catheterization for 9 and 19 days, respectively, and all patients having irritative voiding symptoms for up to two weeks. PSA levels were reduced in eight out of ten. mTHPC is associated with prolonged skin sensitivity, requiring protection of the skin and eyes for up to six weeks. In addition, the drug light interval of days means that separate hospital visits are required for drug and light administration. Due to financial difficulties of the company that was developing this drug, no further work in the prostate has been reported. However, it is a well-established photosensitizer in other fields, particularly head and neck cancers [53,54].

Zaak and colleagues have assessed the use of 5-ALA PDT for prostate cancer [55]. Initial drug distribution work with oral 5-ALA (20 mg/kg) given 4 hours prior to radical prostatectomy showed preferential localization of PpIX in prostate cancer compared to benign tissue. This was followed by a study of six men who underwent PDT in which one then went on to have radical prostatectomy. Histological examination showed necrosis at the site of fiber insertion. Of the five other men, there was no report of post-PDT imaging or biopsy, although PSA reductions were noted.

Motexafin lutetium (MLu, LuTex) has been used in patients with recurrent prostate cancer following radiotherapy [56–58]. A total of 17 patients have been treated, with drug dose escalation from 0.5 to 2 mg/kg, given intravenously, and light doses being escalated from 25 to 150 J/cm. The drug light interval varied from 3 to 24 hours. It was intended to deliver whole-prostate treatment, with the use of computer-aided light dose planning. Posttreatment imaging is not reported. Negative biopsies were seen in three of fourteen patients. Detailed analysis of PSA kinetics showed that, after a transient post procedure rise, a reduction of PSA in comparison to pre-PDT levels only occurred in those receiving high-dose PDT using 2 mg/kg MLu, 150 J/cm and the shortest drug light interval of 3 hours. Toxicity seemed to be limited to grade I or II urinary symptoms.

The palladium bacterioopheophorbide family (WST-09, Tookad, padoporfin and WST-11, Stakel, padeliporfin) has been investigated in both Europe and Canada. The Canadian study [19,59–61] assessed WST-09 (Padoporfin, Tookad) in men with prostate cancer recurrence following radiotherapy. Following initial dose escalation work, a drug dose of 2 mg/kg, given as an intravenous infusion, was established. A light dose of 360 J/cm was also established, following light dose escalation. Computer planning software, based on average optical properties, was developed in order to generate a pre-PDT treatment plan based on MRI imaging. Posttreatment contrast-enhanced MRI and biopsy at 6 months showed a complete response in 60% of the men who had received the highest drug and light dose. Two patients developed rectourethral fistulae and 1 patient was reported to show intraoperative hypotension.

The same photosensitizer has been used in Europe in men with previously untreated prostate cancer. Full results have not been reported, although initial reports [62] have suggested that it is possible to create defined lesions in the prostate by modification of the light dose, with optimal treatment conditions being a drug dose of 2 mg/kg, a light dose of 200 J/cm with light delivery begun during drug infusion. Formal studies [19] showed that skin phototoxicity could not be detected 3 hours after the procedure. This, along with a short drug light interval allowing drug and light delivery in a single session, represents significant advantages over traditional tissue-based photosensitizers. Tookad is a lipid soluble drug that requires a Cremophor-based formulation for intravenous administration; a newer member of the same family, Tookad Soluble, is a water soluble formulation, which does not require Cremophor. It is currently being investigated by the European and Canadian groups in men as a first-line treatment for prostate cancer.

A summary of the clinical work in this area is shown in Table 6.2.

## Renal cancer

Photodynamic techniques have been assessed in a number of different roles in renal cancer. First, as a fluorescent diagnostic technique to help ensure clear margins in nephron-sparing tumor resection. Second, as PDT using a laparoscopic approach. Third, as a pretreatment sensitiser to allow effective radiotherapy treatment. Each of these aspects has undergone early studies, and will be reported briefly here.

### Photodynamic diagnosis

Popken and colleagues report the use of 5-ALA to detect the outer border of renal cell carcinoma in an animal model and in a clinical study [63]. The animal model used subcutaneous and orthotopic implants of human RCC in the subcapsular region of the kidney in nude mice. 5-ALA was administered orally or intravenously, and given between 30 minutes and 6 hours prior to light delivery. All tumors showed fluorescence, with maximum fluorescence at 1.5 hours after intravenous administration of 200 mg/kg 5-ALA, and 4 hours after oral administration of 400 mg/kg 5-ALA.

A clinical study of nine patients with peripheral renal tumors of <4 cm, used 20 mg/kg 5-ALA given 4 to 6 hours prior to retroperitoneal organ preserving tumor resection. The mobilized kidney, prior to resection, the tumor and the postresection site were all examined for fluorescence. There was no fluorescence of the surface of the mobilized kidney, with eight out of nine resected tumors showing good fluorescence, and clear demarcation between the tumor and surrounding healthy tissue. No fluorescence was detected in the postresection site. The only side effect in the clinical study was a transient increase in liver enzyme values. Whether this technique would give additional benefit to the patient over standard techniques for determining the resection limits of a tumor would need to be assessed in further clinical studies.

### Photodynamic therapy

A vascular acting photosensitizer, WST-09, or Tookad, has been assessed in a small study using a pig

**Table 6.2** Comparison of clinical studies of PDT for prostate cancer

| Reference | Photosensitizer (drug dose) | Light delivery: route dose wavelength | Drug–light interval | Target volume | Patient characteristics: Gleason score PSA level primary/salvage setting | Number of patients | Imaging results | Biopsy results | PSA response | Adverse effects | Limitations of the study |
|---|---|---|---|---|---|---|---|---|---|---|---|
| Windahl et al. (1990) [42] | Hematoporphyrin derivative (1.50 mg/kg iv) | Transurethral 15 J/cm² 638 nm | 48 h | Post-TURP remnant | Post-TURP primary setting | 1 | Post-treatment imaging not reported | Post-treatment biopsy not reported | Reduction in PSA level (10.0 to 2.5 μg/l) | No adverse effects reported | Post-treatment imaging and biopsy not reported Only 1 case reported |
| Windahl et al. (1990) [42] | Photofrin (2.50 mg/kg iv) | Transurethral 15 J/cm² 638 nm | 72 h | Post- TURP remnant | Post-TURP primary setting | 1 | Post-treatment imaging not reported | Post-treatment biopsy not reported | Reduction in PSA level (6.0 to 0.2 μg/l) | No adverse effects reported | Post-treatment imaging and biopsy not reported Only 1 case reported |
| Nathan et al. (2002) [51] | Temoporfin (0.15 mg/kg iv) | Transperineal freehand insertion 20 or 50 J/cm² 652 nm | 3 days | Less than whole gland | PSA before radiotherapy up to 37 ng/L Post-radiotherapy setting for T2/3 cancer | 14 | Up to 91% necrosis on cross- sectional CT imaging | Negative biopsies in 3/14 patients | 10/14 patients had a PSA level reduction by up to 96% | 1 patient with rectourethral fistula after rectal biopsy 2 patients with stress urinary incontinence 3 patients with acute urinary retention | Freehand fiber placement Variable timing of post-treatment imaging Variable light dose |
| Moore et al. (2006) [52] | Temoporfin (0.15 mg/kg iv) | Transperineal freehand insertion 50 or 100 J or J/cm 652 nm | 2–5 days | Less than whole gland | Gleason score 3+3 PSA level 1.9–15 ng/L 6 primary treatments 4 repeat treatments | 6 | Up to 51 cm3 necrosis Residual cancer in all patients | Necrosis and fibrosis on biopsy | PSA reduction in 8/10 treatments | 1 patient with gram negative sepsis All patients with irritative voiding symptoms for 2 weeks 2 patients requiring recatheterization 1 patient with mild stress/urge incontinence 1 patient with deterioration in erectile function | Freehand fiber placement Variable timing of post-treatment imaging Variable light dose |

| Reference | Photosensitizer (dose) | Drug–light interval | Light delivery | Target | Patient characteristics | No. of patients | Post-treatment imaging | Biopsy | PSA | Adverse effects | Comments |
|---|---|---|---|---|---|---|---|---|---|---|---|
| Pinthus et al. (2006) [56] Verigos et al. (2006) [57] Patel et al. (2008) [58] | Motexafin lutetium (0.50/1.00/2.00 mg/kg iv) | 3/6/24 h | Perineal template 25–150 J/cm² 732 nm Computer-aided light-dose planning | Whole gland | Postradiotherapy (8 patients external beam, nine patients brachytherapy) | 17[a] | Post-treatment imaging not reported | Negative biopsies in 3/14 patients | Transient procedure-related PSA level rise Post-treatment PSA fall in high-dose PDT only PSA values were analyzed for only 14 of the 17 patients | 1/14 patients with grade II urinary urgency (catheter related) Grade I genitourinary symptoms in many patients | Post-treatment imaging and biopsy not reported Marked variation in PDT doses |
| Zaak et al. (2003) [55] | Aminolaevulinic acid-induced protoporphyrin IX (20.00 mg/kg orally) | 4 h | 1 cm cylindrical diffuser Perineal (n = 2); Transurethral (n = 3); Radical prostatectomy (n = 1) 250 J/cm 633 nm | Variable | Gleason score 5–8 PSA level 4.9–10.6 ng/mL Primary setting | 6 | Post-treatment imaging not reported | Necrosis observed on prostatectomy specimen at fiber insertion | Average decrease 55% for transurethral light delivery; 30% reduction for transperineal light delivery | No adverse effects reported | Post-treatment imaging and biopsy not reported |
| Weersink et al. (2005) [19] Trachtenberg et al. (2008) [59] Trachtenberg et al. (2007) [60] Haider et al. (2007) [61] | Padoporfin (0.10–2.00 mg/kg iv) | 10 min | Perineal template, computer-aided light-dose planning Up to 360 J/cm 763 nm | Whole gland in multifiber patients; single fiber in each of the right and left lobes of the prostate in the earlier part of the study | Organ-confined recurrence after definitive radiotherapy | 24 patients with 2 light fibers; 28 patients with up to 6 fibers | Complete response on MRI in 60% of patients who received high drug and light dose | Complete response on biopsy in 60% of patients who received high drug and light dose | PSA levels decreased in the 8 patients who were biopsy-negative at 6 months | 2 patients with rectourethral fistulae 1 patient with intraoperative hypotension Decreased urinary function until 6 months | Reason for heterogeneity in responses unclear |

iv, intravenous; TURP, transurethral resection of the prostate.

[a] Although 17 patients received PDT, only 14 patients had PSA samples before photodynamic therapy, and so only these 14 patients were evaluable in the PSA paper; at the time of publication of the clinical paper only 14 patients had received PDT.

model of healthy renal tissue [64]. A laparoscopic approach was used, with a modified laparoscopic light source. Following intravenous administration of the photosensitizer at 0.5 or 1 mg/kg, 763 nm light was delivered to the tumor at a dose of 100 or 200 J/cm. Two animals died within minutes of the infusion, and a further animal was sacrificed prior to drug infusion due to an inadvertent bowel injury. Four remaining animals underwent the full PDT procedure and subsequent evaluation with CT, arteriography, pyelography, and EDTA renography, followed by sacrifice and histological evaluation. There was no evidence of urine leakage or effects outside the tumor on any of the post-PDT imaging. Histology showed necrosis of glomeruli with significant hemorrhage and thrombosis of the capillary loops. Significantly, necrosis was not complete in the center of the lesion. As there was some evidence of a dose response effect, it may be that increasing the drug or light dose may lead to more homogenous lesions. In addition, it is possible that tumor tissue may be more sensitive than normal renal tissue. Further studies using this family of photosensitizers are awaited.

As renal cell carcinoma is known to be radioresistant, and some photosensitizers appear to show some effect in increasing the sensitivity of tumors to radiotherapy, one group has assessed the potential of hypericin as a radiosensitizer and photosensitizer in an in vitro model. Wessels and colleagues [15], incubated renal cell derived cell lines with hypericin and confirmed the uptake and intracellular distribution with fluorescence microscopy. They then established that hypericin PDT led to a reduction in metabolic activity of 94–97%, and that the effects of incubation with hypericin prior to irradiation with 2–8 Gy led to a significant reduction in clonogenic survival. This work has not yet been replicated in a preclinical model, but would be an interesting area for further research.

## Future directions

There are a number of potential ways in which photodynamic therapy may be developed in the future. These can be divided into advances in photosensitizers, light delivery systems, and treatment planning and evaluation.

## Photosensitizers

Some groups are assessing the linkage of monoclonal antibodies to photosensitizers in order to improve the tumor specificity of the PDT effect. However, this can lead to a heterogeneous effect within the tumor, due to heterogeneous distribution of the antibody target throughout the tumor. In addition, the linked antibody may reduce the effectiveness of the photosensitizer, and so careful evaluation of each antibody-linked compound is required, in both preclinical and clinical models.

Other groups are looking to increase the effectiveness of photosensitizer by adaptation of established photosensitizers, for example, the work done with 5 5-ALA esters and pegylated mTHPC. Again, each new version requires extensive testing before it is known whether the potential advantages will be realized in clinical practice.

## Light delivery systems

The light dose for PDT can be varied by varying the total light dose, the light dose per unit volume or area, and the rate at which the light dose is given. In addition, some groups have looked at giving the light dose in a fractionated manner, e.g., a few seconds on and a few seconds off, in order to allow recovery of tissue oxygen in between light fractions. This has been shown to result in an increase in PDT effect in experimental models [65,66]. One group assessed the effect of giving the light dose in two fractions, for a single drug dose, using the first light fraction to activate the photosensitizer in the vascular phase, and the second fraction to activate the photosensitizer when it has accumulated in the tissue [67]. Again, this resulted in an increased PDT effect when compared to either light dose given alone.

## Treatment planning and monitoring systems

The complex nature of PDT, which requires sufficient amounts of drug, light, and oxygen to be present at the same time, and each element of which can be "used up" during the treatment period, has led some to look at complex real-time treatment modification devices. For example, a group at the University of Lund, Sweden, are looking at real-time monitoring of photosensitizer, light, oxygen, and temperature within the prostate during mTHPC-mediated PDT, with modification of the light dose throughout the treatment time, in order to maximize PDT effect [68]. Clinical results are awaited from this work. Another group has done extensive modeling in the canine prostate model, and was able to predict necrosis to within 2 mm [69]. This work used the photosensitizer tin etiopurin, which has not been used in any clinical studies of prostate cancer to date.

## Conclusions

The most highly developed applications of photodynamic techniques in urology are photodynamic detection of bladder cancer and photodynamic therapy for prostate cancer. Further research is ongoing, particularly in photodynamic therapy for prostate cancer, although also in other urological malignancies.

## References

1. Bonnett R (1999) Photodynamic therapy in historical perspective. In Reviews in Contemporary Pharmacotherapy, pp. 1–17.
2. Raab O (1900) Ueber die wirkung fluorescierenden stoffe auf infusiorien. Z Biol 39: 524–546.
3. von Tappeiner H, Jodlbauer A (1907) The sensitising action of fluorescent substances. An overall account of investigations on photodynamic phenomena. Leipzig FCW Vogel
4. Lipson RL, Gray MJ, Baldes EJ (1967) Hematoporphyrin derivative for detection and management of cancer. Cancer 20: 2255–2257.
5. Lipson RL, Gray MJ, Baldes EJ (1996) Hematoporphyrin derivative for detection and management of cancer. 9th International Cancer Congress, Tokyo Section II-01-a: 50696. Conference Proceeding, Tokyo, Japan
6. Dougherty TJ et al (1978) Photoradiation for the treatment of tumours. Cancer Res 38: 2628–2635.
7. (TAP) Study Group (1999) Photodynamic therapy of subfoveal choroidal neovascularization in age-related macular degeneration with verteporfin: one-year results of 2 randomized clinical trials–TAP report. Treatment of age-related macular degeneration with photodynamic therapy. Arch Ophthalmol 117: 1329–1345.
8. Dougherty TJ (1993) Photodynamic therapy. Photochem Photobiol 58: 895–900.
9. Oleinick NL, Evans HH (1998) The photobiology of photodynamic therapy: cellular targets and mechanisms. Radiat Res 150: S146–S156.
10. Korbelik M, Stott B, Sun J (2007) Photodynamic therapy-generated vaccines: relevance of tumour cell death expression. Br J Cancer 97(10): 1381–1387.
11. Tralau CJ et al (1989) Mouse skin photosensitivity with dihaematoporphyrin ester (DHE) and aluminium sulphonated phtalocyanien (AlSPc): a comparatove study. Photochem Photobiol 49: 305–312.
12. Uspenskii LV et al (2000) Endobronchial laser therapy in complex preoperative preparation of patients with lung diseases. Khirurgiia (Mosk): 38–40.
13. Sokolov VV et al (1995) The photodynamic therapy of malignant tumors in basic sites with the preparations photohem and photosens (the results of 3 years of observations). Vopr Onkol 41: 134–138.
14. Stranadko EF et al (2001) Photodynamic therapy of recurrent and residual oropharyngeal and laryngeal tumors. Vestn Otorinolaringol 3: 36–39.
15. Wessels JT et al (2008) Photosensitising and radiosensitising effects of hypericin on human renal carcinoma cells in vitro. Photochem Photobiol 84: 228–235.
16. Selman SH et al (2001) Studies of tin ethyl etiopurpurin photodynamic therapy of the canine prostate. J Urol 165; 1795–180117.
17. Hunt DW (2002) Rostaporfin (Miravent Medical Technologies). IDrugs 5(2): 180–186.
18. Scherz A et al (1999) Palladium-substituted bacteriochlorophyll derivatives and use thereof. PCT/IL99/00673. 1999. Ref Type: Patent.
19. Weersink RA et al (2005) Assessment of cutaneous photosensitivity of Tookad (WST09) in oreclinical animal models and patients. Photochem Photbiol 81: 106–113.
20. Fotinos N et al (2006) 5 –Aminolaevulinic acid derivatives in photomedicine: characteristics, application and perspectives. Photochem Photbiol 82: 994–1015.
21. Jocham D, Stepp H, Waidelich R (2008) Photodynamic diagnosis in urology: state of the art. Eur Urol 53: 1138–1150.
22. Alken P et al (2007) A randomised controlled multicentre trial to compare the effects of transurethral resection of bladder carcinomas under 5-ALA induced fuorescence light to conventional white light. EAU Annual Congress poster presentation, March 21-24, 2007, Berlin, Germany.
23. Jichlinski P et al (2003) Hexyl aminolevulinate fluorescence cystoscopy: new diagnostic tool for photodiagnosis of superficial bladder cancer- a multi centre study. J Urol 170: 226–229.
24. Jocham D et al (2005) Improved detection and treatment of bladder cancer using hexaminolevulinate imaging : a prospective, phase III multi center study. J Urol 174: 862–866.
25. Filbeck T et al (2002) Clinically relevant improvement of recurrence free survival with 5 –aminolaevulinic acid

induced fluorescence diagnosis in patients with superficial bladder tumours. J Urol 168: 67–71.

26. Kriegmar M et al (2002) Transurethral resection for bladder cancer using 5-aminolaevulinic acid induced fluorescence endoscopy versus white light endoscopy. J Urol 168: 475–478.

27. Riedl CR et al (2001) Fluorescence endoscopy with 5 aminoleavulinic acid reduces early recurrence rate in superficial bladder cancer. J Urol 165: 1121–1123.

28. Denzinger S et al (2007) Clinically relevant reduction in risk of recurrence of superficial bladder cancer using using 5 aminolaevulinic acid induced fluorescence diagnosis: 8 year results of prospective randomised study. Urology 69: 675–679.

29. Babjuk M et al (2005) 5–aminolaevulinic acid induced fluorescence cystosocopy during transurethra resection reduces the risk of recurrence in stage Ta/T1 bladder cancer. BJU Int 96: 798–802.

30. Daniltchenko DI et al (2005) Long term benefit of 5 amino-laevulinic acid fluorescence assisted transurethral resection of superficial bladder cancer: 5 year results of a prospective randomised study. J Urol 174: 2129–2133.

31. Penkoff H et al (2007) Transurethral detection and resection of bladder carcinomas under white or 5 –ALA induced fluorescence light:results of the first double blind placebo controlled trial [Abstract 1085]. Annual American Urological Association congress, May 19–24, 2007, Annaheim, CA.

32. Denzinger S et al (2007) Does photodynamic transurethral resection of bladder tumour improve the outcome of initial T1 high grade bladder cancer? A long term follow up of a randomised study. BJU Int 101: 566–569.

33. Kelly JF, Snell ME, Berenbaum MC (1975) Photodynamic destruction of human bladder carcinoma. Br J Cancer 31(2): 237–244.

34. Kreigmar M et al (1997) Early clinical experience with 5-amino laevulinic acid for photodynamic therapy of superficial bladder cancer. BJU Int. 77: 667–671.

35. D'Hallewin MA, Star W, Baert L (1997) Initial evaluation of whole bladder wall photodynamic therapy after intravesical ALA sensitisation for carcinoma in situ of the bladder. SPIE 3191: 210–213.

36. Waidelich R et al (2001) Clinical experience with 5 amino – laevulinic acid and photodynamic therapy for refractory superficial bladder cancer. J Urol 165: 1904–1907.

37. Shackley DC et al (2002) Photodynamic therapy for superficial bladder cancer under local anaesthetic. BJU Int 89(7): 665–67038.

38. Waidelich R et al (2003) Whole bladder photodynamic therapy with 5 amino-laevulinic acid using a white light source. Urology 61: 332–337.

39. Berger AP et al (2003) Photodynamic therapy with intravesical instillation of 5 amino-laevulinic acid for patients with recurrent superficial bladder cancer: a single center study. Urology 61: 338–341.

40. Jichlinski P, Leisinger HJ (2001) Photodynamic therapy in superficial bladder cancer: past, present and future. Urol Res 29: 396–405.

41. Walther Mc M (2000) The role of photodynamic therapy in the treatment of recurrent superficial bladder cancer. Urol Clin North Am 27: 163–170.

42. Windahl T, Andersson SO, Lofgren L (1990) Photodynamic therapy of localised prostatic cancer. Lancet 336: 1139.

43. Chang SC et al (1996) Interstitial and transurethral photodynamic therapy of the canine prostate using meso-tetra-(m-hydroxyphenyl) chlorin. Int J Cancer 67: 555–562.

44. Chang SC et al (1997a) Interstitial photodynamic therapy in the canine prostate with disulfonated aluminum phthalocyanine and 5-aminolevulinic acid-induced protoporphyrin IX. Prostate 32: 89–98.

45. Selman SH, Keck RW (1994) The effect of transurethral light on the canine prostate after sensitization with the photosensitizer tin (II) etiopurpurin dichloride: a pilot study. J Urol 152: 2129–2132.

46. Selman SH, Keck RW, Hampton JA (1996) Transperineal photodynamic ablation of the canine prostate. J Urol 156: 258–260.

47. Lee LK et al (1997) Interstitial photodynamic therapy in the canine prostate. Br J Urol 80: 898–902.

48. Shetty SD et al (1997) Evaluation of prostatic optical properties and tissue response to photodynamic therapy in a canine model. SPIE 2078. Conference Proceeding, San Diego, CA

49. Chen Q et al (2002) Preclinical studies in normal canine prostate of a novel palladium-bacteriopheophorbide (WST09) photosensitizer for photodynamic therapy of prostate cancers. Photochem Photobiol 76: 438–445.

50. Hsi RA et al (2001) Photodynamic therapy in the canine prostate using motexafin lutetium. Clin Cancer Res 7: 651–660.

51. Nathan TR et al (2002) Photodynamic therapy for prostate cancer recurrence after radiotherapy: a phase I study. J Urol 168: 1427–1432.

52. Moore CM et al (2006) Photodynamic therapy using meso tetra hydroxy phenyl chlorin (mTHPC) in early prostate cancer. Lasers Surg Med 38: 356–363.

53. Lou PJ et al (2004) Interstitial photodynamic therapy as salvage treatment for recurrent head and neck cancer. Br J Cancer 91: 441–446.

54. Lou PJ, Jones L, Hopper C (2003) Clinical outcomes of photodynamic therapy for head-and-neck cancer. Technol Cancer Res Treat 2: 311–317.

55. Zaak D et al (2003) Photodynamic therapy by means of 5-ALA induced PPIX in human prostate cancer – preliminary results. Medical Laser Application 18: 91–95.

56. Pinthus JH et al (2006) Photodynamic therapy for urological malignancies: past to current approaches. J Urol 175: 1201–1207.

57. Verigos K et al (2006) Updated results of a phase I trial of motexafin lutetium-mediated interstitial photodynamic therapy in patients with locally recurrent prostate cancer. J Environ Pathol Toxicol Oncol 25: 373–387.

58. Patel H et al (2008) Motexafin lutetium-photodynamic therapy of prostate cancer: short- and long-term effects on prostate-specific antigen. Clin Cancer Res 14: 4869–4876.

59. Trachtenberg J et al (2008) Vascular-targeted photodynamic therapy (padoporfin, WST09) for recurrent prostate cancer after failure of external beam radiotherapy: a study of escalating light doses. BJU Int 102: 556–562.

60. Trachtenberg J et al (2007) Vascular targeted photodynamic therapy with palladium-bacteriopheophorbide photosensitizer for recurrent prostate cancer following definitive radiation therapy: assessment of safety and treatment response. J Urol 178: 1974–1979.

61. Haider MA et al (2007) Prostate gland: MR imaging appearance after vascular targeted photodynamic therapy with palladium-bacteriopheophorbide. Radiology 244: 196–204.

62. Moore C et al (2006) Vascular-targeted photodynamic therapy in organ confined prostate cancer–report of a novel photosensitiser [Abstract #434]. Eur Urol 5 (suppl.): 131.

63. Popken G, Wetterauer U, Schultze-Seeman W (1999) Kidney preserving tumour resection in renal cell carcinoma with photodynamic detection by 5 amino laevulinic acid: pre clinical and preliminary clinical results. BJU Int 83: 578–582.

64. Matin SF et al (2008) A pilot trial of vascular targeted photodynamic therapy for renal tissue. J Urol 180: 338–342.

65. Curnow A et al (2006) Comparing and combining light dose fractionation and iron chelation to enhance experimental photodynamic therapy with aminolevulinic acid. Lasers Surg Med 38: 325–331.

66. Togashi H et al (2006) Fractionated photodynamic therapy for a human oral squamous cell carcinoma xenograft. Oral Oncol 42: 526–532.

67. Dolmans DE et al (2002) Targeting tumor vasculature and cancer cells in orthotopic breast tumor by fractionated photosensitizer dosing photodynamic therapy. Cancer Res 62: 4289–4294.

68. Johansson A et al (2007) Realtime light dosimetry software tools for interstitial photodynamic therapy of the human prostate. Med Phys 34: 4309–4321.

69. Jankun J et al (2005) Diverse optical characteristic of the prostate and light delivery system: implications for computer modelling of prostatic photodynamic therapy. BJU Int 95: 1237–1244.

# 7

# Perspectives on nanotechnology

*Aleksandar F. Radovic-Moreno*[1]*, Kai P. Yuet*[1]*,*
*Robert S. Langer*[1]*, and Omid C. Farokhzad*[2]

[1]Harvard-MIT Division of Health Sciences and Technology, MIT Department of Chemical Engineering, Cambridge, MA, USA
[2]Department of Anesthesia, Brigham and Women's Hospital, Harvard Medical School, Boston, MA, USA

## Introduction

"Nanomedicine," or the application of nanotechnology to medicine, is a rapidly growing field that has benefited greatly from our increasing ability to manufacture from the "top-down" or self-assemble from the "bottom-up" objects or features on surfaces that are of the same scale as proteins in the body. This field has provided us with the unprecedented ability to more precisely engineer interactions between nanomaterials and biomolecules to provide more targeted and potent effects. In contrast to small molecule agents, which are typically limited to performing a single action at a specific site, nanotechnology products can be engineered to interact with cells or proteins by performing multiple functions at several sites. Certain nanotechnology products, such as quantum dots, have significantly more potent properties by virtue of their size and chemical composition than equivalent small molecule agents. Nanotechnology products can even be engineered to interact with their environment to trigger changes in their own properties, such as stimulating drug release in response to local environmental cues or aggregating to provide contrast enhancement for more sensitive imaging.

Despite all of these interesting advances, nanomedicine is still in a relative state of infancy, with its particular niche in clinical practice still being defined. The potential of this field to make a positive impact in urological oncology in the future is really limited only by our imagination. However,

with greater sophistication comes greater complexity. As small molecule drugs almost invariably have "side effects," it too will be important to understand thoroughly how nanomaterials interact with components of the body. Nanotechnology is also likely to produce challenges from a regulatory and drug approval point of view, which must be overcome prior to effective clinical translation. The focus of this chapter will be on providing an overview of the major concepts that have emerged from decades of research in the lab setting, highlighted by interesting examples from the current literature. Our objective is to introduce the urological oncologist to the field of nanomedicine and perhaps inspire new research directions or applications that will help realize the potential of nanotechnology.

We begin the tour of nanomedicine by first considering how the various properties of a nanomaterial affect its biodistribution. This is of critical importance to designing all major categories of nanoparticles (diagnostic, therapeutic, and combined or "theranostic"). Following this, we survey some of the major types of therapeutic nanoparticles, highlighting advantages and disadvantages of each. We end by considering future directions for this exciting field, in the hope that you are able to contribute!

## Biodistribution of nanomaterials

One of the most important properties of a nanomaterial as it relates to in vivo use is how that material

*Interventional Techniques in Uro-oncology*, First Edition. Edited by Hashim Uddin Ahmed, Manit Arya, Peter T. Scardino & Mark Emberton. © 2011 Blackwell Publishing Ltd. Published 2011 by Blackwell Publishing Ltd.

distributes itself through the body and its residence time within the body's tissues—its biodistribution. Several parameters play a significant role in determining the biodistribution of a nanomaterial: (1) method of administration and dose [1], (2) size [2], (3) surface charge [3], (4) surface hydrophobicity, (5) degree of surface coverage of poly(ethylene glycol) (PEG) or other stabilizing agent [4], (6) presence and density of targeting ligand [5,6], (7) ability to repel adsorption of opsonizing proteins, such as complement proteins, albumin, or apolipoproteins, and (8) nanoparticle shape [7]. In some special circumstances, other properties of a nanomaterial can have a significant impact, as would be the case with magnetically guided nanoparticles or particles that can be triggered to degrade in response to an external stimulus, such as heat [8], pH [9], or enzyme concentration [10].

## Nanoparticle size and interactions with organs

To appreciate how the size of a nanomaterial will impact how it distributes throughout the body, it is instructive to consider the route that nanomaterials take as they distribute through the body from an intravenous injection. Nanoparticles will flow towards the right heart in the low-pressure venous circulation, collect in the right ventricle, and then proceed through the pulmonary artery to the capillaries in the lung, which are generally 7 to 8 μm in diameter. At this point, nanomaterials that have aggregated together due to the relatively high ionic strength of the body (~150 mEq/L) or due to adsorption of opsonizing proteins, will be not be able to pass effectively through the capillaries to reach the pulmonary veins. From the left heart, nanoparticles will distribute to various organs in the body depending on the relative amount of cardiac output that each organ receives, and in the case of the liver, the additional blood flow that comes from the portal vein. The organs that have the greatest capacity to alter the biodistribution of a nanoparticle are the liver, kidneys, spleen, and bone marrow.

### Liver
Teleologically, an important function of the liver is to clear blood of food-borne toxins and microorganisms that have entered the mesenteric circulation before that blood re-enters the general circulation. The microarchitecture of the liver reflects this function by having a fenestrated endothelial layer, which allows blood contents to come into intimate contact with hepatocytes and macrophages known as Kupffer cells [11]. Nanoparticles that are smaller than ~50 nm are able to enter the space between endothelial cells (known as the space of Disse). Those that do not escape will reside there until they are metabolized by hepatocytes or Kupffer cells and are eliminated into the bile. Nanoparticles that are larger than ~200 nm are most effectively cleared from the circulation by Kupffer cells which can reach into the sinusoidal space, since the relatively low flow conditions of the liver sinusoids allows plenty of time for phagocytosis or macropinocytosis to occur. Liver uptake can be greatly enhanced if the nanomaterial has adsorbed elements of the plasma onto its surface, particularly, complement proteins, albumin, or apolipoproteins. Macrophages are more able to phagocytose nanomaterials when they are covered with the complement protein C3b, a fragment of C3 when the latter undergoes spontaneous hydrolysis (alternative pathway) or, if the nanomaterial has been recognized by antibodies, by the classical pathway C3 convertase (the C4b2b complex). Hepatocytes express various receptors for apolipoproteins, such as the low density lipoprotein receptor (LDL-R). Nanomaterials that have been covered by these proteins and lipids can thus accumulate more readily in the liver [12]. In addition, it is important to appreciate that the high degree of cardiac output that the liver receives together with the intimate contact between hepatocytes and blood components, and the presence of blood clearing Kupffer cells makes the liver the major site of accumulation of many nanomaterial constructs, and that nanoparticle size plays a significant role in modulating the degree of accumulation in the liver as well as the major cell type within the liver that is targeted.

### Kidneys
In parallel to the liver, blood is distributed to the kidneys through the renal arteries, which also receive a significant quantity of cardiac output. The kidneys have a specialized capillary network, the glomerulus, which is fenestrated and will filter into the tubular fluid anything in the plasma that is less than approximately 5 nm in diameter. Due to the fixed charges present on the endothelial cells and the glomerular basement membrane, cationic materials are more likely to be filtered than a neutral or negatively charged material of the same size [13]. Most nanomaterials are too

**103**

large to be excreted through the renal system, but it is important to consider that certain components of nanomaterials that are not biodegradable, such as the commonly used polyether PEG, should be small enough to promote renal clearance to enhance overall biocompatibility.

*Spleen*

The spleen is another important organ to be considered in designing nanomaterials that are to be injected into the systemic circulation due to its purifying effect on the blood. The microcirculation of the spleen is divided into two major pathways: (1) the closed-circuit pathway whereby blood flows directly from capillaries to the splenic veins and (2) the open pathway, which is characterized by capillaries with a discontinuous endothelium, allowing contact of blood components with the extracellular matrix and tissue macrophages that normally function to clear the blood of aged red blood cells [14]. Similar to the liver, nanoparticles that are larger than ~200 nm will accumulate in the phagocytic cells of the spleen [15].

*Bone marrow*

Similarly, the bone marrow is a site of discontinuous basement membrane and large numbers of macrophages, which function to remove aged and defective red blood cells from the circulation, as well as other debris [14]. Collectively, the liver, spleen, and bone marrow account for a significant portion of the injected dose of most nanomaterials, particularly if they have not been engineered to resist the adsorption of plasma proteins (Figures 7.1 and 7.2).

## Nanoparticle tumor targeting

Tumor targeting is thought to be achieved by a combination of two major mechanisms: (1) passive accumulation and (2) active targeting. An important phenomenon that has been observed repeatedly in small animal studies is the passive accumulation of nanoscale objects (~50–500 nm) in certain types of solid tumors, known as the enhanced permeability and retention (EPR) effect [16]. In order to expand beyond a certain critical size and meet elevated metabolic demands, solid tumors often secrete soluble factors, such as vascular endothelial growth factor (VEGF), to promote localized angiogenesis. It is believed that the rate of formation of the microcirculation of a tu-

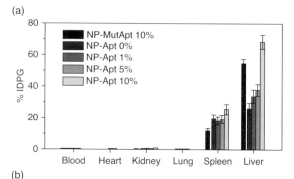

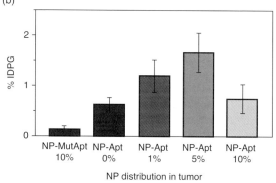

**Fig 7.1** (a) Biodistribution of PLGA-PEG polymeric nanoparticles approximately 150–200 nm in size in mice administered intravenously by retro-orbital injection. %IDPG, percent initial dose per gram of tissue. NP, nanoparticle; NP-Apt, anti-PSMA aptamer conjugated to the surface of a nanoparticle; NP-MutApt, nonfunctional aptamer conjugated to the surface of a nanoparticle. (b) NP accumulation in tumors, the percentage indicates a relative amount of aptamer on the surface of the nanoparticles. Note that an optimal amount of surface coverage of targeting ligand (Apt, anti-PSMA aptamer) was observed; further increases in targeting ligand surface density resulted in increased accumulation in the liver. Obtained from [5]. (Copyright 2008 National Academy of Sciences, USA.)

mor is so rapid that the endothelium does not form properly, leading to enhanced permeability. In addition, the lymphatic drainage of the tumor is defective for similar reasons, leading to an inability to properly drain the tumor effectively. The net effect of increased permeability and reduced drainage is accumulation, particularly of larger macromolecules and nanomaterials. In small animal studies, EPR is the principal mechanism by which nanomaterials accumulate in solid tumors. The other major form of tumor targeting is through an "active" mechanism,

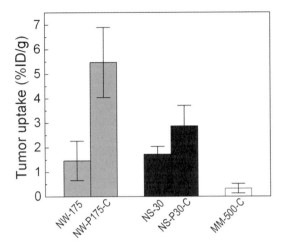

Fig 7.2 Tumor targeting of nanoworms as compared to nanospheres in mice administered nanoparticles intravenously. Note that the combined effect of using a PEG spacer plus a targeting ligand increases tumor localization in these samples, and that this effect is more prominent in nanoworms than in nanospheres. %ID/g, percent initial dose per gram of tissue. NW-175, nanoworm with 175 amine groups on the surface per particle. NW-P175-C, Nanoworm with 175 amine groups per particle to which the targeting ligand peptide CREKA is attached using a PEG spacer. NS-30, nanosphere with 30 amine groups on the surface per particle. NS-P30-C, Nanosphere with 30 amine groups on the surface per particle to which CREKA is attached using a PEG spacer. MM-500-C, commercially available iron oxide nanoparticle with 500 amine groups on the surface per particle with CREKA conjugated to the surface without a PEG spacer. Obtained from [7]. (Copyright Wiley-VCH Verlag GmbH & Co. KGaA. Reproduced with permission.)

whereby some component of the nanomaterial, usually a surface conjugated targeting ligand, "actively" alters the biodistribution pattern. Currently in the literature there is some controversy regarding whether a targeting ligand actually changes macroscale organ accumulation. The effect of conjugating a targeting ligand to the surface of a nanoparticle will depend on the size of nanomaterial, the affinity of the targeting ligand for its receptor, the integrity of the microcirculation and the lymphatic drainage, the osmotic pressure of the tumor interstitium, the accessibility of the targeted protein, and other parameters that will affect the probability of the nanoparticle encountering the targeted antigen. In some studies in small animals, it

has been observed that the effect of a targeting ligand is simply to enhance intracellular delivery without affecting macroscale biodistribution significantly [17,18]. Others have shown that a targeting ligand does indeed alter the biodistribution, with the targeting ligand leading to greater accumulation in sites of expression of the targeted antigen [6]. It also stands to reason in a thought experiment: if one imagines the size of a nanoparticle approaching that of the Fc portion of an antibody, it is clear that the presence of the targeting portion (the Fab region) makes a significant difference in the biodistribution of a nanoscale system (in this particular case, the nanoscale system is an antibody). To what extent conjugating a targeting ligand on the surface has on biodistribution, as well as how the size of the nanoparticle system affects this analysis, has not yet been fully elucidated. However, in general, the biodistribution of smaller nanoparticles ($\lesssim$ 50 nm) and macromolecules will be more likely to be affected by addition of a targeting ligand because of their increased permeability through tissues. Larger nanoparticles ($\gtrsim$ 200 nm) are more likely to be trapped in tumors or other compartments, reducing the effect of the targeting ligand on biodistribution.

## Surface physicochemical characteristics

### Zeta potential

The surface physicochemical characteristics of a nanomaterial greatly impact the biodistribution independent of size. The zeta potential, a measure of the degree of surface charge relative to that of the dispersion medium, plays a significant role in biodistribution [19,20]. Nanoparticles with positive surface charges (zeta potential $\gtrsim$+15 mV) are more likely to aggregate and to be cleared by tissue macrophages from the blood stream due to the abundance of negatively charged materials in the plasma [21,22]. In addition, positively charged materials are more likely to be excreted renally [13], and more likely to interact nonspecifically with various types of cells in the body. In general, positively charged nanomaterials will tend to accumulate in the liver, lung, and kidney [23–25]. From a microscopic viewpoint, this accumulation in the lung is due to the formation of large aggregates that transiently occlude the capillary network in the lung, although some degree of delivery to specific cell types within the lung has been observed

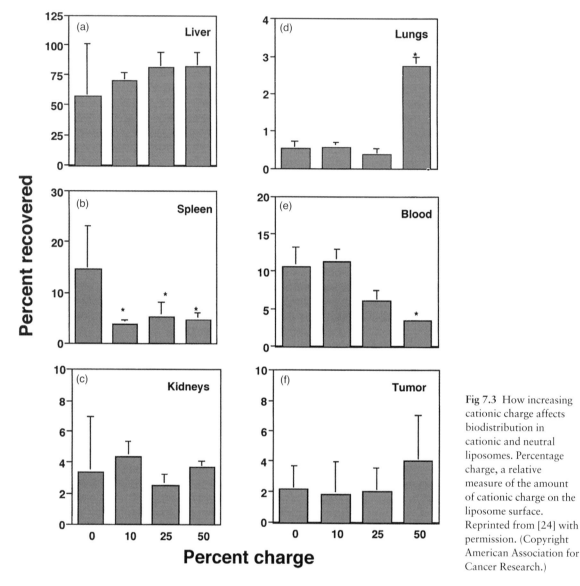

**Fig 7.3** How increasing cationic charge affects biodistribution in cationic and neutral liposomes. Percentage charge, a relative measure of the amount of cationic charge on the liposome surface. Reprinted from [24] with permission. (Copyright American Association for Cancer Research.)

[26]. Cationic nanomaterials will tend to accumulate in the Kupffer cells of the liver, although accumulation in hepatocytes is also possible, particularly if the internalization efficiency of the cationic material is very high. Negatively charged materials (zeta potential $\lesssim$ -15 mV) are less likely to interact with plasma proteins. However, highly negatively charged nanoparticles have been shown to be more likely to be phagocytosed by macrophages [27,28] (Figure 7.3). It appears that a relatively neutral surface charge (zeta potential $\sim 0 \pm 10$ mV) has the most desirable biodistribu-

tion to date. It is important to point out that neutral nanoparticles are more likely to aggregate, so it is important to have another method of stabilizing these nanoparticles, e.g., using steric hindrance via surface modification with PEG.

*PEGylation*

Surface conjugating a nanoparticle with PEG is a widespread method of improving biocompatibility, circulation half-life, organ biodistribution, and the interaction between targeting ligand and receptor [29]. When conjugated to the surface of biodegradable PLGA nanoparticle dispersed in aqueous medium, PEG behaves as if it were free in solution [30], with low energy rotation around carbon-carbon and carbon-oxygen bonds providing excellent flexibility. The flexibility of PEG chains makes it energetically unfavorable that a protein adsorbs, since it would greatly reduce the conformational freedom of the PEG chains [31]. In addition, the flexibility of PEG allows it to act like a steric barrier, which protects the surface of the nanoparticles from protein adsorption. The ability of PEG to reduce nonspecific protein binding to nanomaterial surfaces depends on the density of the PEG layer and, to a limited extent, on the length of the PEG chain [4,32,33]. Studies have shown that as few as 6 repetitions of the PEG structural unit are required to provide an effective steric barrier [31]. As far as density is concerned, there is an optimal level of PEG coverage. At low levels of PEG coverage, there is insufficient PEG to provide protection from protein adsorption. However, if the PEG density is too high, adjacent PEG chains restrict freedom of movement, lowering the free energy change of adsorption and making nonspecific adsorption more likely. PEG also improves the interaction between the targeting ligand and the targeted antigen. The flexibility of the PEG chains allows the targeting ligand to sample a greater degree of conformations, making it more likely that it will find the optimal confirmation for binding to the target antigen. PEG is also an excellent hydrogen bond acceptor, which makes it very well hydrated in water. This increases the hydrophilicity of the nanoparticle surface, which also reduces the binding of relatively hydrophobic proteins, such as albumin or apolipoproteins.

## Nanoparticle shape and frontiers

Frontiers in understanding and improving biodistribution are in investigating how nanoparticle shape affects biodistribution, as well as devising advanced methods for improving tumor targeting. The role of nanoparticle shape in biodistribution is just beginning to be appreciated and studied. Recently, it was found that the shape of a material plays a significant role in whether the particulate can be phagocytosed, with rod-shaped materials being less likely to be phagocytosed at the same volume as spherical materials [34]. However, small rod-shaped materials were shown to have higher internalization rates into nonphagocytic cells [35]. Using magnetic nanoparticles as imaging agents, it was shown that rod-shaped nanomaterials could target tumors more effectively in vivo [7]. Novel methods of improving accumulations in tumors are being explored. An interesting platelet-mimetic amplification method for improving nanoparticle accumulation in tumors was recently reported. In this manuscript, nanoparticles were developed that bound to sites of thrombosis, triggering more binding of nanoparticles, which triggered more thrombosis in a positive feedback loop. It was proposed that these nanoparticles could be used to selectively thrombose tumor vasculature [36] (Figure 7.4).

## Nanoparticle cancer vaccines

Activating the body's innate and adaptive immune responses to clear tumors is an exciting but challenging area of research, and one where nanomaterials may prove to have the advantages necessary to provide significant breakthroughs. Traditional vaccines generally consist of live attenuated viruses, purified protein derivatives, or killed whole pathogens plus an aluminum salt as an adjuvant material. While traditional vaccines are both safe and effective infectious diseases, they have been relatively disappointing in stimulating anticancer responses. In addition, these traditional approaches are somewhat limited as to the types of antigens that can one can vaccinate against. Nanotechnology has the potential to produce novel vaccine carriers or adjuvant agents that can generate a more potent response against a wider variety of antigens, including the weakly immunogenic cancer antigens.

Cancerous cells use a variety of techniques to evade the immune system, including down regulating MHC I complexes, secreting anti-inflammatory cytokines such as IL-10 and TGF-beta, and recruiting regulatory T cells [37]. In addition, it has been proposed that solid tumors undergo "immune editing" whereby the immune system selects for nonimmunogenic clones by eliminating those that it can recognize [38]. In theory, using a patient's own immune system to eliminate neoplastic foci is attractive in that one could induce remission with minimal side effects, disseminated tumors could be targeted, and the surveillance

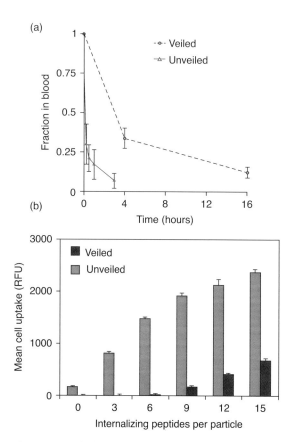

Fig 7.4 Using the local tumor environment to increase tumor accumulation by removing a PEG coating and exposing a cell-penetrating peptide. (a) Exposing the cell-penetrating peptide (unveiled) results in increased cell uptake. (b) Keeping particles PEGylated (veiled) results in significantly increased blood circulation time. Modified from [10]. (Copyright Wiley-VCH Verlag GmbH & Co. KGaA. Reproduced with permission.)

functions of the immune system could be used to prevent recurrence. Alternative approaches to nanomaterials for generating CD8+ CTL responses against urological cancers have been explored, particularly involving ex vivo manipulations of autologous antigen presenting cells (APCs), including dendritic cells [39], which have produced promising immune responses [40]. However, there have been problems translating cell-based vaccine technology to the clinic. A recent trial involving a granulocyte monocyte-colony stimulating factor (GM-CSF)-secreting prostate cancer cell used as a therapeutic vaccine (GVAX, Cell Genesys)

was terminated prematurely due to a low probability of improving overall survival. Indeed, the response rate for cancer vaccines in general is low. It is clear that a need exists for developing novel vaccination strategies that could harness the unique advantages of nanotechnology.

Nanomaterials have the potential to play a significant role in developing novel vaccines by more effectively targeting components of the immune system, encapsulating antigens to deliver them at more controlled rates, improving cytosolic delivery for improved antigen presentation in MHC I complexes, and delivering DNA for sustained expression of antigens within APCs. The major types of nanomaterials that have been explored for eliciting immune responses have been polymer nanoparticles, nondegradable nanoparticles, and liposomes.

## Biodegradable nanoparticle vaccines

Polymeric nanoparticles composed of poly(lactic-co-glycolic acid) (PLGA) have been evaluated extensively as vaccine carriers [41]. PLGA is an attractive polymer for vaccination due to its extensive track record of safety in humans in controlled release formulations and in biodegradable sutures, as well as the well-defined methods of encapsulating both hydrophobic and hydrophilic antigens. PLGA has been used as a polymer to deliver DNA vaccines and shown to protect against challenge with tumor cells. In this study, it was shown that blending a lipophilic agent, such as a lipid-PEG conjugate, to the PLGA helped to improve DNA encapsulation and also the consistency and potency of the immune response, which included both cellular and humoral responses [42]. Co-delivering a Toll-like receptor 4 (TLR-4) ligand with the melanoma antigen tyrosinase-related protein 2 (TRP2) using PLGA nanoparticles ~400 nm in size resulted in induction of tumor-specific CD8+ T cells that led to a therapeutic anti-tumor effect [43]. PLGA nanoparticles have also been evaluated as delivery vehicles for oral immunization due to uptake at the lymphoid follicles present in the gut, also known as Peyer's patches [44,45]. One study considered the effect of PLGA particle size on production of IgG titers against bovine serum albumin (BSA). They found that for their particular system, larger (1000 nm) particles generally elicited more potent antibody titers, although this was complicated by the fact that these larger particles also encapsulated more protein [46]. PLGA is thus developing as an attractive candidate material for vaccine delivery.

## Nondegradable nanoparticle vaccines

Solid, nondegradable nanoparticles have been explored for vaccine delivery. Gold nanoparticles were used as a platform onto which the cationic carbohydrate polymer chitosan was conjugated in order to deliver a DNA vaccine. This system showed potent humoral and CD8+ T cell responses in mice after intramuscular injection [47]. Patterning alternating striations of anionic hydrophilic with hydrophobic groups onto gold nanoparticles showed enhanced cell membrane penetration for cytosolic delivery of nanoparticles [48]. In addition, pH-responsive nanoparticle materials have been engineered to enhance cytosolic delivery based on increased endosomal membrane disruption [49]. It is hypothesized that by increased delivery to the cytoplasm, antigen can be delivered for presentation on MHC I complexes for more potent initiation of CD8+ T cell responses, such as is relevant for cancer immunotherapy. Fluorescent polystyrene nanoparticles were used to study the effect of size on targeting to draining lymph nodes after mouse footpad injection. It was found that smaller nanoparticles (<200 nm) could freely drain into lymph nodes, whereas larger nanoparticles (>500 nm) were carried to lymph nodes following phagocytosis and transport by epidermal and dermal dendritic cells, not significantly by free diffusion [50]. This may be significant for targeting specific populations of immune cells, which may have applications in eliciting certain types of immune responses.

## Liposome vaccines

Liposomes have shown considerable progress in developing nanoparticle-based vaccines due to their ability to co-deliver antigen plus adjuvant effectively to APCs [51]. Various routes of entry have been probed for liposome-based vaccines. Liposomes have been used to successfully deliver antigen plus a TLR-9 agonist CpG oligodeoxynucleotide (ODN) motif intravenously for targeting APCs in the spleen [52]. In addition, liposomes were used to vaccine against a tumor-associated antigen by co-delivering CpG ODN using the more traditional subcutaneous injection technique [53]. The field of nanoparticle-based vaccine design is relatively young, but these early reports of successful vaccination in animals provides optimism about the prospects of this type of technology and its potential role in cancer therapy in the future.

## Nanoparticles for cancer therapy

One of the most exciting aspects of nanotechnology is its potential impact on cancer therapy. The majority of emphasis in this space has been in developing materials for drug delivery, but effort has also gone towards developing nanomaterials that can generate high temperatures locally to kill cells by hyperthermia [54], as well as engineering particles that can perform multiple functions including drug delivery, targeted hyperthermia, imaging, or "smart" sensing, such as increasing fluorescence following drug release.

In the last thirty years, many different materials have been synthesized or adapted as drug delivery vehicles. From a drug formulation perspective, it makes a lot of sense to think about the drug and the encapsulating material in terms of their physicochemical characteristics, as these are often the most important parameters used to develop a nanoparticle drug delivery system. The simple principles of "like dissolves like" and "oppositely charged materials attract" are usually enough to understand the motivation behind formulating certain drugs with certain types of materials.

### Drug encapsulation

Encapsulation strategies and the optimal material vary between different types of drugs. The most commonly used nanoscale drug delivery vehicles are liposomes, polymers, dendrimers, quantum dots, gold nanoparticles, and nanoshells, but many examples do not necessarily fit within these broad categories. The goals of encapsulating drugs are to improve solubility, increase drug circulation half-life, increase target organ drug concentration, deliver drugs intracellularly, target a specific receptor or transport mechanism to improve delivery, and reduce incidence or severity of side effects.

Generally, one would consider encapsulating a drug in the following scenarios:

1 Insoluble in water.

2 Toxic to cells but is not particularly toxic to hepatocytes, splenocytes, or bone marrow cells.

3 Cleared very rapidly from the body.

4 Degraded in the presence of serum.

5 Active only inside a cell and is unable to diffuse across the cell membrane.

6 Delivering the drug over an extended period of time in a controlled fashion would significantly improve treatment outcome.

Drugs that have been encapsulated in nanoscale drug delivery vehicles are thus generally proteins, small molecule hydrophobic drugs, or nucleic acids. Proteins are generally relatively small, and would be cleared renally relatively quickly if not encapsulated. Hydrophobic drugs must usually be dissolved in a surfactant formulation, before they can be administered at therapeutic levels. Encapsulating the drug inside of a nanoparticle with a hydrophobic core can provide altered biodistribution and pharmacokinetics, characterized by increased half-life and the possibility of less toxic components. Nucleic acids are generally unable to cross the cell membrane efficiently, and so must be formulated with a transfection agent to produce a biological effect.

## Liposomes

Liposomes are the earliest to be developed and most thoroughly studied and widely used nanoparticle drug delivery systems in the clinic to date. Liposomes generally exist as spherical structures, about 100 nm in diameter, with a bilayer structure delimiting the exterior from an internal aqueous compartment. Liposome size can be tightly controlled by processing conditions to yield relatively monodisperse nanoparticle populations. The thin lipid bilayer can be used to carry hydrophobic materials, such as lipophilic drugs or imaging agents. The types of lipids used can alter important properties of the liposome. For example, incorporating lipids with PEG conjugated to the polar head group helps to extend the circulation half-life and biocompatibility of the liposome [55]. In general, the advantage of using liposomes over other drug delivery formulations is that they boast long circulation timescales, incorporate both hydrophilic and hydrophobic materials, have a track record of safety in humans, many important pharmacokinetic and biocompatibility properties have already been evaluated, and there

is an extensive body of knowledge surrounding their development and use. The major drawback to using liposomes is that there is little control over when the drug is released from the liposome carrier, even if the liposome reaches the target destination. Drug release from a liposome usually occurs as a burst—a relatively rapid release over a short period of time—as the liposome structure falls apart.

Liposomes have been modified in multiple ways to provide additional functionality and to overcome some of their shortcomings. As with other nanomaterials, liposomes have been modified with targeting ligands to improve intracellular delivery. PEGylated liposomes have been modified with antibodies to bind to sites of HER2/neu over-expression for delivery of drugs to breast cancer cells in vivo [56]. Of interest to urological oncology, liposomes have been modified with the prostate cancer-specific monoclonal antibody 5D4 to enhance the cytotoxicity of liposomal doxorubicin [57]. Liposomes have also been used to target gene therapy to prostate specific membrane antigen (PSMA) expressing cells using a monoclonal antibody [58]. More recently, liposomes have slowly become increasingly sophisticated, with more recent embodiments boasting the ability to respond to local environments to alter their physical properties in order to improve tumor targeting or to trigger drug delivery. For example, liposomes have been generated that use changes in pH to trigger a change in their fusogenic potential to enhance drug delivery [59]. At the physiologic pH of 7.4, the liposomes are coated with PEG and display a cell-specific targeting ligand. Once they have bound to an antigen and have been internalized into a compartment that acidifies, or in the low pH of an acidic tumor interstitium, an acid-sensitive link is hydrolyzed, revealing the fusogenic peptide motif TAT that can increase the amount of liposome internalization into cells. One can understand the value of this type of technology by considering the path that a drug delivery vehicle must take in order to deliver drugs to the interior of cells. Initially, during the circulation, desirable properties are a nonfouling surface that will interact specifically with the targeted cell type. Once the targeted cell type has been reached, a fundamental shift occurs in desirable properties—the nanoparticle should ideally interact avidly with cells in order to promote the most efficient uptake. By having the ability to "double target" using environmentally responsive nanoparticles, these two goals can potentially both be met in a single nanoparticle delivery device.

Perhaps one of the most exciting aspects of liposomes is that they have had excellent success translating to the clinic. Several liposome formulations are now in clinical use. Doxil (Johnson & Johnson) is a liposomal formulation of doxorubicin typically used in the treatment of acquired immunodeficiency syndrome (AIDS)-related Kaposi's sarcoma, multiple myeloma, or ovarian cancer. A liposome formulation of the antifungal agent amphotericin B (Ambisome, Gilead) has also been approved for systemic fungal infections and in the case of Cryptococcal meningitis in HIV-infected patients. Although these formulations are not directly relevant to urological cancers, they highlight that liposomes have had the correct blend of safety and efficacy to yield a clinically relevant vehicle, which may facilitate clinical translation of future technologies using this nanoparticle platform.

Polymers

Various types of polymer architectures have been evaluated for drug delivery. Depending on the properties of the polymer, different types of nanoparticle structures are possible. Some of the major structures include: polymer micelles, polymer nanoparticles, single polymer chains, and cross-linked hydrogels. Polymer micelles are aggregated structures of block co-polymers that consist of hydrophilic and hydrophobic segments. These self-assemble into spherical nanoscale structures where the hydrophobic segments cluster, forming a hydrophobic core with the hydrophilic segments protruding out into the solution phase. Polymer micelles are equilibrium structures that exhibit a critical micelle concentration (CMC), above which micellization occurs. These types of systems have been developed extensively, particularly for the delivery of small molecule hydrophobic drugs and for gene delivery [60]. The work on small molecule hydrophobic drugs has culminated in the recent entry of a polymer micelle consisting of paclitaxel encapsulated in poly(lactic acid)-block-poly(ethylene glycol) (PLA-PEG) into phase II clinical trials in the United States for the treatment of metastatic pancreatic cancer (Genexol-PM, Samyang). Lupron Depot$^®$, a polymeric sustained release formulation of a gonadotropin-releasing hormone agonist, is currently approved for androgen deprivation therapy (ADT) in advanced prostate cancer. Other polymeric systems have been under continued development for gene delivery by becoming more sophisticated in their release mechanisms. Polymer micelles are currently being engineered to respond specifically to conditions in tumors or endolysosomes to trigger drug release or to enhance intracellular delivery. For example, a block copolymer of PEG-poly[($N'$-citraconyl-2-aminoethyl)aspartamide] was synthesized, which reverses its charge from overall negative at pH 7.4 to positive at pH 5.5 in order to release a relatively positively charged drug in response to distribution to acidified compartments, such as the interstitium of certain tumors or endolysosomes [61]. Continuing with this theme of switchable properties for more effective delivery, a PEG-poly(3-[(3-aminopropyl)amino]propylaspartamide) block copolymer was synthesized with a side chain with a pKa selected in order to provide enhanced intracellular delivery for improved small interfering RNA (siRNA) delivery [62]. Mixed micelles of PEG-poly(L-histidine) and PEG-poly(L-lactide) have been formulated for pH sensitive drug delivery. The side chain of the amino acid histidine has a pKa of 6, allowing it to become protonated and facilitates endosome disruption as the pH of the solution drops below 6 via a combination of osmotic lysis and cationic interaction with the negatively charged membrane components [63]. This blend of polymers was shown to improve drug delivery to tumors with lowered pH of the interstitium [64].

Polymeric nanoparticles arise from block copolymers when the hydrophobic segment is large relative to the hydrophilic segment, resulting in a precipitation of the hydrophobic segment to form a solid nanoparticle core. These types of polymer systems originally began their development as controlled release microparticle formulations, which encapsulated a variety of different drugs, ranging from small hydrophobic molecules to hydrophobic proteins to hydrophilic proteins. In these types of systems, drug can be incorporated into the polymer through two main procedures: nanoprecipitation for encapsulating hydrophobic materials and double emulsion for encapsulating hydrophilic materials. In both cases, the drug is dispersed in a matrix of polymer, allowing drug release to occur through two mechanisms: (1) degradation of the polymer matrix, and (2) diffusion down the concentration gradient [65]. These systems were shown to release encapsulated macromolecules over very long time periods [66,67]. Drug release rates were shown to be tunable depending on the crystallinity of the polymer, and the type of chemical bonds used to keep the polymer backbone together. These microparticle systems were scaled down to produce nanoparticles, which had a couple of interesting effects. First, it was shown that surface conjugating PEG greatly extended the circulating half-life of the nanoparticle [29]. Second, drug release rates were accelerated tremendously due to the increase in surface area per unit volume. Release rates of docetaxel, a hydrophobic drug used in metastatic hormone refractory prostate cancer, from polymeric nanoparticles consisting of poly(lactic-co-glycolic acid)-block-poly(ethylene glycol) (PLGA-PEG) was shown to be in the order of hours to days. Nanoparticle controlled release polymer formulations also benefit from systemic administration. In fact, PLGA-PEG nanoparticles have been developed that target PSMA for drug delivery to PSMA+ prostate cancers [68,69]. In addition to showing that adding a targeting ligand increases intracellular delivery, it was shown that the density of targeting ligand on the nanoparticle surface plays a significant role in biodistribution [5] and therefore, presumably, in treatment efficacy. During in vitro studies, it was shown that, in general, the higher the targeting ligand density, the more effective nanoparticle uptake became. However, when nanoparticles made with different density of targeting ligand were injected systemically into mice bearing tumors, it was found that there was an optimal density. It was hypothesized that above a certain density, the steric repulsion effects of the PEG corona became less effective, and the nanoparticles became more visible to the cells of the mononuclear phagocytic system (MPS) in the liver, spleen, and bone marrow, and thus were able to target tumors less effectively. This same PSMA-targeting PLGA-PEG nanoparticle system was also used to target a cisplatin prodrug to PSMA+ cells for the treatment of metastatic prostate cancers [70]. A lipid-polymer hybrid nanoparticle system for drug delivery was recently developed. This system was composed of a hydrophobic PLGA core stabilized with lipid and PEG-conjugated lipid (lipid-PEG) surfactant. This hybrid lipid-polymer nanoparticle system showed excellent stability and ability to deliver drugs to prostate cancer cells in vitro [71,72].

## Dendrimers

Dendrimers are branched polymer structures that are produced by divergent or convergent synthetic techniques to yield very regular, virtually monodisperse macromolecules with rotational symmetry. Dendrimers are typically grown in "generations" with precisely defined chemical structures leading to nanoscale macromolecules, typically ~5 nm in diameter. Drugs or other medically relevant molecules can be incorporated into the dendrimer structure between the different branches, conjugated chemically, or adsorbed onto the surface [73]. The most commonly used dendrimer structure, the polyamido amine (PAMAM) dendrimer, has a net positive charge on its surface due to the presence of primary amine groups at the distal end of each dendrimer branch. It is possible, however, to modify those end groups to change the physicochemical nature of the dendrimer surface or to facilitate conjugation of other molecules. Dendrimers have been evaluated in a number of contexts for drug delivery. Due to their size and chemical groups, they have been evaluated extensively for nucleic acid delivery [74]. The presence of tertiary amines at junction points in the PAMAM dendrimer structure are hypothesized to be sites of protonation at the low pH of endosomes and lysosomes, which facilitates endosome escape and nuclear or cytoplasmic delivery of drugs. Dendrimers have also been shown to facilitate intracellular drug delivery by transiently perforating the plasma membrane [75]. Dendrimers have been shown to be toxic to cells at relatively low concentrations, particularly to red blood cells in vivo especially at higher generations [76], although through certain modifications, it is possible to reduce their cytotoxicity.

Various types of dendrimers have been developed for gene and siRNA delivery due to their inherent transfection potential. Amphiphilic dendrimers with a hydrophobic core and a hydrophilic exterior were shown to be more effective than many commercially available in vitro transfection reagents [77]. Another interesting architecture was a linear-dendritic hybrid polymer, which was developed to improve gene delivery. It is hypothesized that the dendrimer segment serves to condense the nucleic acid, while the linear segment was made of PEG functionalized with a targeting ligand at the distal end to provide selective uptake in cells [78]. Dendrimers have also been used to deliver boron-10 for boron neutron capture therapy. These dendrimers were targeted to the epidermal growth factor receptor (EGFR) expressing gliomas using boronated EGF [79].

## Nucleic acid delivery

Due to the particular challenges inherent in nucleic acid delivery, development of materials for this particular class of drugs has diverged from that of other drugs. Nucleic acids, from a physicochemical properties point of view, are large, negatively charged, and have defined secondary structures that are important functionally. The most relevant types of nucleic acid from a drug delivery perspective are DNA plasmids for gene therapy or DNA vaccines; antisense oligonucleotides; and double stranded RNAs, such as small interfering RNAs (siRNA) for activation of the RNA interference (RNAi) pathway. Many materials have been developed for nucleic acid delivery [80]; here, in broad strokes, we highlight some of the major trends, along with some illustrative examples from the recent literature.

Due to the physicochemical nature of these molecules, most nucleic acid delivery approaches have involved condensing the nucleic acid using a cationic material, such as cationic polymers, cationic lipids, or dendrimers. However, cationic materials tend to be toxic to cells due to their ability to damage the cell membrane, in addition to their relatively poor biodistribution, so some of these materials have been limited to in vitro cell transfections [81]. Many of these materials have been modified to improve biocompatibility, reduce toxicity, and improve in vivo circulation properties, but in many cases these modifications have also gone hand-in-hand with a reduction in the efficacy of the delivery system. Cationic lipid-like materials, known as "lipidoids," have been synthesized through combinatorial chemistry techniques into large libraries of materials with slightly different chemical functionalities [82]. This library of materials was screened in vitro for efficacy of siRNA delivery, with the most promising formulations being tested in various animal models all the way through nonhuman primates for delivery efficacy [83]. Perhaps not surprisingly, these lipidoid materials had excellent tropism for the liver, showing excellent ability to deliver a siRNA targeted to a protein produced in hepatocytes. These materials distributed according to their size and physicochemical properties only,

as they lacked any specific targeting ligand. This approach may make it difficult to target sites other than the liver, though using this approach, it may be possible to address this problem directly in the future. Cyclodextrin-containing polycations have been developed and studied extensively for targeted siRNA delivery to transferring receptors [84]. After showing effective target gene silencing in vitro, these nanoparticles were evaluated in vivo, showing a relatively modest but statistically significant reduction in tumor growth rate [85]. A multilamellar vesicle encapsulating siRNA targeted to cyclin D1 was targeted to $\beta_7$ integrins to use RNAi to reduce signs of intestinal inflammation [86]. Nucleic acid delivery will continue to be an area of active interest, as the advantages and potential of DNA vaccines RNAi and gene therapy will continue to motivate and inspire researchers to make an impact in this important field.

## Future directions

A more recent trend has been to design nanoparticles that have multiple biological functions, such as combining drug delivery with providing contrast for imaging (for more in depth discussion, please see specialized reviews [87,88]). The benefits of this type of approach are that more information can be obtained by having the tandem of imaging and drug delivery or localized hyperthermia, and that in some instances, this information can be used to improve treatment efficacy.

An important concept when designing multifunctional nanoparticles is that more is not necessarily better. The key attributes that make a good therapeutic nanoparticle are sometimes at odds with those that make a good contrast enhancing nanoparticle for imaging. In general, good attributes of a therapeutic nanoparticle are high drug loading per nanoparticle, a size that is both large enough and small enough to avoid excessive accumulation in the liver (~50–200 nm in diameter), extended blood circulation half-life to improve accumulation in target tissues or organs, and construction with materials that are nontoxic and biodegradable. Nanoparticles that have good properties for providing contrast enhancement will vary depending on the application. In general, they are relatively small in size (<50 nm) so that they can have good tissue distribution and are cleared relatively rapidly from the circulation so that contrast enhancement is maximal. In addition, one can tolerate use of slightly more toxic materials since the amount of nanoparticles administered for imaging applications are much smaller than that needed for therapeutic purposes.

For example, a multifunctional nanoparticle system that can deliver a drug and simultaneously report back when the drug has been released from the nanocarrier has been developed [89]. Other possible functions that can be engineered into a single nanoparticle carrier are in the case of remotely actuated nanoparticle systems, where drug release occurs following an external stimulus. In this setting, imaging can be used to provide feedback in real-time as to whether the drug has been released from a nanocarrier. This information could be used to alter the intensity of the external stimulus. For example, nanoparticles have been engineered to release a DNA intercalating agent in response to hyperthermia by using double-stranded DNA as a carrier [90]. As the nanoparticle is heated in a magnetic field, the annealing temperature of the DNA is exceeded, leading to denaturation of the double strand and release of the DNA-intercalating agent. Another interesting combination was near infrared (NIR) plasmon resonance activating gold nanoshells encapsulating magnetic iron oxide nanoparticles to provide simultaneous hyperthermia plus MRI contrast [91]. These nanoparticles were targeted to HER2/neu expressing breast cancer cells using an antibody and showed efficacy with relatively little power input.

## Conclusions

Nanotechnology has the potential to revolutionize the way that urological oncology is practiced by producing more potent vaccines for immunotherapy, enabling real-time monitoring of therapy using multifunctional nanoparticles, enhancing treatment efficacy while reducing side effects using nanoparticle delivery systems, and by increasing the sensitivity and specificity of imaging modalities to detect cancer using contrast enhancement with various imaging modalities. The common denominator to making these technologies clinically relevant lies in improving biocompatibility and biodistribution, which can be understood by recognizing that the important parameters are size,

physicochemical characteristics, PEGylation, and targeting ligand density. These variables affect how the nanomaterial interacts with several important organs in the body, particularly the liver, kidneys, spleen, and bone marrow. Enhanced permeability and retention is an important effect that leads to the accumulation of nanoscale materials in vascularized tumors. Over the next few years, we can expect more novel materials and perhaps more biomimetic, multifunctional materials as well as extension of current technologies to other diseases, including urological neoplasms.

## References

1. Panagi Z et al (2001) Effect of dose on the biodistribution and pharmacokinetics of PLGA and PLGA-mPEG nanoparticles. Int J Pharm 221(1–2): 143–152.
2. De Jong WH et al (2008) Particle size-dependent organ distribution of gold nanoparticles after intravenous administration. Biomaterials 29(12): 1912–1919.
3. Li SD, Huang L (2008) Pharmacokinetics and biodistribution of nanoparticles. Mol Pharm 5(4): 496–504.
4. Gref R et al (2000) 'Stealth' corona-core nanoparticles surface modified by polyethylene glycol (PEG): influences of the corona (PEG chain length and surface density) and of the core composition on phagocytic uptake and plasma protein adsorption. Colloids Surf B Biointerfaces 18(3–4): 301–313.
5. Gu F et al (2008) Precise engineering of targeted nanoparticles by using self-assembled biointegrated block copolymers. Proc Natl Acad Sci USA 105(7): 2586–2591.
6. Pirollo KF, Chang EH (2008) Does a targeting ligand influence nanoparticle tumor localization or uptake? Trends Biotechnol 26(10): 552–558.
7. Park JH et al (2009) Systematic surface engineering of magnetic nanoworms for in vivo tumor targeting. Small 5(6): 694–700.
8. Cheng C et al (2008) Functionalized thermoresponsive micelles self-assembled from biotin-PEG-b-P(NIPAAm-co-HMAAm)-b-PMMA for tumor cell target. Bioconjug Chem 19(6): 1194–1201.
9. Lee ES, Na K, Bae YH (2005) Super pH-sensitive multifunctional polymeric micelle. Nano Lett 5(2): 325–329.
10. Harris TJ et al (2008) Protease-triggered unveiling of bioactive nanoparticles. Small 4(9): 1307–1312.
11. Alberts B et al (2007) *Molecular Biology of the Cell*, 5th edn. New York: Garland Science
12. Alexis F et al (2008). Factors affecting the clearance and biodistribution of polymeric nanoparticles. Mol Pharm 5(4): 505–515.

13. Rennke H, Denker B, Rose B (2006) *Renal Pathophysiology*, 2nd edn. Baltimore, MD: Lippincott Williams & Wilkins

14. Kumar V, Fausto N, Abbas A (2004) *Robbins & Cotran Pathologic Basis of Disease*, 7th edn. Philadelphia, PA: Saunders

15. Desjardins M, Griffiths G (2003) Phagocytosis: latex leads the way. Curr Opin Cell Biol 15(4): 498–503.

16. Maeda H et al (2000) Tumor vascular permeability and the EPR effect in macromolecular therapeutics: a review. J Control Release 65(1–2): 271–284.

17. Kirpotin DB et al (2006) Antibody targeting of long-circulating lipidic nanoparticles does not increase tumor localization but does increase internalization in animal models. Cancer Res 66(13): 6732–6740.

18. Bartlett DW et al (2007) Impact of tumor-specific targeting on the biodistribution and efficacy of siRNA nanoparticles measured by multimodality in vivo imaging. Proc Natl Acad Sci U S A 104(39): 15549–15554.

19. Ishiwata H et al (2000) Characteristics and biodistribution of cationic liposomes and their DNA complexes. J Control Release 69(1): 139–148.

20. Neal JC et al (1998) Modification of the copolymers poloxamer 407 and poloxamine 908 can affect the physical and biological properties of surface modified nanospheres. Pharm Res 15(2): 318–324.

21. Ochietti B et al (2002) Altered organ accumulation of oligonucleotides using polyethyleneimine grafted with poly(ethylene oxide) or pluronic as carriers. J Drug Target 10(2): 113–121.

22. Jeong GJ et al (2007) Biodistribution and tissue expression kinetics of plasmid DNA complexed with polyethylenimines of different molecular weight and structure. J Control Release 118(1): 118–125.

23. Bragonzi A et al (2000) Biodistribution and transgene expression with nonviral cationic vector/DNA complexes in the lungs. Gene Ther 7(20): 1753–1760.

24. Campbell RB et al (2002) Cationic charge determines the distribution of liposomes between the vascular and extravascular compartments of tumors. Cancer Res 62(23): 6831–6836.

25. Boyd BJ et al (2006) Cationic poly-L-lysine dendrimers: pharmacokinetics, biodistribution, and evidence for metabolism and bioresorption after intravenous administration to rats. Mol Pharm 3(5): 614–627.

26. Brown MD, Schatzlein AG, Uchegbu IF (2001) Gene delivery with synthetic (non viral) carriers. Int J Pharm 229(1–2): 1–21.

27. Stossel TP et al (1972) Quantitative studies of phagocytosis by polymorphonuclear leukocytes: use of emulsions to measure the initial rate of phagocytosis. J Clin Invest 51(3): 615–624.

28. Heck JD, Costa M (1983) Influence of surface charge and dissolution on the selective phagocytosis of potentially carcinogenic particulate metal compounds. Cancer Res 43(12 Pt 1): 5652–5656.

29. Gref R et al (1994). Biodegradable long-circulating polymeric nanospheres. Science 263(5153): 1600–1603.

30. Hrkach JS et al (1997) Nanotechnology for biomaterials engineering: structural characterization of amphiphilic polymeric nanoparticles by 1H NMR spectroscopy. Biomaterials 18(1): 27–30.

31. Li L et al (2005) Protein adsorption on oligo(ethylene glycol)-terminated alkanethiolate self-assembled monolayers: The molecular basis for nonfouling behavior. J Phys Chem B 109(7): 2934–2941.

32. Sofia SJ, Premnath VV, Merrill EW (1998) Poly(ethylene oxide) grafted to silicon surfaces: grafting density and protein adsorption. Macromolecules 31(15): 5059–5070.

33. Pasche S et al (2005) Effects of ionic strength and surface charge on protein adsorption at PEGylated surfaces. J Phys Chem B 109(37): 17545–17552.

34. Champion JA, Mitragotri S (2009) Shape induced inhibition of phagocytosis of polymer particles. Pharm Res 26(1): 244–249.

35. Gratton SE et al (2008) The effect of particle design on cellular internalization pathways. Proc Natl Acad Sci USA 105(33): 11613–11618.

36. Simberg D et al (2007) Biomimetic amplification of nanoparticle homing to tumors. Proc Natl Acad Sci USA 104(3): 932–936.

37. Mesa C, Fernandez LE (2004) Challenges facing adjuvants for cancer immunotherapy. Immunol Cell Biol 82(6): 644–650.

38. Bitton RJ (2004) Cancer vaccines: a critical review on clinical impact. Curr Opin Mol Ther 6(1): 17–26.

39. Fong L, Engleman EG (2000) Dendritic cells in cancer immunotherapy. Annu Rev Immunol 18: 245–273.

40. Lehrfeld TJ, Lee DI (2008) Dendritic cell vaccines for the treatment of prostate cancer. Urol Oncol 26(6): 576–580.

41. Caputo A et al (2008) Functional polymeric nano/microparticles for surface adsorption and delivery of protein and DNA vaccines. Curr Drug Deliv 5(4): 230–242.

42. McKeever U et al (2002) Protective immune responses elicited in mice by immunization with formulations of poly(lactide-co-glycolide) microparticles. Vaccine 20(11–12): 1524–1531.

43. Hamdy S et al (2008) Co-delivery of cancer-associated antigen and Toll-like receptor 4 ligand in PLGA nanoparticles induces potent CD8+ T cell-mediated anti-tumor immunity. Vaccine 26(39): 5046–5057.

44. Gupta PN et al (2007) M-cell targeted biodegradable PLGA nanoparticles for oral immunization against hepatitis B. J Drug Target 15(10): 701–713.

45. Garinot M et al (2007) PEGylated PLGA-based nanoparticles targeting M cells for oral vaccination. J Control Release 120(3): 195–204.

46. Gutierro I et al (2002) Size dependent immune response after subcutaneous, oral and intranasal administration of BSA loaded nanospheres. Vaccine 21(1–2): 67–77.

47. Zhou X et al (2008) The effect of conjugation to gold nanoparticles on the ability of low molecular weight chitosan to transfer DNA vaccine. Biomaterials 29(1): 111–117.

48. Verma A et al (2008) Surface-structure-regulated cell-membrane penetration by monolayer-protected nanoparticles. Nat Mater 7(7): 588–595.

49. Hu Y et al (2007) Cytosolic delivery of membrane-impermeable molecules in dendritic cells using pH-responsive core-shell nanoparticles. Nano Lett 7(10): 3056–3064.

50. Manolova V et al (2008) Nanoparticles target distinct dendritic cell populations according to their size. Eur J Immunol 38(5): 1404–1413.

51. Fenske DB, Chonn A, Cullis PR (2008) Liposomal nanomedicines: an emerging field. Toxicol Pathol 36(1): 21–29.

52. Wilson KD et al (2009) The combination of stabilized plasmid lipid particles and lipid nanoparticle encapsulated CpG containing oligodeoxynucleotides as a systemic genetic vaccine. J Gene Med 11(1): 14–25.

53. de Jong S et al (2007) Encapsulation in liposomal nanoparticles enhances the immunostimulatory, adjuvant and anti-tumor activity of subcutaneously administered CpG ODN. Cancer Immunol Immunother 56(8): 1251–1264.

54. Huang X et al (2006) Cancer cell imaging and photothermal therapy in the near-infrared region by using gold nanorods. J Am Chem Soc 128(6): 2115–2120.

55. Torchilin VP et al (1994) Poly(ethylene glycol) on the liposome surface: on the mechanism of polymer-coated liposome longevity. Biochim Biophys Acta 1195(1): 11–20.

56. Goren D et al (1996) Targeting of stealth liposomes to erbB-2 (Her/2) receptor: in vitro and in vivo studies. Br J Cancer 74(11): 1749–1756.

57. Sawant RM et al (2008) Prostate cancer-specific monoclonal antibody 5D4 significantly enhances the cytotoxicity of doxorubicin-loaded liposomes against target cells in vitro. J Drug Target 16(7): 601–604.

58. Ikegami S et al (2006) Targeting gene therapy for prostate cancer cells by liposomes complexed with antiprostate-specific membrane antigen monoclonal antibody. Hum Gene Ther 17(10): 997–1005.

59. Sawant RM et al (2006) "SMART" drug delivery systems: double-targeted pH-responsive pharmaceutical nanocarriers. Bioconjug Chem 17(4): 943–949.

60. Otsuka H, Nagasaki Y, Kataoka K (2003) PEGylated nanoparticles for biological and pharmaceutical applications. Adv Drug Deliv Rev 55(3): 403–419.

61. Lee Y et al (2007) A protein nanocarrier from charge-conversion polymer in response to endosomal pH. J Am Chem Soc 129(17): 5362–5363.

62. Itaka K et al (2004) Supramolecular nanocarrier of siRNA from PEG-based block catiomer carrying diamine side chain with distinctive pKa directed to enhance intracellular gene silencing. J Am Chem Soc 126(42): 13612–13613.

63. Yin H et al (2008) Physicochemical characteristics of pH-sensitive poly(L-histidine)-b-poly(ethylene glycol)/poly(L-lactide)-b-poly(ethylene glycol) mixed micelles. J Control Release 126(2): 130–138.

64. Lee ES, Gao Z, Bae YH (2008) Recent progress in tumor pH targeting nanotechnology. J Control Release 132(3): 164–170.

65. Saltzman WM, Langer R (1989) Transport rates of proteins in porous materials with known microgeometry. Biophys J 55(1): 163–171.

66. Langer R, Folkman J (1976) Polymers for the sustained release of proteins and other macromolecules. Nature 263(5580): 797–800.

67. Creque HM, Langer R, Folkman J (1980) One month of sustained release of insulin from a polymer implant. Diabetes 29(1): 37–40.

68. Farokhzad OC et al (2004) Nanoparticle-aptamer bioconjugates: a new approach for targeting prostate cancer cells. Cancer Res 64(21): 7668–7672.

69. Cheng J et al (2007) Formulation of functionalized PLGA-PEG nanoparticles for in vivo targeted drug delivery. Biomaterials 28(5): 869–876.

70. Dhar S et al (2008) Targeted delivery of cisplatin to prostate cancer cells by aptamer functionalized Pt(IV) prodrug-PLGA-PEG nanoparticles. Proc Natl Acad Sci U S A 105(45): 17356–17361.

71. Zhang L et al (2008) Self-assembled lipid–polymer hybrid nanoparticles: a robust drug delivery platform. ACS Nano 2(8): 1696–1702.

72. Chan JM et al (2009) PLGA-lecithin-PEG core-shell nanoparticles for controlled drug delivery. Biomaterials 30(8): 1627–1634.

73. Lee CC et al (2005) Designing dendrimers for biological applications. Nat Biotechnol 23(12): 1517–1526.

74. Dufes C, Uchegbu IF, Schatzlein AG (2005) Dendrimers in gene delivery. Adv Drug Deliv Rev 57(15): 2177–2202.

75. Hong S et al (2006) Interaction of polycationic polymers with supported lipid bilayers and cells: nanoscale

hole formation and enhanced membrane permeability. Bioconjug Chem 17(3): 728–734.

76. Malik N et al (2000) Dendrimers: relationship between structure and biocompatibility in vitro, and preliminary studies on the biodistribution of 125I-labelled polyamidoamine dendrimers in vivo. J Control Release 65(1–2): 133–148.

77. Joester D et al (2003) Amphiphilic dendrimers: novel self-assembling vectors for efficient gene delivery. Angew Chem Int Ed Engl 42(13): 1486–1490.

78. Wood KC et al (2005) A family of hierarchically self-assembling linear-dendritic hybrid polymers for highly efficient targeted gene delivery. Angew Chem Int Ed Engl 44(41): 6704–6708.

79. Barth RF et al (2002) Molecular targeting of the epidermal growth factor receptor for neutron capture therapy of gliomas. Cancer Res 62(11): 3159–3166.

80. Nguyen DN et al (2009) Polymeric materials for gene delivery and DNA vaccination. Advanced Materials 21(8): 847–867.

81. Hunter AC (2006) Molecular hurdles in polyfectin design and mechanistic background to polycation induced cytotoxicity. Adv Drug Deliv Rev 58(14): 1523–1531.

82. Akinc A et al (2008) A combinatorial library of lipid-like materials for delivery of RNAi therapeutics. Nat Biotechnol 26(5): 561–569.

83. John M et al (2007) Effective RNAi-mediated gene silencing without interruption of the endogenous microRNA pathway. Nature 449(7163): 745–747.

84. Bartlett DW, Davis ME (2007) Physicochemical and biological characterization of targeted, nucleic acid-containing nanoparticles. Bioconjug Chem 18(2): 456–468.

85. Bartlett DW, Davis ME (2008) Impact of tumor-specific targeting and dosing schedule on tumor growth inhibition after intravenous administration of siRNA-containing nanoparticles. Biotechnol Bioeng 99(4): 975–985.

86. Peer D et al (2008) Systemic leukocyte-directed siRNA delivery revealing cyclin D1 as an anti-inflammatory target. Science 319(5863): 627–630.

87. Torchilin VP (2006) Multifunctional nanocarriers. Adv Drug Deliv Rev 58(14): 1532–1555.

88. Torchilin V (2009) Multifunctional and stimuli-sensitive pharmaceutical nanocarriers. Eur J Pharm Biopharm 71(3): 431–444.

89. Bagalkot V et al (2007) Quantum dot-aptamer conjugates for synchronous cancer imaging, therapy, and sensing of drug delivery based on bi-fluorescence resonance energy transfer. Nano Lett 7(10): 3065–3070.

90. Derfus AM et al (2007) Remotely triggered release from magnetic nanoparticles. Advanced Materials. 19(22): 3932–3936.

91. Kim J et al (2006) Designed fabrication of multifunctional magnetic gold nanoshells and their application to magnetic resonance imaging and photothermal therapy. Angew Chem Int Ed Engl 45(46): 7754–7758.

**117**

# Imaging in diagnosis and staging of urologic cancers: magnetic resonance imaging

*Jurgen J. Fütterer*[1] *and Stijn T.W.P.J. Heijmijnk*[2]

[1]Department of Interventional Radiology, Nijmegen Medical Center, Radboud University, Nijmegan, The Netherlands
[2]Department of Radiology, Nymegen Medical Center, Radboud University, Nymegen, The Netherlands

## Introduction

Imaging has given radiology a significant role in the diagnosis and staging of urinary tract tumors. Magnetic resonance imaging (MRI) offers advantages in imaging urinary tumors due to superior soft-tissue contrast. This chapter will review the role of MRI in imaging malignant lesions of the urinary tract.

## Kidney

Renal cell carcinoma (RCC) is a large socioeconomic problem, accounting for more than 3% of the estimated new cancer cases in men [1]. The worldwide incidence of RCC is increasing [6]. Most renal tumors arise from the renal parenchyma ($\pm$90%) [7], with smaller numbers arising from the mesenchyma or the urothelium of the renal collecting system. RCC occurs twice as often in men as in women. Cigarette smoking contributes to the development of RCC in one-third of the patients [8]. This chapter will mainly focus on the RCC. The classic triad of flank pain, hematuria, and a palpable flank mass occurs in less than 5% to 15% of patients with RCC [9,10]. Initial presentation with clinical symptoms like anorexia, weight loss, tiredness, varicocele, or paraneoplastic syndromes are seen. It is estimated, that 10% to 40% of patients with RCC will develop a paraneoplastic syndrome. Hypercalcemia is the most common of the paraneoplastic syndromes (13% to 20% of patients [11–13]).

Of those with hypercalcemia and RCC, approximately 75% have high-stage lesions [10,14].

The widespread availability of cross-sectional imaging modalities in clinical practice, particularly computed tomography (CT) and MRI, led to an increased detection rate of renal masses. Up to 30% to 40% of RCCs are discovered at imaging [15]. Accurate characterization of renal masses is essential for adequate patient management. Ultrasonography and multidetector CT are commonly used for renal imaging. MR imaging can particularly be used to characterize renal lesions. Correlating the anatomical findings and MR signal intensity characteristics with the clinical features allows optimal diagnosis and staging.

### Clinical staging

The goal of any staging system is to combine available data about malignant disease to assess prognosis and survival characteristics, as well as to stratify appropriate treatment modalities. The tumor, nodes, and metastases (TNM) staging system is the most often used staging system in patients with RCC. RCC was first categorized by the TNM staging system in 1974 [32]. The current version of the 2002 TNM staging of the American Joint Committee on cancer is presented in Table 1 of [33]. Prognosis is generally reflected in staging severity, with lower-stage disease being associated with longer survival rates. The prognosis is clearly adversely affected by spread of the tumor beyond the renal fascia and into the retroperitoneum, i.e., stage

*Interventional Techniques in Uro-oncology*, First Edition. Edited by Hashim Uddin Ahmed, Manit Arya, Peter T. Scardino & Mark Emberton. © 2011 Blackwell Publishing Ltd. Published 2011 by Blackwell Publishing Ltd.

T3a and higher. The 5-year cancer-specific survival of patients with pT4 RCC and lymph node metastases are 20% and 5% to 30%, respectively [34].

Regional lymph node involvement, with or without distant metastases, is present in less than 10% of the patients who undergo surgery as their first line of treatment. Twenty-five percent to thirty-three percent of the patients who present with RCC have metastases at presentation [35,36]. The most common sites of metastases are the lung (75%), bone (40%), liver (40%), soft tissues, and brain [7]. Uncommon sites are thyroid, skin, gallbladder, pancreas, orbits, and bladder [7,35,37,38]. Clinical data have shown that the localization and number of metastases have an independent prognostic value distinct form other clinical and pathologic variables. Bone or liver metastases are associated with worse prognosis compared with lung metastases. Furthermore, large tumors tend to be associated with more advanced dissemination.

## MR technique

The imaging protocol for effective MRI of the kidney should include maximal soft-tissue contrast, exploit the sensitivity of MRI to contrast material enhancement, and make use of the multiplanar capability of this modality. Due its intrinsic high soft-tissue contrast, MR imaging has many advantages over other imaging modalities in the detection and staging of RCC [39].

MR imaging is performed with a multiarray coil with the patient in supine position. The basic protocol of the kidneys includes a single-shot T2-weighted sequence, turbo or fast spin-echo T2-weighted fat-suppressed sequence in two directions (preferably, coronal and axial), and T1-weighted images acquired as non-suppressed and fat-suppressed sequences. Images are supplemented by coronal dynamic contrast-enhanced 3-dimensional spoiled gradient-echo sequences (arterial, nephrogenic [20 seconds after corticomedullary phase], and pyelographic phases [30 seconds after nephrogenic phase]) with fat-suppression. MR urography can be helpful in the evaluation of pathology in the collecting duct [40]. Both heavily T2-weighted images and gadolinium-enhanced T1-weighted images can be used to evaluate the collecting system. The former technique can be obtained with fast single-shot T2-weighted MR imaging techniques and respiratory-gated 3D turbo or fast spin-echo techniques. Gadolinium-enhanced MR urography can be performed using a high-resolution 3D T1-weighted sequence or breath-hold 3D fat-saturated T1-weighted gradient-echo sequence after administration of gadolinium contrast material.

Fast acquisition, single-shot MRI techniques can be used in patients with poor breath-hold capacity. The kidneys have restricted motion during respiration due to their retroperitoneal location. This is the reason why renal MR images are frequently insensitive to movements. Drawbacks of single-shot acquisition techniques (e.g., single-shot half-Fourier turbo spin-echo or single-shot fast spin-echo) are signal-to-noise limitations and some blurring of the MR images.

The normal kidney has a relatively long T2 time. The renal medulla is hyperintense to the renal cortex on T2-weighted MR images. The renal parenchyma is hyperintense relative to the liver, and close in signal intensity to the spleen. The renal cortex is slightly higher in signal intensity than the medulla on T1-weighted MR images. The medulla has a similar signal intensity compared with muscle. Most renal cysts are high in signal on T2-weighted images and low in signal on T1-weighted images due to their long relaxation time (Figure 8.1). High signal intensity on T1-weighted images and low signal intensity on T2-weighted images can be seen within cysts when they are complicated by hemorrhage or contain proteinaceous fluid. Solid tumors can demonstrate variable signal intensity on T2-weighted images, and have slightly lower signal intensity than that of the renal cortex on T1-weighted images. Fat-containing lesions, like angiomyolipoma, have high signal intensity compared to the renal cortex. T1-weighted sequences with fat suppression can be applied to confirm the diagnosis of angiomyolipoma (macroscopic fat within the angiomyolipoma will be suppressed). In- and opposed-phase T1-weighted MR imaging can be used to reliably diagnose angiomyolipoma (macroscopic fat). Clear cell renal carcinoma (intracellular fat) can be confirmed with the latter technique. This will result in a relative focal or diffuse loss of signal intensity on opposed-phase images.

Coronal T2-weighted, pre- and postcontrast T1-weighted MR images are frequently helpful to evaluate the superior and inferior borders of the renal lesion, characterize the lesion as cystic or solid, or demonstrate perirenal extension. The dynamic contrast-enhanced 3-dimensional spoiled gradient-echo

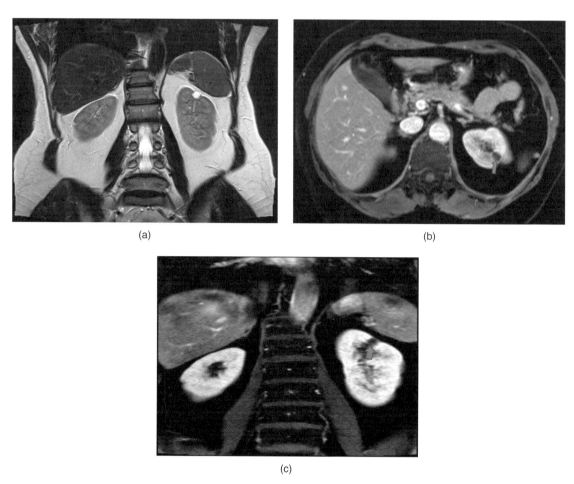

(a)

(b)

(c)

**Fig 8.1** MRI in man who had an indeterminate lesion on cross-sectional contrast-enhanced CT and B-mode ultrasound image. MRI demonstrates a fluid-filled lesion (a) with no enhancement of wall or septations indicating a simple cyst (b and c). (Courtesy of Hashim U Ahmed, University College London.)

sequences may aid to further delineate the primary tumor, liver lesions, and to evaluate any vascular thrombus identified.

### Tumor localization

RCC is a heterogeneous disease with multiple subtypes that differ in their histopathologic features. These histopathologic entities differ in their prognosis and biologic behavior. In addition, these entities differ in their response to therapies.

Clear cell carcinoma commonly appears heterogeneous at imaging due to the presence of hemorrhage, necrosis, and cysts (Figures 8.2 and 8.3). Clear cell

RCC originates from the renal cortex and typically exhibits an expansile growth pattern. Multicentricity and bilaterality are rare (<5%) in sporadic cases [41–46]. Clear cell carcinoma is hypo- to isointense on T1-weighted MR images, and iso- to hyperintense on T2-weighted MR images [41,43]. Clear cell tumors typically show hypervascularity on contrast-enhanced MR imaging. This hypervascularity has been ascribed to inactivation of tumor suppressor genes and subsequent elaboration of vascular and other growth factors [47]. The degree of enhancement may help to differentiate clear cell carcinoma from nonclear cell variants [45,46]. Lesions with microscopic lipid content show a conspicuous drop in signal intensity on

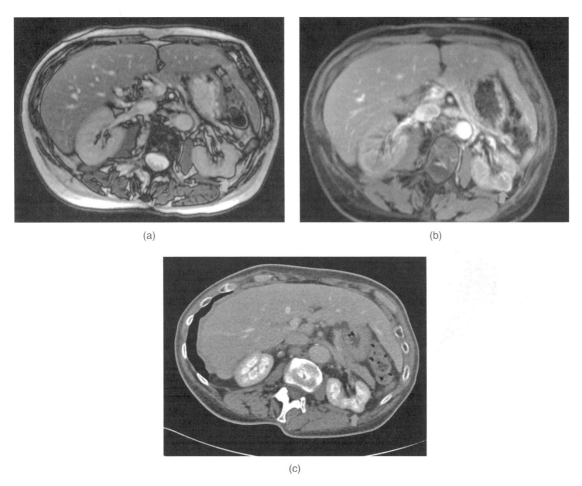

(a)

(b)

(c)

**Fig 8.2** Renal lesion in left kidney indeterminate on cross-sectional CT imaging. T2W MRI is also indeterminate (a), but on enhancement with gadolinium, the lesion and wall demonstrate suspicious enhancement (b and c). Histology from surgery demonstrated clear cell renal carcinoma. (Courtesy of Hashim U Ahmed, University College London.)

images obtained at an opposed-phase echo time compared to in-phase gradient-echo images. Clear cell carcinoma may demonstrate considerable signal intensity drop on opposed-phase echo time MR images due to the presence of abundant microscopic fat [44].

Papillary RCC commonly demonstrates low signal intensity on T2-weighted scans due to the presence of byproducts of hemorrhage and necrosis [42]. Larger tumors demonstrate heterogeneity due to necrosis, hemorrhage, and calcification. Unlike clear cell carcinoma, papillary RCC typically demonstrates relative hypovascularity at MRI. Papillary tumors demonstrate lesser degree of contrast-enhancement than clear

cell tumors at contrast-enhanced MR imaging. An important feature of papillary RCC is that bilateral and multifocal tumors are more common than in other subtypes of RCC.

Chromophobe RCC may present as a low signal intensity on T2-weighted images. Chromophobe RCC demonstrates relatively homogeneous enhancement at MRI. Recently, a spoke-wheel pattern of contrast-enhancement classically associated with oncocytomas has recently been described in association with chromophobe RCC [48]. Oncocytomas develop from type B intercalated cells of the cortical collecting duct, and are indistinguishable from RCC on MR imaging.

**121**

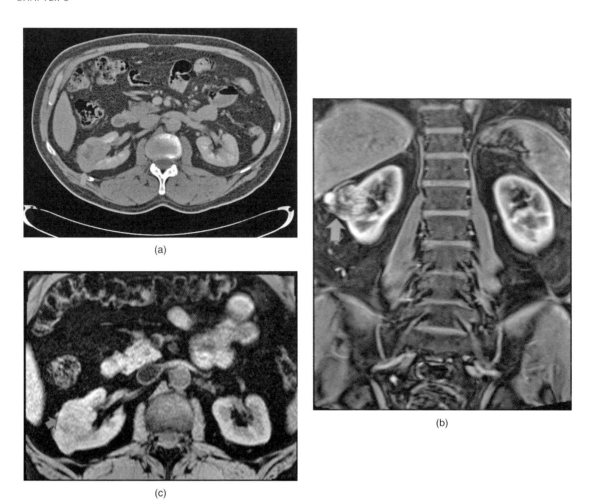

(a)

(b)

(c)

**Fig 8.3** Renal lesion in right kidney indeterminate on cross-sectional CT imaging with the possibility of oncocytoma raised (a). MRI enhancement with gadolinium shows the lesion and wall demonstrate suspicious enhancement, (b) although diffusion weighting is less conclusive (c). Histology from surgery demonstrated clear cell renal carcinoma. (Courtesy of Hashim U Ahmed, University College London.)

Collecting duct carcinoma is characterized by an infiltrative growth pattern at MR imaging. Collecting duct carcinoma commonly demonstrates low signal intensity on T2-weighted MRI and hypovascularity with contrast-enhancement.

### Local staging

Accurate presurgical measurement of tumor size is possible with MR imaging. The presence of a pseudo-capsule surrounding the tumor predicts the absence of perinephric fat involvement (capsular invasion) [49].

This pseudocapsule is seen as a linear low signal intensity on T1- and T2-weighted images in 66% of patients with RCC $\leq$ 4 cm in diameter. Aggressive tumors are usually poorly marginated and a pseudocapsule is not visualized. Opposed-phase MRI can be applied to detect perinephric extension. The renal contour is artificially accentuated by the black line (India ink artifact) at renal-retroperitoneal fat interface caused by the chemical shift artifact in these images [50].

Venous tumor thrombus can also be demonstrated. The inferior vena cava is involved in 3% to 22.5% of patients with RCC. Vena cava inferior thrombus is not a contraindication for surgical resection. The 5-year survival rates as high as 68% are found in patients with RCC and venous thrombus extending into the inferior vena cava [51].

The histologic presence of tumor necrosis has been correlated with a poor prognosis [22]. Macroscopic tumor necrosis can be appreciated on contrast-enhanced MR imaging. However, some necrotic features are beyond the resolution of current imaging techniques. While microscopically tumor necrosis has been associated with a worse prognosis in clear cell and chromophobe RCC; this correlation has not been found in papillary RCC [22].

Lymph node metastases have a significant impact on the prognosis of patients with malignancies. Lymph node involvement occurs in approximately 10% to 20% of the patients with RCC without evidence of distant metastases. Since benign and malignant lymph nodes have similar signal intensities in conventional MR imaging, metastatic lymph nodes are mainly identified by node enlargement. This may result in missing small metastases in normal-sized nodes, resulting in false-negative metastasis. Routine cross-sectional imaging modalities, such as CT and conventional nonenhanced MR imaging, have a limited sensitivity in identifying lymph node metastases. Using a cut-off of 1 cm for short-axis nodal size, sensitivity and specificity of 83% and 88% have been reported, respectively.

## Local recurrence

Surgical resection is the only effective means of cure for clinically localized renal tumors [52]. Total nephrectomy and partial nephrectomy (nephron-sparing) are equally effective in selected groups. Local recurrence in the nephrectomy bed occurs in 20% to 40% of the patients, within the first 5 years after surgery [53]. Isolated recurrences in the nephrectomy bed are uncommon [54]. MRI can be used as a follow-up imaging tool, however CT is the most sensitive imaging technique for follow-up in the abdomen.

## Diffusion-weighted imaging

The risk of nephrogenic systemic fibrosis (NSF) in patients with significantly impaired renal function, which is considered to be associated with some gadolinium-based contrast agents, should be considered carefully when staging with MRI [55,56]. Diffusion-weighted MRI provides both qualitative and quantitative tissue characterization without the need for intravenous contrast material. The use of diffusion-weighted imaging has been investigated for various renal diseases, such as infection, ischemia, chronic renal disease, and parenchymal diseases [57–61]. Currently, there are limited reports available on the use of diffusion-weighting in renal mass characterization and localization [62–65]. This type of imaging has equivalent performance to that of the enhancement ratio in the diagnosis of nonfat containing T1 hyperintense renal lesions [66]. Renal solid masses demonstrate lower apparent diffusion coefficients compared to simple cysts ($1.7 \pm 0.48 \times 10^{-3}$ mm$^2$/s vs. $3.65$ $0.09 \times 10^{-3}$ mm$^2$/s) [62,64]. The apparent diffusion coefficient of normal renal tissue was $2.19 \pm 0.17 \times 10^{-3}$ mm$^2$/s, which was significantly higher compared to solid benign and malignant lesions ($1.55 \pm 0.20 \times 10^{-3}$ mm$^2$/s) [63]. Diffusion-weighted MR imaging can provide additional information to that acquired with contrast-enhancement for the diagnosis of oncocytoma, and may be used to characterize histologic subtypes of RCC [67].

## Dynamic-contrast imaging

Accurate characterization of complex renal masses is based primarily on the presence or absence of enhancement on dynamic contrast-enhanced MR imaging [68]. The presence of enhancement generally indicates a diagnosis of RCC. A 15% increase in signal intensity within a renal lesion at 2 to 4 minutes after administration of contrast material has been proposed as an optimal threshold for distinguishing benign cysts from malignancies [69]. Recent developments in the understanding of the biology of RCC have substantial therapeutic implications. Some subtypes of RCC are less responding to tyrosine inhibiting treatment options, for example patients with papillary or chromophobe RCC [70,71]. With MR imaging, enhancement can be assessed by measuring signal intensity changes or evaluated visually with or without image subtraction [67]. Hyper- (e.g., clear cell carcinomas) and relative hypovascular lesions (e.g., papillary RCCs) demonstrate different enhancement patterns using dynamic contrast-enhanced MR imaging [69]. Measurement of relative enhancement in renal masses, by placing manually defined ROIs within the lesion, on the basis of percentage increase in signal intensity following intravenous gadolinium contrast administration can be applied. Applying this strategy resulted in a sensitivity of 100% and specificity of 94% for distinguishing cysts from solid renal masses (>15% enhancement ratio) [72]. Enhancement ratios obtained with MR imaging are arbitrary and depend on the coil system and pulse sequence used. Both quantitative and qualitative methods are sensitive in the detection of enhancement within a renal mass [73]. The characterization of T1-weighted hyperintense lesions (which include hemorrhagic or proteinaceous cysts and RCC) can be problematic in the determination of enhancement owing to high signal intensity on precontrast MR images. Hence, in lesions that are hyperintense on T1-weighted unenhanced MR images, qualitative assessment based on image subtraction should be performed to avoid false-negative quantitative results [73].

## Bladder

Bladder cancer is the most expensive of all malignancies treated in the United States from diagnosis to death [74,75]. Carcinoma of the urinary bladder, after prostate cancer, is the most common malignant tumor of the urinary tract and accounts for 2% of all malignancies. Bladder cancer is more common in males than in females with a ratio of approximately 4:1, and is predominantly seen in the sixth and seventh decades of life [76]. Bladder cancer is rare in the first decade of life.

### Clinical staging

Clinical staging is not reliable for determining tumor extension. Imaging modalities are needed to determine tumor extension beyond the bladder wall [77]. Differentiation between superficial and invasive bladder tumors is essential. Preoperative MRI is the modality of choice for imaging the urinary bladder due to the superior soft-tissue contrast (Figure 8.4).

Clinical management of urinary bladder cancer is determined primarily on the basis of distinguishing superficial tumors from invasive ones (stage ≤ T1 vs. stage T2 and higher; Table 2 of [33]). The treatment options differ considerably. Noninvasive tumors are treated with transurethral resection alone, whereas invasive tumors are treated with radical cystectomy, radiation therapy, chemotherapy, or a combination [87,88]. Approximately 66% to 80% of all bladder cancers are noninvasive and associated with a 5-year survival of 81%.

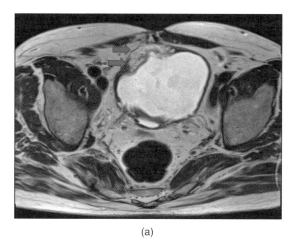

(a)

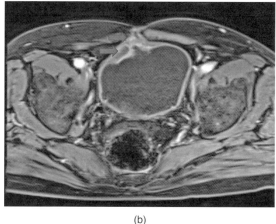

(b)

**Fig 8.4** A man with a long-term suprapubic catheter in situ for urethral injury refractory to multiple repairs. Presented with bleeding and recurrent urinary tract infections. Examination revealed a hard indurated mass around the suprapubic catheter site. Bladder biopsies demonstrated keratinizing squamous metaplasia with a small focus of moderately differentiated mucin-producing adenocarcinoma. MRI shows an infiltrating mass on unenhanced (a) and enhanced images (b) suspicious for malignancy. Radical cystectomy with excision of skin around suprapubic catheter site was performed. (Courtesy of Hashim U Ahmed, University College London.)

Invasive bladder cancer initially spreads through the inner bladder wall and then circumferentially through the muscular layer. Depending on the location of the bladder tumor, it may invade perivesical fat, prostate, obturator internus muscle, or seminal vesicle. In women, it rarely invades the cervix or uterus. Invasion of or growth into the urethra or ureter is common when the tumor originates near one of these structures [89]. Lymphatic spread is found in 25% of invasive tumors, and is seen in the three major lymphatic trunks that drain into the external iliac groups. Hematogenous spread of urinary bladder cancer is infrequently seen. If it occurs, these metastases usually appear in the bones, lungs, and liver. Bony metastases predominantly are seen in, in order of frequency, pelvic bones, upper femora, ribs, and skull, and are always osteolytic [99].

## MR technique

MR imaging is superior to CT for staging carcinoma of the urinary bladder, and offers several advantages over CT. The imaging protocol for effective MR imaging of the bladder should include maximal soft-tissue contrast, exploit the sensitivity of MR imaging to contrast material enhancement, and make use of the multiplanar capability of this modality. This allows improved evaluation of the location and extent of the tumor, as well as improved characterization of the lesion.

MR imaging is performed with a multiarray coil with the patient in supine position. The basic protocol of the bladder includes turbo or fast spin-echo, or gradient-recalled echo T1-weighted sequence and turbo or fast spin-echo T2-weighted sequence in two directions. The direction of the planes depends on the site of the lesion. A plane perpendicular to the wall at the base of the tumor can be acquired. This allows better delineation of muscle involvement. The coronal plane is helpful for visualizing tumor arising from the base, dome, and lateral bladder wall. The sagittal plane can be used to visualize anterior and cranially located tumors and tumors at the bladder sphincter. A short tau inversion recovery sequence through the pelvis is included in the protocol. Images are supplemented by dynamic contrast-enhanced fat-suppressed 3-dimensional spoiled gradient-echo sequences before at 20 seconds (arterial phase), and at 70 seconds (venous phase) after administration of gadolinium contrast material (0.1 mmol/kg). Adequate distension of

the bladder will improve evaluation of the bladder wall and allows visualization of focal lesions. However, if the bladder is too distended, this may result in overlooking small lesions. Optimally, the patient is asked to void 2 hours before the MRI scan acquisition [91].

The urine has a low signal intensity on T1-weighted images, and a high signal intensity on T2-weighted images. The normal bladder wall has an intermediate signal intensity equal to skeletal muscle on T1-weighted images, and a low signal intensity on T2-weighted images. On fat-saturated T1-weighted images the bladder wall has a slightly higher signal intensity than urine or perivesical fat [91,92]. On fat-saturated T2-weighted images, perivesical fat and bladder wall have low signal intensity. Perivesical vessels and the vas deferens appear as low signal intensity tubular structures on T1-weighted sequences.

Immediately after injection of gadolinium contrast material the urinary bladder wall demonstrates rapid enhancement. The inner mucosa and submucosa (more vascular) shows early enhancement, while the muscular layer (less vascular) enhances later [93]. The imaging plane can be preselected on the previously performed T1- or T2-weighted sequences.

## Local staging

Both T1- and T2-weighted images are useful in staging bladder cancers [94–98]. Urinary bladder cancer has intermediate signal intensity, equal to that of the muscle on T1-weighted images. T1-weighted MR images are used to assess perivesical fat invasion, involvement of surrounding organs (except for the prostate), lymph node involvement, and bone marrow. On T2-weighted images, bladder tumors have the same or slightly higher signal intensity as the bladder wall. T2-weighted images are recommended for assessment of the extent of tumor invasion into the muscle layer of the bladder wall and prostate. Mr staging accuracies ranged from 72% to 95% reported in literature. The addition of contrast agent to the imaging protocol also increased the staging accuracy (9% to 14% increase) compared to unenhanced MR imaging [99–101]. The most accurate staging results are obtained using intravenous gadolinium contrast material and fast T1-weighed sequences.

Currently, there are limited reports available on the use of diffusion-weighted MR imaging in bladder cancer localization and staging [102–104]. Diffusion-weighted images are a highly reliable imaging method for identification of bladder tumors in patients with gross hematuria [103]. The staging accuracy significantly increased adding diffusion-weighting to T2-weighted and dynamic contrast-enhanced MRI [104].

Papillary transitional cell carcinoma of the bladder has a loose connective tissue stalk. The stalk is defined as a structure that extends from the bladder wall to the center of the tumor with signal intensity different from that of the tumor [105]. Most stalks show lower signal intensity than tumor on T2-weighted images, less enhancement on early contrast-enhanced MR imaging, and stronger enhancement on delayed-enhancement MR images. The identification of the stalk is an important finding to exclude muscle wall invasion of the tumor [105].

An intact, low signal intensity muscle layer of the bladder wall at the base of the tumor is classified as stage Ta or T1 disease. The use of gadolinium contrast agents has improved the imaging of bladder carcinomas. Bladder carcinoma tends to enhance more than the surrounding bladder wall early after injection of contrast agent. Early contrast-enhanced images may help to recognize muscle wall infiltration. Findings suggesting superficial tumors (stage T1 and lower) are, smooth muscle layer, tenting of the bladder wall, fernlike vasculature, and uninterrupted submucosal enhancement. Differentiation between Ta tumor from T1 is problematic, and can be better delineated on contrast-enhanced studies.

A disrupted low signal intensity muscle layer without infiltration of perivesical fat is classified as stage T2b disease. Muscle wall invasion is divided into superficial and deep (stage T2a vs. T2b). Differentiation of stage T2a and stage T2b with MR imaging is usually not possible.

A focal, irregular decrease in fat signal intensity on T1- and T2-weighted images is classified as stage T3b disease (macroscopic perivesical fat infiltration). On contrast-enhanced T1-weigthed images, a lesion with an irregular, shaggy outer border, and streaky areas of the same signal intensity of the tumor in perivesical fat is classified as stage T3b.

Invasion of the tumor into an adjacent organ or abdominal and pelvic sidewall may be inferred from the extension of abnormal tumor signal intensity through fat planes into adjacent structures. Contrast-enhanced MR imaging demonstrate these findings well.

## Lymph node staging

CT and MR imaging are comparable regarding staging of lymph nodes. Accuracies ranging from 73% to 98% are found with MR imaging. Lymph node metastasis in patients with superficial tumors is rare. When the deep muscle layer is involved or if extravesical invasion is seen, the incidence of lymph node metastasis rises to 30% and 60%, respectively. CT and MR imaging have a low sensitivity (76%) as metastases in normal-sized lymph nodes are still missed.

## Prostate

MR imaging is the most widely used cross-sectional imaging technique for prostate cancer. While ultrasound provides real-time data, it is also highly operator-dependent and experience is needed in order to perform it. In addition, it provides little by way in information that can differentiate tumor from benign tissue in the modern era in which tumors are smaller. MR imaging allows for a more standardized examination of the prostate, and with the addition of functional imaging techniques [106] such as diffusion-weighting, proton MR spectroscopy, and dynamic contrast-enhancment a unique insight can be obtained in the cancer characteristics.

Currently, at a field strength of 1.5 tesla (T), the use of an endorectal coil (ERC) in combination with an external phased-array coil is the set up of choice for optimal imaging of the prostate [107,108]. At 3 T it is possible to perform the local prostate imaging using only an ERC [109–111], although multichannel external coil set up may be an alternative [112].

### T2-weighted imaging

The intrinsic high soft-tissue contrast on MR imaging allows for the differentiation between healthy tissue and cancer within the prostate [118]. Conventionally, prostate cancer was defined as an area of low signal intensity on T2-weighted imaging. Other common causes of low signal on T2-weighted imaging are postbiopsy hemorrhage [119] and prostatitis. Ideally, it is advised to perform MR imaging at least three weeks (optimally six weeks) after biopsy to prevent false-positive findings due to biopsy artifacts [120]. Recently, it was shown that the signal intensity on T2-weighted imaging as compared with that of adjacent muscle was correlated with the Gleason score of the cancer, whereby a lower signal intensity was indicative of a more aggressive cancer [121].

However, in the current PSA (semi)screening era, it appears that more cancer foci will be less conspicuous due to the shift towards less aggressive cancers [122]. T2-weighted images at 1.5T using the integrated external pelvic phased-array coil and ERC provided a sensitivity of 52–67% [123]. At 3T using an ERC, the sensitivity of localizing prostate cancer for experienced readers was 53–58% [111]. Thus, it appears that the use of a higher field strength does not aid in localizing prostate cancer and that additional information such as functional imaging is necessary in order to obtain a higher accuracy in localizing prostate cancer.

In order to prevent false-positive findings, high-specificity reading is currently the reading mode of choice for reporting prostate cancer stage [124,125]. Signs with 98–100% specificity of extracapsular cancer extension have been, in order of descending sensitivity): overt extracapsular tumor, tumor signal intensity within the periprostatic fat, neurovascular bundle asymmetry, and obliteration of the rectoprostatic angle [110]. A sign of seminal vesicle invasion is the presence of an area of low signal intensity on T2-weighted imaging in one or both seminal vesicles [126].

For staging of prostate cancer (Table 3 of [33]), it was shown that at 1.5 T the use of an integrated pelvic phased-array coil and ERC had a significantly higher staging performance compared with using an external coil only, particularly by increasing staging specificity [107,108,127]. Other significant factors were the use of multiple imaging planes, the use of contrast agent [127], and the application of cross-referencing between different imaging series [128]. In a meta-analysis, the summary receiver operating characteristic curve had a joint maximum sensitivity and specificity of 71% for determining extracapsular extension, and 82% for determining seminal vesicle invasion [127] (Figure 8.5). Recent studies showed that compared with 1.5T, imaging at 3T with an ERC improved sensitivity with remaining high specificity [110,111]: staging sensitivity with 3T ERC imaging was 80–88% for experienced readers.

### Diffusion-weighted imaging

Diffusion-weighted imaging is a noninvasive MR technique that visualizes and quantifies the motion of water molecules within the extracellular space of tissues [129]. In biologic tissues, diffusion is lowest in tissues with a high cellular density thus causing smaller extracellular spaces [130]. By adapting the traditional T2-weighted spin-echo sequence using gradients, the diffusivity of water molecules within tissue can be determined. Quantitatively, the degree of diffusivity can be expressed in apparent diffusion coefficient (ADC) values [129]. A number of studies have been performed using diffusion-weighted MR imaging in prostate cancer [131]. Diffusion-weighted imaging can be applied at various field strengths using external coils or an endorectal coil [132–138]. It was found that the average ADC values of prostate cancer tissue were significantly lower than those of healthy prostatic tissue. However, there is still considerable overlap between the values in individual patients. The ADC value may also be related to the Gleason score of the prostate cancer. Addition of diffusion-weighting to T2-weighted imaging in localizing prostate cancer was shown to increase the localization performance [139]. Diffusion-weighted imaging may be better in localizing and detecting prostate cancer compared with T2-weighted imaging [136]. Although larger studies need to be performed. It was also shown that diffusion-weighting may be of value in detecting local recurrence after radiation therapy [138] (Figure 8.6).

### Proton MR spectroscopic imaging

Proton MR spectroscopic imaging (MRSI) depicts metabolic processes within the prostate gland by determining the amounts of citrate, choline, and creatine at various locations in the gland [140–142]. Choline and creatine levels are markers for cell turnover. Per voxel these substances are plotted in spectra. Healthy prostatic tissue shows high citrate levels and low choline and creatine levels. During malignant transformation and dedifferentiation the citrate level decreases while the choline and creatine levels increase; thus the ratio between citrate/choline+creatine is a marker for cancer localization [141]. The advantage of MRSI is the fact that the metabolite levels can be expressed quantitatively. Thereby, established thresholds will not vary amongst individuals and quantitative scoring can be established [123,143].

At various field strengths, MRSI can be performed using external coils or an ERC alone, or using a combination of the two [123,144–146]. Recently, it was

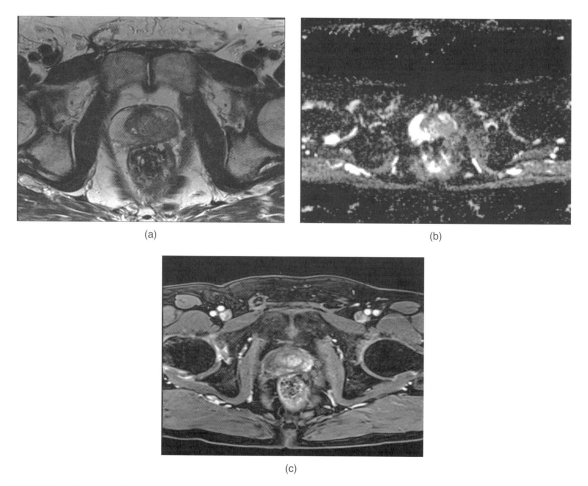

(a)

(b)

(c)

**Fig 8.5** A multiparametric MRI in a man with high-risk prostate cancer (PSA 20 ng/nL, Gleason 4 + 3 with tertiary pattern 5, 9/10 cores positive, maximum cancer core length involvement 15 mm, perineural involvement). The images demonstrate extracapsular extension on the left side visible on all sequences (arrows). These images were taken prior to biopsies. (Courtesy of Hashim U Ahmed, University College London.)

shown that a qualitative approach to MRSI in routine clinical practice by qualitatively interpreting the metabolite spectra is feasible [147]. Most studies have focused on MRSI of the peripheral zone. Nevertheless, MRSI of the central gland is also feasible [143,146]. However, due to more overlap in spectra between benign prostatic hyperplasia and prostate cancer the differentiation between these two is slightly more difficult [146]. At 1.5T using an ERC, using a standardized threshold approach an accuracy of 81%, specificity of 81–88%, and sensitivity of 75–92% was found

[143]. A recent multi-institutional American College of Radiology Imaging Network (ACRIN) study examining MRSI in the peripheral zone revealed equal localization performance of MRSI compared with T2-weighted imaging with areas under the ROC curves between 0.58–0.60 [148].

Recently, a systematic review and meta-analysis concluded that the use of a combination of T2-weighted imaging and MRSI could be a rule-in test for patients at low risk of prostate cancer [149]. MRSI may play a role in identifying patients suitable for

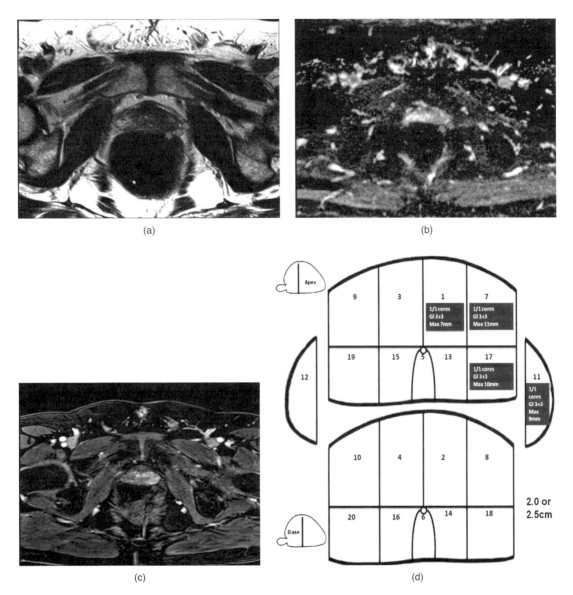

(a)

(b)

(c)

(d)

**Fig 8.6** Multiparametric MRI in a man who has biochemical recurrence after primary external beam radiation therapy a number of years prior. Apical disease on the right side is not visible on axial T2W images, (a) but obvious on coronal T2W images (b) as well as on diffusion (c) and dynamic contrast-enhanced scans (d). This was confirmed histologically on template mapping biopsies (e) (green and yellow zones). (Courtesy of Hashim U Ahmed, University College London.) *See also plate 8.6.*

active surveillance by estimating the cancer volume [150,151] and in establishing local recurrence in patients [152–155]. However, larger studies need to be performed in these patient populations. Generally, it is assumed that MRSI is most valuable if one takes into consideration that its strength lies in the high specificity; thus if an abnormal metabolic area is observed its positive predictive value is high.

**129**

## Contrast-enhanced MR imaging

Contrast-enhanced MR imaging provides an insight into the cancer vasculature and its permeability [156]. Intravenously administered gadolinium-based contrast agents [157] will diffuse into the extracellular interstitial space and accumulate up to a certain concentration before—also by diffusion—returning to the intraluminal vascular space. Since these agents cause increased signal relaxation on T1-weighted imaging, this sequence can track such signal changes. T1-weighted imaging of the entire prostate can be obtained several times after contrast administration. This can be performed qualitatively by reviewing the images before and after contrast administration and observing foci of increased signal gain. By using a subtraction technique it is possible to construct an imaging set in which only the contrast-related signal intensity changes are visible.

An ever more widely used approach is to perform imaging at multiple time points after gadolinium administration and from this analyze the signal changes using compartment models, of which the Tofts model has been most frequently used [158]. This method is often referred to as dynamic contrast-enhanced (DCE) MR imaging [123,155,159–161]. Using these models the permeability of the vasculature in the tissue can be expressed, (often using parameters such as $K^{trans}$ or $K^{ep}$), as well as an estimation of the extracellular volume ($V_e$). If one images long enough to observe the downslope of the signal intensity curve, one can determine the rate of decline in the signal (washout). A disadvantage is the fact that many institutions use in house software based on these models, which increases the difficulty of comparing studies. Likewise, no objective threshold for the aforementioned parameters has yet been proposed. These techniques can be used at various field strengths, as well as using both external coils and an ERC. Using an ERC can increase the spatial and/or temporal imaging resolution. While temporal resolution at 1.5 T was described at two seconds, at 3T this could be improved to one second [109].

DCE was shown to significantly improve cancer localization (Figures 8.7 and 8.8). Using an ERC at 1.5T, the area under the ROC curve increased from 0.68 with T2-weighted imaging and 0.80 with MRSI to 0.91 with DCE [123]. In this study, the separate parameters were analyzed and the washout parame-ter was observed to have the highest specificity, while the extracellular interstitial volume parameter had the highest sensitivity. DCE can aid in localizing cancer foci after previous negative transrectal ultrasound biopsy [112,162]. Recently, high performance was observed in using this sequence to detect local recurrence both after curative radical prostatectomy [155,163] and radiation therapy [164,165].

It was shown that at 1.5 T, administration of contrast agent significantly increased the staging performance for less experience readers [159]. The area under the ROC curve increased from 0.66 with unenhanced MR imaging to 0.82 with enhanced MR imaging. Thus, application of DCE MR imaging may be an advantage for readers at the start of the learning curve of reading prostate MR imaging.

## MR-guided biopsy

The advantage of MR imaging lies in the fact that all the features described above can be used in combination in order to localize prostate cancer. This new paradigm is called multiparametric MRI, and can now be directly used in order to localize prostate cancer for direct MR-guided biopsy [166–169]. The combination of diagnostic MR imaging and MR-guided biopsy (MRGB) may increase the tumor detection rate [112]. The current literature on MRGB of the prostate however is limited, and the few studies available have included a small number of patients [166,170,171]. Beyersdorff et al performed an MR-guided biopsy in twelve patients with elevated PSA levels and previous negative transrectal ultrasound-guided biopsy round [166]. In seven of these patients the suspicious regions could be defined with the fast sequence, in the other five cases the areas of interest were clearly visible in the prebiopsy images and could be marked on the images obtained during biopsy. These are promising data and demonstrate the potential clinical value of MR-guided biopsies [112,166,170,171]. One group has shown a very high negative predictive value for the presence of clinically significant cancer volume of 85% and 95% for ≥ 0.2 cc and ≥0.5 cc lesions, respectively, if DCE is used prior to a first prostate biopsy [187]. The University College London team have proposed that there is sufficient evidence that warrants the use of multiparametric MRI prior to biopsy in men with a raised PSA [188] (Figure Prostate-Right-Lesion). This will need evaluating carefully in a prospective study that uses

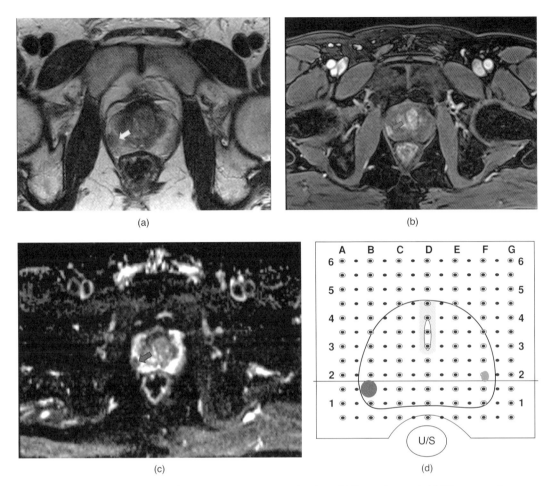

(a)

(b)

(c)

(d)

**Fig 8.7** Axial images taken on a 1.5 Tesla MRI using a pelvic phased-array coil in a man with intermediate-risk prostate cancer on TRUS-guided biopsies. (a) T2-weighted image shows a low-signal area in the left lobe, although not clear. (b) Dynamic contrast-enhanced image shows enhancement in the left lobe consistent with cancer. (c) Diffusion-weighted image confirms the same area has poor signal on ADC map (arrows). (d) The man underwent template transperineal mapping biopsies using a 5-mm sampling frame, which confirmed the area on the MRI in the left lobe (red areas). A total of 24 cores were taken. (Courtesy of Hashim U Ahmed, University College London.) *See also plate 8.7.*

detailed mapping biopsies of the prostate as a reference standard in this group of men. At the time of this chapter going to press, such a study is under way in the United Kingdom.

## Scrotum and testes

The first step in diagnosing testicular cancer is usually through self-examination. Testicular cancer most commonly presents as a painless scrotal mass. Testic-

ular cancer, although representing 1% of all cancer in males, is the most common neoplasm in boys and young adults from 15 to 34 years old [3]. The incidence of testicular cancer has doubled in the last forty years. Bilateral tumors are found in 0.7% of men with germ cell tumors at diagnosis, and 1.5% of patients develop metachronous lesions within 5 years [4].

Once the leading cause of cancer deaths in men between 15 and 35 years of age, it has now proved to be a model of success with a 5-year survival rate exceeding 95% [176]. This success in treatment is related

**131**

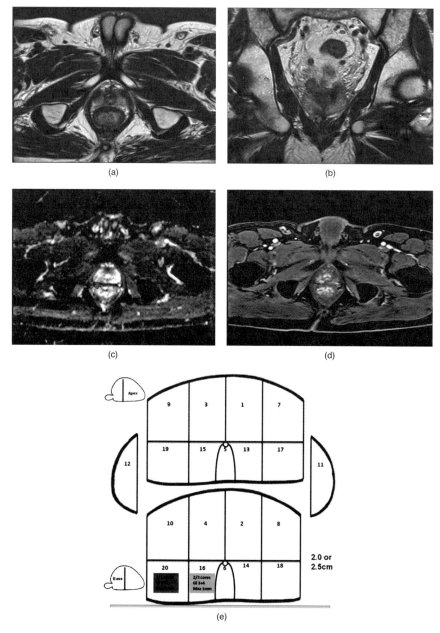

**Fig 8.8** Axial images taken on a 1.5 Tesla MRI using a pelvic phased-array coil in a man with a PSA of 6.5 ng/mL. (a) T2-weighted image shows a low-signal area in the right-peripheral zone although this is far from clear. (b) Dynamic contrast-enhanced image shows enhancement in the right-peripheral zone lesion consistent with cancer. (c) Diffusion-weighted image confirms the same area has poor signal on ADC map. (d) The man underwent template transperineal mapping biopsies using a 5-mm sampling frame rather than transrectal biopsies (arrows). The template biopsies confirmed the area on the MRI in the right-peripheral zone (red) with 2 cores positive for Gleason score 4 + 3, 3 mm and 5-mm cancer core length. A smaller, presumed insignificant area was also shown on the left (blue) with 1 mm of Gleason 6 cancer. A total of 66 cores were taken. (Courtesy of Hashim U Ahmed, University College London.) *See also plate 8.8.*

to improved staging and treatment methods. Imaging plays a central role in assessment of tumor bulk, sites of metastases, monitoring response to therapy, surgical planning, and accurate assessment of disease at relapse [177].

Serum tumor markers are especially helpful to differentiate germ cell tumors from each other and from other malignancies. Serum concentrations of alphafetoprotein (AFP) and/or beta-human chorionic gonadotropin (beta-hCG) are elevated in 80% to 85% of nonseminomas. In contrast, serum beta-hCG is elevated in fewer than 25% of testicular seminomas, and AFP is not elevated in pure seminomas. However, these tumor markers cannot accurately assess disease bulk or locate sites of tumor spread [177].

## Clinical staging

As soon as the diagnosis of germ cell cancer has been pathologically confirmed, further staging examinations are warranted to examine the extent of disease. Staging is of utmost importance as it is the cornerstone for further treatment after orchiectomy. The European Germ Cell Cancer Consensus Group (EGCCCG) recommended that TNM staging should be used [33] (Table 4). Today, CT of the abdomen and chest is the standard technique in initial staging.

The most common sites for metastases are via the lymphatic system to the retroperitoneal nodes, and via the hematogenous route to the lungs and less common to the liver, brain, and bone. In general, advanced stage disease will be treated primarily with chemotherapy. Nonseminomatous germ cell tumors appear as multiple small peripheral nodules, whereas seminoma metastases tend to be larger masses [177]. Other sites of hematogenous metastases, though rarely seen and usually only in the setting of advanced disease, include the adrenals, kidneys, spleen, pleura, pericardium, and peritoneum [177].

Lymphatic spread occurs via lymphatic channels (from spermatic cord and testicular vessels to retroperitoneal lymph nodes). Usually, right-sided testicular neoplasms spread to the right side of the retroperitoneum. Lymph node metastases can be identified around the inferior vena cava, and between the level of right renal hilum and the aortic bifurcation. Lymph node metastases of left-sided testicular cancer may be found adjacent to the abdominal aorta and just below the left renal vein. Contralateral involvement is

uncommon, but may occur with a larger disease burden [178]. Pelvic lymph adenopathy is uncommon in the absence of bulky disease [179].

## MR technique

MR imaging is performed in the supine position and surface coils (phased-array) are positioned above the testicles. The scrotum is elevated by means of a support between the tights (folded towel is placed between the tights) to ensure that both testes are in the same horizontal plane for proper coronal imaging. The penis is angled to the side and the whole region is draped.

T1- and T2-weighted sequences in at least two planes are acquired (coronal and axial). The coronal plane is the ideal plane for imaging the scrotum. The coronal series covers from the posterior aspect of the scrotum to the anterior aspect of the external inguinal ring. DCE subtraction MR imaging can be used to differentiate testicular diseases from scrotal disorders [180]. In general, contrast-enhanced MR imaging is reserved for patients with subtle, atypical, or complex findings. For staging purposes, T1-weighted axial images of the abdomen should be obtained to search for adenopathy.

The normal testis is a sharply demarcated oval structure of intermediate homogeneous signal intensity to muscle on T1-weighted images and homogeneous higher signal intensity (less than fluid signal intensity) on T2-weighted images. Signal intensity of the epididymis is low signal intensity on both T1- and T2-weighted images. The epididymis is more clearly differentiated from the testis on T2-weighted images because it is lower in signal intensity than the adjacent testis. The testis is completely surrounded by the tunica albuginea, a thick layer of dense fibrous tissue. The tunica albuginea and testicular septa appear as low signal intensity structures [181]. The mediastinum testis can be identified as a low signal intensity band within the posterior testis on T2-weighted images.

## MR imaging

Ultrasonography is currently the primary imaging modality in the assessment of scrotal disease. However, because of its wide field of view, multiplanar capabilities, and intrinsic high soft-tissue contrast, MRI may represent an efficient supplemental technique for scrotal imaging [182–187]. Tumors are typically isointense with normal testis on T1-weighted MR images, becoming inhomogeneous and slightly darker on proton-density-weighted MR images and moderately darker on T2-weighted images.

The MR imaging appearance of seminoma, like its histology, has been consistent. Seminoma is usually homogeneous in appearance and relatively isointense to the normal testicular parenchyma on T1-weighted images and low signal intensity on T2-weighted images. However, MRI cannot reliably predict the histological type [188]. Although, atypical, some seminomatous lesions may bleed internally, resulting in a focus of different signal dependent on the age of the hemorrhage.

Nonseminomatous germ cell tumors are more likely to have cystic areas than seminomas. The former tumors, given their histologic patterns, are markedly inhomogeneous on MR images, which represent their most distinctive feature when compared with seminomatous lesions. These tumors are usually iso- to hyperintense on T1-weighted MR and hypointense on T2-weighted MR. The overall heterogeneous appearance is mostly due to the presence of mixed cell types, hemorrhage, and necrosis.

On occasion, primary testicular tumors may undergo spontaneous regression. These lesions are usually termed "burnt-out" germ cell tumors. At MR imaging, T2-weighted images demonstrate a focal low signal intensity area of distortion of the normal testicular architecture, without a visible mass. The appearance can resemble segmental infarction.

## Future directions

As the risk of radiation increases, the value of MRI in imaging urological cancers will grow. Novel protocols incorporating blood oxygen level dependent (BOLD) MRI is able to provide additional functional information, and may be useful in assessing tumor necrosis and aggressiveness as well as posttreatment evaluation. Novel contrast agents based on molecular imaging are also emerging, and will be able to provide not only localization information, but also characterization of suspicious lesions.

Once images are achieved, registration or fusion will be important to deliver therapy in real-time to the areas of tumor in order to achieve good ablation but also with an appropriate margin. Work in this area

is particularly pertinent for prostate cancer and focal therapy.

## Conclusions

The role of MRI in urological oncology seems most eminent in prostate cancer. With this gland, MRI has the potential to detect clinically important cancer to a high degree of accuracy. Importantly, it may identify those men with a clinical suspicion of prostate cancer who need to have biopsies with the conduct of those biopsies improved with targeting. Furthermore, with novel ablative techniques now able to treat cancer in a focal manner, MRI can allow the delivery of precision ablation in order to reduce toxicity while retaining cancer control efficacy.

## References

1. Jemal A et al (2008) Cancer statistics. CA Cancer J Clin 58: 71–96.
2. Baade PD, Youlden DR, Krnjacki LJ (2009) International epidemiology of prostate cancer: geographic distribution and secular trends. Mol Nutr Food Res 53: 171–184.
3. Garner MJ et al (2005) Epidemiology of testicular cancer: an overview. Int J Cancer 116: 331–339.
4. Comiter CV et al (1995) Nonpalpable intratesticular masses detected sonographically. J Urol 154: 1367–1369.
5. Ries LAG et al (eds.) (2008) *SEER Cancer Statistics Review*, 1975–2005, National Cancer Institute. Bethesda, MD, http://seer.cancer.gov/csr/1975_2005.
6. Mathew A et al (2002) Global increases in kidney cancer incidence, 1973–1992. Eur J Cancer Prev 11: 171–178.
7. Eble JN, Sauter G, Epstein JI, Sesterhenn IA (eds.) (2004) *Pathology and Genetics of Tumours of the Urinary System and Male Genital Organs.* Lyon, France: IARC Press.
8. Motzer RJ, Bander NH, Nanus DM (1996) Renal-cell carcinoma. N Engl J Med 335: 865–875.
9. Ng CS et al (2008) RCC: diagnosis, staging, and active surveillance. Am J Roentgenol 191: 1220–1232.
10. Palapattu GS, Kristo B, Rajfer J (2002) Paraneoplastic syndromes in urologic malignancy: the many faces of RCC. Rev Urol 4: 163–170.
11. Muggia FM (1990) Overview of cancer-related hypercalcemia: epidemiology and etiology. Semin Oncol 17: 3–9.

12. Warren WD, Utz DC, Kelalis PP (1971) Concurrence of hypernephroma and hypercalcemia. Ann Surg 174: 863–865.

13. Mundy GR et al (1984) The hypercalcemia of cancer. N Engl J Med 310: 1718–1727.

14. Buckle RM, McMillan M, Mallinson C (1970) Ectopic secretion of parathyroid hormone by a renal adenocarcinoma in a patient with hypercalcemia. Br Med J 4: 724–726.

15. Leslie JA, Prihoda T, Thompson IM (2003) Serendipitous RCC in the post-CT era: continued evidence in improved outcomes. Urol Oncol 21: 39–44.

16. Chesbrough RM et al (1989) Gerota versus Zuckerkandl: the renal fascia revisited. Radiology 173: 845–846.

17. Semelka RC (2002) Kidneys, testes. In: RC Semelka (ed.) *Abdominal-Pelvic MRI*, 1st edn. New York: Wiley-Liss, pp. 741–1007.

18. Kovacs G et al (1997) The Heidelberg classification of renal cell tumors. J Pathol 183: 131–133.

19. Storkel S et al (1997) Classification of RCC: Workgroup No. 1. Union International Contre le Cancer (UICC) and the American Joint Committee on Cancer (AJCC). Cancer 80: 987–989.

20. Novara G et al (2007) Grading systems in RCC. J Urol 177: 430–436.

21. Bostwick DG, Murphy GP (1998) Diagnosis and prognosis of RCC: highlights from an international consensus workshop. Semin Urol Oncol 16: 46–52.

22. Cheville JC et al (2003) Comparisons of outcome and prognostic features among histologic subtypes of RCC. Am J Surg Pathol 27: 612–624.

23. Sukosd F et al (2003) Deletion of chromosome 3p14.2-p25 involving VHL and FHIT genes in conventional RCC. Cancer Res 63: 455–457.

24. Presti JC Jr et al (1991) Histopathological, cytogenetic, and molecular characterization of renal cortical tumors. Cancer Res 51: 1544–1552.

25. Ishikawa I, Kovacs G (1993) High incidence of papillary renal cell tumours in patients on chronic haemodialysis. Histopathology 22: 135–139.

26. Delahunt B et al (2001) Morphologic typing of papillary RCC: comparison of growth kinetics and patient survival in 66 cases. Hum Pathol 32: 590–595.

27. Delahunt B, Eble JN (1997) Papillary RCC: a clinicopathologic and immunohistochemical study of 105 tumors. Mod Pathol 10: 537–544.

28. Rumpelt HJ et al (1991) Bellini duct carcinoma: further evidence for this rare variant of RCC. Histopathology 18: 115–122.

29. Polascik TJ, Bostwick DG, Cairns P (2002) Molecular genetics and histopathologic features of adult distal nephron tumors. Urology 60: 941–946.

30. Srigley JR, Elbe JN (1998) Collecting duct carcinoma of kidney. Semin Diagn Pathol 15: 54–67.

31. Prasad SR et al (2006) Common and uncommon histologic subtypes of RCC: imaging spectrum with pathologic correlation. Radiographics 26: 1795–1810.

32. Harmer M (1974) *TNM Classification of Malignant Tumors*, 3rd edn. Geneva: International Union Against Cancer.

33. Sobin LH, Wittekind CH (2002) *UICC: TNM Classification of Malignant Tumours*, 6th edn. New York: Wiley-Liss.

34. Lane BR, Kattan MW (2005) Predicting outcomes in RCC. Curr Opin Urol 15: 289–297.

35. Figlin RA (1999) RCC: management of advanced disease. J Urol 161: 381–386.

36. Staudenherz A et al (1999) Is there a diagnostic role for bone scanning of patients with a high pretest probability for metastatic RCC? Cancer 85: 153–155.

37. Zagoria RJ, Bechtold RE (1997) The role of imaging in staging renal adenocarcinoma. Semin Ultrasound CT MR 18: 91–99.

38. Ng CS et al (1999) Metastases to the pancreas from RCC: findings in three-phase contrast-enhanced helical CT. Am J Roentgenol 172: 1555–1559.

39. Pretorius ES, Wickstrom ML, Siegelman ES (2000) MR imaging of renal neoplasms. Magn Reson Imaging Clin N Am 8: 813–836.

40. Nolte-Ernsting CC et al (1998) Gadolinium-enhanced excretory MR urography after low-dose diuretic injection: comparison with conventional excretory urography. Radiology 209: 147–157.

41. Cheng WS, Farrow GM, Zincke H (1991) The incidence of multicentricity in RCC. J Urol 146: 1221–1223.

42. Shinmoto H et al (1998) Small RCC: MRI with pathologic correlation. J Magn Reson Imaging 8: 690–694.

43. Soyer P et al (1997) RCC of clear type: correlation of CT features with tumor size, architectural patterns, and pathologic staging. Eur Radiol 7: 224–229.

44. Yoshimitsu K et al (2004) MR imaging of RCC: its role in determining cell type. Radiat Med 22: 371–376.

45. Kim JK et al (2002) Differentiation of subtypes of RCC on helical CT scans. AJR Am J Roentgenol 178: 1499–1506.

46. Jinzaki M et al (2000) Double-phase helical CT of small renal parenchymal neoplasms: correlation with pathologic findings and tumor angiogenesis. J Comput Assist Tomogr 24: 835–842.

47. Cohen HT, McGovern FJ (2005). Renal-cell carcinoma. N Engl J Med 353: 2477–2490.

48. Kondo T et al (2004) Spoke-wheel-like enhancement as an important imaging finding of chromophobe RCC: a retrospective analysis on computed tomography and

magnetic resonance imaging studies. Int J Urol 11: 817–824.

49. Yamashita Y et al (1996) Detection of pseudocapsule of RCC with MR imaging and CT. AJR Am J Roentgenol 166: 1151–1155.

50. Krestin GP (1999) Genitourinary MR: kidneys and adrenal glands. Eur Radiol 9: 705–714.

51. Vaidya A, Ciancio G, Soloway M (2003) Surgical techniques for treating a renal neoplasm invading the inferior vena cava. J Urol 169: 435–444.

52. Russo P (2000) RCC: presentation, staging, and surgical treatment. Semin Oncol 27: 160–176.

53. Chin AI et al (2006) Surveillance strategies for RCC patients following nephrectomy. Rev Urol 8: 1–7.

54. Itano NB et al (2000) Outcome of isolated RCC fossa after nephrectomy. J Urol 164: 322–325.

55. Broome DR et al (2007) Gadodiamide-associated nephrogenic systemic fibrosis: why radiologists should be concerned. Am J Roentgenol 188: 586–592.

56. Grobner T (2006) Gadolinium: a specific trigger for the development of nephrogenic fibrosing dermopathy and nephrogenic systemic fibrosis? Nephrol Dial Transplant 21: 1104–1108.

57. Muller MF et al (1994) Functional imaging of the kidney by means of measurement of the apparent diffusion coefficient. Radiology 193: 711–715.

58. Siegel CL et al (1995) Feasibility of MR diffusion studies in the kidney. J Magn Reson Imaging 5: 617–620.

59. Naminoto T et al (2000) Measurement of the apparent diffusion coefficient in diffuse renal disease by diffusion-weighted echo-planar MR imaging. J Magn Reson Imaging 11: 156–160.

60. Thoeny HC et al (2005) Diffusion-weighted MR imaging of the kidney in healthy volunteers and patients with parenchymal disease: initial experience. Radiology 18: 377–382.

61. Ries M et al (2001) Diffusion tensor MRI of the human kidney. J Magn Reson Imaging 14: 42–49.

62. Squillaci E et al (2004) Diffusion-weighted MR imaging in the evaluation of renal tumors. J Exp Clin Cancer Res 23: 39–45.

63. Cova M et al (2004) Diffusion-weighted MRI in the evaluation of renal lesions: preliminary results. Br J Radiol 77: 851–857.

64. Yoshikawa T et al (2006) ADC measurement of abdominal organs and lesions using parallel imaging technique. AJR Am J Roentgenol 187: 1521–1530.

65. Zhang J et al (2008) Renal masses: characterization with diffusion-weighted MR imaging-a preliminary experience. Radiology 247: 458–464.

66. Kim S et al (2009) T1 hyperintense renal lesions: characterization with diffusion-weighted MR imaging versus contrast-enhanced MR imaging. Radiology 251: 796–807.

67. Taouli B et al (2009) Renal lesions: characterization with diffusion-weighted imaging versus contrast-enhanced MR imaging. Radiology 251(2): 398–407

68. Israel GM, Bosniak MA (2003) Renal imaging for diagnosis and staging of RCC. Urol Clin North Am 30: 499–514.

69. Scialpi M et al (2000) Small renal masses: assessment of lesion characterization and vascularity on dynamic contrast-enhanced MR imaging with fat suppression. AJR Am J Roentgenol 175: 751–757.

70. Motzer RJ et al (2007) Sunitinib versus interferon alfa in metastatic renal-cell carcinoma. N Engl J Med 356: 115–224.

71. Escudier B et al (2007) Sorafenib in advanced clear-cell renal-cell carcinoma. N Engl J Med.

72. Ho VB et al (2002) Renal masses: quantitative assessment of enhancement with dynamic MR imaging. Radiology 224(3): 695–700.

73. Hecht EM et al (2004) Renal masses: quantitative analysis of enhancement with signal intensity measurements versus qualitative analysis of enhancement with image subtraction for diagnosing malignancy at MR imaging. Radiology 232: 373–378.

74. Riley GF et al (1996) Medicare payments from diagnosis to death for elderly cancer patients by stage at diagnosis. Med Care 33: 828–841.

75. Botteman MF et al (2003) The health economics of bladder cancer: a comprehensive review of published literature. Pharmacoeconomics 21: 1315–1330.

76. Barentsz JO, Debruyne FMJ, Ruijs SHJ (eds.) (1990) *Magnetic Resonance Imaging of Carcinoma of the Urinary Bladder*. Dordrecht: Kluwer Academic Publishers.

77. Barentsz JO et al (1996) Evaluation of chemotherapy in advanced urinary bladder cancer with fast contrast-enhanced MR imaging. Radiology 207(3): 791–797.

78. Banson ML (1996) Normal MR anatomy and technique for imaging the male pelvis. Magn Reson Imaging Clin N Am 4: 481–496.

79. Fritzsche PJ, Wilbur MJ (1989) The male pelvis. Semin Ultrasound CT MR 10: 11–28.

80. Ross MH, Romrell LJ, Kaye GI (eds.) (1995) GI: Urinary system. In: *Histology: A Text and Atlas*, 3rd edn. Philadelphia: William & Wilkins, pp. 582–583.

81. Fawcett DW, Jensh RP (eds.) (1998) Histology of the urinary system. In: *Concise Histology*. London: Chapman & Hall, pp. 240–251.

82. Rosai J (1996) Bladder and male urethra. In: J Rosai (ed.) *Ackerman's Surgical Pathology*. Baltimore: Mosby, pp. 1195–1196.

83. Woolf N (1998) Urinary bladder. In: N Woolf (ed.) *Pathology Basic and System*. Philadelphia: WB Saunders, pp. 713–717.

84. Messing EM, Catalona WJ (1998) Urothelial tumors of the urinary tract. In: PC Walsh (ed.) *Cambell's Urology*. Philadelphia: Saunders, pp. 2343–2348.

85. Ghoneim MA (1994) Nontransitional cell bladder cancer. In: MK Smith (ed.) *Clinical Urology*. Philadelphia: Lippincott, pp. 680–681.

86. Chan TY, Epstein JL (2001) In situ adenocarcinoma of the bladder. Am J Surg Pathol 25: 892–899.

87. Josephson D, Pasin E, Stein JP (2007) Superficial bladder cancer. II. Management. Expert Rev Anticancer Ther 7: 567–581.

88. Sherif A, Jonsson MN, Wiklund NP (2007) Treatment of muscle-invasive bladder cancer. Expert Rev Anticancer Ther 7: 1279–1283

89. Heiken JP, Fofman HP, Brown JJ (1994) Neoplasms of the bladder, prostate and testis. Radiol Clin North Am 32: 81–98.

90. Elkin M (1980) Tumors of urinary tract. In: M Eiken (ed.) *Radiology of the Urinary System*. Vol I. Boston: Little Brown, pp. 296–426.

91. Barentsz JO, Ruijs JHJ, Strijk SP (1993) The role of MR imaging in carcinoma of the urinary bladder. AJR Am J Roentgenol 160: 937–947.

92. Barentsz JO, Witjes JA, Ruijs JH (1997) What is new in bladder cancer imaging. Urol Clin North Am 24: 538–602.

93. Siegelman ES, Schnall MD (1996) Contrast-enhanced MR imaging of the bladder and prostate. Magn Reson Imaging Clin N Am 4: 153–169.

94. Fischer MR, Hricak H, Tanagho EA (1985) Urinary bladder MR imaging. Part II. Neoplasms. Radiology 157: 471–477.

95. Amendola MA et al (1986) Staging of bladder carcinoma: MRI-CT-surgical correlation. Am J Roentgenol 146: 1179–1183.

96. Husband JE et al (1989) Bladder cancer: staging with CT and MR imaging. Radiology 173: 435–440.

97. Persad R et al (1993) Magnetic resonance imaging in the staging of bladder cancer. Br J Urol 71: 566–573.

98. Bryan PJ et al (1987) CT and MR imaging in staging bladder neoplasms. J Comput Assist Tomogr 11: 96–101.

99. Tekes A et al (2005) Dynamic MRI of bladder cancer: evaluation of staging accuracy. AJR Am J Roentgenol 184: 121–127.

100. Hayashi N et al (2000) A new staging criterion for bladder carcinoma using gadolineum-enhanced magnetic resonance imaging with an endorectal surface coil: a comparison with ultrasonography. BJU Int 85: 32–36.

101. Narumi Y et al (1993) Bladder tumors: staging with gadolineum-enhanced oblique MR imaging. Radiology 187: 145–150.

102. Matsuki M et al (2007) Diffusion-weighted MR imaging for urinary bladder carcinoma: initial results. Eur Radiol 17(1): 201–204.

103. Abou-El-Ghar M et al (2009) Bladder cancer: diagnosis with diffusion-weighted MR imaging in patients with gross hematuria. Radiology 251: 415–421.

104. Takeuchi M *et al*. Urinary bladder cancer: diffusion-weighted MR imaging-accuracy for diagnosing T stage and estimating histologic grade. Radiology 251: 112–121.

105. Saito W et al (2000) Histopathological analysis of bladder cancer stalk observed on MRI. Magn Reson Imaging 18: 411.

106. Choi YJ et al (2007) Functional MR imaging of prostate cancer. Radiographics 27: 63–75.

107. Hricak H et al (1994) Carcinoma of the prostate gland: MR imaging with pelvic phased-array coils versus integrated endorectal–pelvic phased-array coils. Radiology 193: 703–709.

108. Fütterer JJ et al (2007) Prostate cancer: comparison of local staging accuracy of pelvic phased-array coil alone versus integrated endorectal-pelvic phased-array coils : Local staging accuracy of prostate cancer using endorectal coil MR imaging. Eur Radiol 17: 1055–1065.

109. Fütterer JJ et al (2004) Initial experience of 3 tesla endorectal coil magnetic resonance imaging and 1H-spectroscopic imaging of the prostate. Invest Radiol 39: 671–680.

110. Fütterer JJ et al (2006) Prostate cancer: local staging at 3-T endorectal MR imaging–early experience. Radiology 238: 184–191.

111. Heijmink SW et al (2007) Prostate cancer: body-array versus endorectal coil MR imaging at 3 T–comparison of image quality, localization, and staging performance. Radiology 244: 184–195.

112. Hambrock T et al (2008) Thirty-two-channel coil 3T magnetic resonance-guided biopsies of prostate tumor suspicious regions identified on multimodality 3T magnetic resonance imaging: technique and feasibility. Invest Radiol 43: 686–694.

113. Myers RP, Goellner JR, Cahill DR (1987) Prostate shape, external striated urethral sphincter and radical prostatectomy: the apical dissection. J Urol 138: 543–550.

114. Fuse H et al (1992) Evaluation of seminal vesicle characteristics by ultrasonography before and after ejaculation. Urol Int 49: 110–113.

115. Villeirs GM, De Meerleer GO (2007) Magnetic resonance imaging (MRI) anatomy of the prostate and

application of MRI in radiotherapy planning. Eur J Radiol 63: 361–368.

116. Barry MJ. Clinical practice. (2001) Prostate-specific-antigen testing for early diagnosis of prostate cancer. N Engl J Med 344: 1373–1377.

117. McNeal JE (1981) Normal and pathologic anatomy of prostate. Urology 17: 11–16.

118. Coakley FV, Hricak H (2000) Radiologic anatomy of the prostate gland: a clinical approach. Radiol Clin North Am 38: 15–30.

119. White S et al (1995) Prostate cancer: effect of post-biopsy hemorrhage on interpretation of MR images. Radiology 195: 385–390.

120. Ikonen S et al (2001) Optimal timing of post-biopsy MR imaging of the prostate. Acta Radiol 42: 70–73.

121. Wang L et al (2008) Assessment of biologic aggressiveness of prostate cancer: correlation of MR signal intensity with Gleason grade after radical prostatectomy. Radiology 246: 168–176.

122. Derweesh IH et al (2004) Continuing trends in pathological stage migration in radical prostatectomy specimens. Urol Oncol 22: 300–306.

123. Fütterer JJ et al (2006) Prostate cancer localization with dynamic contrast-enhanced MR imaging and proton MR spectroscopic imaging. Radiology 241: 449–458.

124. Jager GJ et al (1996) Primary staging of prostate cancer. Eur Radiol 6: 134–139.

125. Jager GJ et al (2000) Prostate cancer staging: should MR imaging be used?–a decision analytic approach. Radiology 215: 445–451.

126. Sala E et al (2006) Endorectal MR Imaging in the evaluation of seminal vesicle invasion: diagnostic accuracy and multivariate feature analysis. Radiology 238: 929–937.

127. Engelbrecht MR et al (2002) Local staging of prostate cancer using magnetic resonance imaging: a meta-analysis. Eur Radiol 12: 2294–2302.

128. Wang L et al (2007) Incremental value of multiplanar cross-referencing for prostate cancer staging with endorectal MRI. AJR Am J Roentgenol 188: 99–104.

129. Koh DM, Collins DJ (2007) Diffusion-weighted MRI in the body: applications and challenges in oncology. AJR Am J Roentgenol 188: 1622–1635.

130. Zelhof B et al (2009) Correlation of diffusion-weighted magnetic resonance data with cellularity in prostate cancer. BJU Int 103: 883–888.

131. Somford DM et al (2008) Diffusion and perfusion MR imaging of the prostate. Magn Reson Imaging Clin N Am 16: 685–695.

132. Gibbs P, Pickles MD, Turnbull LW (2006) Diffusion imaging of the prostate at 3. 0 tesla. Invest Radiol 41: 185–188.

133. Choi YJ, Kim JK, Kim N, Kim KW, Choi EK, Cho KS (2007) Functional MR imaging of prostate cancer. Radiographics 27: 63–75.

134. Kim CK et al (2007) Value of diffusion-weighted imaging for the prediction of prostate cancer location at 3T using a phased-array coil: preliminary results. Invest Radiol 42: 842–847.

135. Kim CK et al (2007) Diffusion-weighted imaging of the prostate at 3 T for differentiation of malignant and benign tissue in transition and peripheral zones: preliminary results. J Comput Assist Tomogr 31: 449–454.

136. Miao H, Fukatsu H, Ishigaki T (2007) Prostate cancer detection with 3-T MRI: comparison of diffusion-weighted and T2-weighted imaging. Eur J Radiol 61: 297–302.

137. Mazaheri Y et al (2008) Prostate cancer: identification with combined diffusion-weighted MR imaging and 3D 1H MR spectroscopic imaging–correlation with pathologic findings. Radiology 246: 480–488.

138. Kim CK, Park BK, Lee HM (2009) Prediction of locally recurrent prostate cancer after radiation therapy: incremental value of 3T diffusion-weighted MRI. J Magn Reson Imaging 29: 391–397.

139. Lim HK et al (2009) Prostate cancer: apparent diffusion coefficient map with T2-weighted images for detection–a multireader study. Radiology 250: 145–151.

140. Kurhanewicz J et al (1995) Citrate as an in vivo marker to discriminate prostate cancer from benign prostatic hyperplasia and normal prostate peripheral zone: detection via localized proton spectroscopy. Urology 45: 459–466.

141. Heerschap A et al (1997) In vivo proton MR spectroscopy reveals altered metabolite content in malignant prostate tissue. Anticancer Res 17: 1455–1460.

142. Heerschap A et al (1997) Proton MR spectroscopy of the normal human prostate with an endorectal coil and a double spin-echo pulse sequence. Magn Reson Med 37: 204–213.

143. Fütterer JJ et al (2007) Standardized threshold approach using three-dimensional proton magnetic resonance spectroscopic imaging in prostate cancer localization of the entire prostate. Invest Radiol 42: 116–122.

144. Cunningham CH et al (2005) Sequence design for magnetic resonance spectroscopic imaging of prostate cancer at 3 T. Magn Reson Med 53: 1033–1039.

145. Scheenen TW et al (2005) Optimal timing for in vivo 1H-MR spectroscopic imaging of the human prostate at 3T. Magn Reson Med 53: 1268–1274.

146. Scheenen TW et al (2007) Three-dimensional proton MR spectroscopy of human prostate at 3 T without endorectal coil: feasibility. Radiology 245: 507–516.

147. Villeirs GM, Oosterlinck W, Vanherreweghe E, De Meerleer GO (2010) A qualitative approach to combined magnetic resonance imaging and spectroscopy in the diagnosis of prostate cancer. Eur J Radiol 73(2): 352–356

148. Weinreb JC et al (2009) Prostate cancer: sextant localization at MR imaging and MR spectroscopic imaging before prostatectomy–results of ACRIN prospective multi-institutional clinicopathologic study. Radiology 251: 122–133.

149. Umbehr M et al (2009) Combined magnetic resonance imaging and magnetic resonance spectroscopy imaging in the diagnosis of prostate cancer: a Systematic Review and Meta-analysis. Eur Urol 55(3): 575–590

150. Cabrera AR et al (2008) Prostate cancer: is inapparent tumor at endorectal MR and MR spectroscopic imaging a favorable prognostic finding in patients who select active surveillance? Radiology 247: 444–450.

151. Kumar R et al (2008) Potential of magnetic resonance spectroscopic imaging in predicting absence of prostate cancer in men with serum prostate-specific antigen between 4 and 10 ng/ml: a follow-up study. Urology 72: 859–863.

152. Coakley FV et al (2004) Endorectal MR imaging and MR spectroscopic imaging for locally recurrent prostate cancer after external beam radiation therapy: preliminary experience. Radiology 233: 441–448.

153. Pickett B et al (2004) Use of MRI and spectroscopy in evaluation of external beam radiotherapy for prostate cancer. Int J Radiat Oncol Biol Phys 60: 1047–1055.

154. Pucar D et al (2005) Prostate cancer: correlation of MR imaging and MR spectroscopy with pathologic findings after radiation therapy-initial experience. Radiology 236: 545–553.

155. Sciarra A et al (2008) Role of dynamic contrast-enhanced magnetic resonance (MR) imaging and proton MR spectroscopic imaging in the detection of local recurrence after radical prostatectomy for prostate cancer. Eur Urol 54: 589–600.

156. Ocak I et al (2007) The biologic basis of in vivo angiogenesis imaging. Front Biosci 12: 3601–3616.

157. Burtea C et al (2008) Contrast agents: magnetic resonance. Handb Exp Pharmacol (185 Pt 1): 135–165.

158. Tofts PS (1997) Modeling tracer kinetics in dynamic Gd-DTPA MR imaging. J Magn Reson Imaging 7: 91–101.

159. Fütterer JJ et al (2005) Staging prostate cancer with dynamic contrast-enhanced endorectal MR imaging prior to radical prostatectomy: experienced versus less experienced readers. Radiology 237: 541–549.

160. Bloch BN et al (2007) Prostate cancer: accurate determination of extracapsular extension with high-spatial-resolution dynamic contrast-enhanced and T2-weighted MR imaging–initial results. Radiology 245: 176–185.

161. Franiel T et al (2009) Prostate MR imaging: tissue characterization with pharmacokinetic volume and blood flow parameters and correlation with histologic parameters. Radiology 252: 101–108.

162. Cheikh AB et al (2009) Evaluation of T2-weighted and dynamic contrast-enhanced MRI in localizing prostate cancer before repeat biopsy. Eur Radiol 19: 770–778.

163. Casciani E et al (2008) Endorectal and dynamic contrast-enhanced MRI for detection of local recurrence after radical prostatectomy. AJR Am J Roentgenol 190: 1187–1192.

164. Rouviere O et al (2004) Recurrent prostate cancer after external beam radiotherapy: value of contrast-enhanced dynamic MRI in localizing intraprostatic tumor–correlation with biopsy findings. Urology 63: 922–927.

165. Haider MA et al (2008) Dynamic contrast-enhanced magnetic resonance imaging for localization of recurrent prostate cancer after external beam radiotherapy. Int J Radiat Oncol Biol Phys 70: 425–430.

166. Beyersdorff D et al (2005) MR imaging-guided prostate biopsy with a closed MR unit at 1. 5 T: initial results. Radiology 234: 576–581.

167. Zangos S et al (2005) MR-guided transgluteal biopsies with an open low-field system in patients with clinically suspected prostate cancer: technique and preliminary results. Eur Radiol 15: 174–182.

168. Pondman KM et al (2008) MR-guided biopsy of the prostate: an overview of techniques and a systematic review. Eur Urol 54: 517–527.

169. Yakar D et al (2008) Magnetic resonance-guided biopsy of the prostate: feasibility, technique, and clinical applications. Top Magn Reson Imaging 19: 291–295.

170. Anastasiadis AG et al (2006) MRI-guided biopsy of the prostate increases diagnostic performance in men with elevated or increasing PSA levels after previous negative TRUS biopsies. Eur Urol 50: 738–748.

171. Engelhard K et al (2006) Prostate biopsy in the supine position in a standard 1.5-T scanner under real time MR-imaging control using a MR-compatible endorectal biopsy device. Eur Radiol 16: 1237–1243.

174. National Cancer Institute. SEER Cancer Statistics Review, 1975–2001. Bethesda, MD, 2004. Available at: http://seer.cancer.gov/csr/1975_2001/ Accessed June 15, 2009.

175. Dalal PU, Sohaib SA, Huddart R (2006) Imaging of testicular germ cell tumours. Cancer Imaging 6: 124–134.

176. Donohue JP, Zachary JM, Maynard BR (1982) Distribution of nodal metastases in nonseminomatous testis cancer. J Urol 128: 315–320.

177. Mason MD et al (1991) Inguinal and iliac lymph node involvement in germ cell tumours of the testis: implications for radiological investigation and for therapy. Clin Oncol 3: 147–150.

178. Watanabe Y et al (2000) Scrotal disorders: evaluation of testicular enhancement patterns at dynamic contrast-enhanced subtraction MR imaging. Radiology 217: 219–227.

179. Schultz-Lampel D et al (1991) MRI for evaluation of scrotal pathology. Urol Res 19: 289–292.

180. Baker LL et al (1987) MR imaging of the scrotum: normal anatomy. Radiology 163: 89–92.

181. Baker LL et al (1987) MR imaging of the scrotum: pathologic conditions. Radiology 163: 93–98.

182. Seidenwurm D et al (1987) Testes and scrotum: MR imaging at 1.5T. Radiology 164: 393–398.

183. Rholl KS et al (1987) MR imaging of the scrotum with a high resolution surface coil. Radiology 163: 99–103.

184. Thurnher S et al (1988) Imaging of the testis: comparison between MR imaging and US. Radiology 167: 631–636.

185. Schnall M (1993) Magnetic resonance imaging of the scrotum. Semin Roentgenol 28: 19–30.

186. Cramer BM, Schlegel EA, Thueroff JW. MR imaging in the differential diagnosis of scrotal and testicular disease. Radiographics 1991: 11; 9–21.

187. Puech P et al (2009) Dynamic contrast-enhanced-magnetic resonance imaging evaluation of intraprostatic prostate cancer: correlation with radical prostatectomy specimens. Urology 74(5): 1094–1099.

188. Ahmed HU et al (2009) Is it time to consider a role for MRI before prostate biopsy? Nat Rev Clin Oncol 6(4): 197–206.

# 9

# Imaging in diagnosis and staging of urological cancers: ultrasound, CT, and PET

*Jorge Rioja[1], Charalampos Mamoulakis[1], Stavros Gravas[2], and Jean de la Rosette[1]*

[1]Department of Urology, AMC University Hospital, Amsterdam, The Netherlands
[2]Department of Urology, University Hospital of Larissa, Larissa, Greece

## Introduction

Imaging is the cornerstone in the management of all human malignancies including those arising from the urogenital system. At primary diagnosis, and during the follow-up period, it is of utmost importance to accurately assess the disease stage in order to decide the most effective treatment strategy for patients with urological malignancies. Ultrasound plays a major role principally in the initial diagnosis, but is also very useful in guiding a variety of interventional diagnostic and therapeutic procedures. Technological advances including the employment of contrast agents might enhance the value of this modality in the field of uro-oncology.

CT scans have played an important role in oncologic imaging since the very early period of its application. Technical innovations, however, have further improved precision, accuracy, and speed of acquisition. Recently, the traditionally morphology-based modalities have been complemented with functional and molecular imaging capabilities. One such modern and most promising imaging modality is PET, which allows noninvasive determination of various physiological and pathological processes in vivo, including tissue energy consumption and metabolism, cell proliferation, tissue perfusion, and hypoxia. The combination of PET with CT (PET-CT) provides metabolic and functional information alongside anatomical detail.

## Ultrasound

Ultrasound has a central role in the diagnostic armamentarium of uro-oncology. It is one of the most popular imaging modalities in medicine due to being rapid, noninvasive, safe, relatively inexpensive, and portable. Modern ultrasound imaging is primarily based on the application of a pulse-echo approach with a brightness-mode (B-mode) display. During the past years it has undergone refinements that have expanded its role through diagnosis to management and follow-up of uro-oncology patients. These technical improvements have brought about advances in the position of ultrasound in guiding urological procedures with higher precision in order to minimize morbidity, implement new treatment options (percutaneous tumor ablation), and monitor therapy response. The recent innovations that have improved the performance of modern ultrasound equipment, which are applicable in urology are schematically presented in Table 9.1. This section focuses mainly on the potential application of elasticity imaging, contrast-enhanced ultrasound (CE-US), and novel tissue characterization algorithms that have come to the fore in uro-oncology.

### Elastography

Elastography is a real-time, noninvasive method to image tissue hardness. It measures tissue motion caused by a force (excitation stress), to reconstruct tissue elastic parameters. Ultrasound detects the resulting tissue

*Interventional Techniques in Uro-oncology*, First Edition. Edited by Hashim Uddin Ahmed, Manit Arya, Peter T. Scardino & Mark Emberton. © 2011 Blackwell Publishing Ltd. Published 2011 by Blackwell Publishing Ltd.

Derby Hospitals NHS Foundation Trust
Library and Knowledge Service

**Table 9.1** Technical advances in ultrasonography: An overview.

**(A) Main advantages/aims: Improved resolution**
  Digital beam formers (programmability function, wide frequency range, dynamic apperture, apodization)
  Larger channel count (greater number of beam formers, i.e., crystal elements per data line)
  Coded pulse excitation technology (increases signal-to-noise ratio, preserves spatial resolution at larger depths)
  Harmonic imaging (higher than the transmitted frequencies received, artifacts eliminated/improved)
  Spatial compound imaging (multiple beams oriented along different directions image tissue multiple times)
  Electronic focusing by using array and matrix transducers
  Endoscopic and intraoperative ultrasonography (direct contact of transducer on the organ allows higher frequency use)

**(B) Main advantages/aims: Improved lesion detection and differentiation**
  Elasticity imaging
  Contrast-enhanced ultrasonography

**(C) Other technical innovations (main advantages)**
  Extended field of view imaging (inclusion of an entire large lesion in one image)
  Three- and four-dimensional imaging (whole volume view of solid structures and real-time delivery)

displacement by the excitation stress, which can be either mechanical (static; slight compression by the transducer or dynamic; mechanical vibrators) or the radiation force of an ultrasound source.

Hard tissues move as a unit and are displaced about the same amount when compressed, i.e., their displacement rate-of-change versus depth (strain values) are minimal. Softer tissues present much more displacement closer to the source of the excitation force than far away, i.e., larger displacement rate-of-change versus depth. Therefore, harder areas within soft tissues show low strain values and are displayed dark, while softer areas show higher strain values and are displayed bright on the elastogram. Two classic parameters are used to describe tissue stiffness: the Young elastic modulus, which is the change in length of a material in relation to the stretching/compressive force applied; and the shear modulus, which relates the deformability of a material in response to the force applied parallel to one of its surfaces.

*Contrast-enhanced ultrasound*
Contrast agents consist of microbubbles with a diameter of 1–10μm, injected intravenously that are small enough to pass through the pulmonary circulation and penetrate into the smallest microvessels. Their introduction along with new functional imaging techniques and special perfusion software permits imaging tumor neovascularity (10–50μm) [1].

Microbubbles have evolved from the first generation such as Levovist® (Schering; Berlin, Germany) into the "modern" second-generation agents. These consist of an immunologically inert lipoprotein shell filled in with an inert gas. Currently, the most commonly used agents include SonoVue® (Bracco Imaging, Milan, Italy), Optison® (Amersham Health AS, Oslo, Norway), and Definity® (Bristol-Myers Squibb, Billerica, Massachusetts), which differ in their physical properties. They are generally safe and only minor side effects have been associated with their use (alteration of taste, general/facial flush, local pain at the injection site) [2].

Contrast agents are very efficacious ultrasound scatters by contracting and expanding in response to the ultrasound beam energy. Due to the extremely large differences between the acoustic impedance of the gas and the surrounding liquid, a much stronger backscatter than blood or normal tissue is produced. Therefore, contrast agents provide the ideal way to image prostate or kidney tumors by means of microvessel imaging.

Contrast agents are imaged by two basic methods: (a) color or power doppler (CD/PD) ultrasound and (b) gray-scale harmonic imaging. Conventional harmonic imaging has been further improved with the implementation of different techniques such as pulse inversion, intermittent imaging, flash-replenishment, and cadence contrast-pulse sequence (CPS) allowing better visualization of the microvasculature [3].

The improved resolution achieved to date due to the recent advances in ultrasound technology, together with the sufficient computing power presently available, has made possible three-dimensional (3D) renderings of ultrasound images and their real-time delivery (4D imaging). This produces whole volume views of solid structures, allowing an increased measuring accuracy of volumes, better appreciation of relationship to surrounding structure, and elimination of user-dependent scanning variation.

### Prostate cancer

Prostate cancer shows an increase in both cell density and vascularization. The increased cell density leads to changes in tissue elasticity and may be visualized with elasticity imaging while the increased vascularization can be visualized with CE-US (Figure 9.1).

#### Elastography
The use of elasticity imaging for the detection of prostate cancer (PCa) is based on the fact that these tumors are firmer than the surrounding normal

parenchyma. The prostate was the first organ to be considered for elasticity imaging [4].

A number of studies have recently been conducted in order to evaluate the role of this imaging modality in the detection of prostate cancer [5]. These studies can be divided into two categories: (a) Group A (Table 9.2) in which the technique was evaluated solely on images (no targeted biopsies obtained) [6], (b) Group B: studies that evaluated the method as a tool to support or replace gray-scale transrectal ultrasound (TRUS)-guided systematic biopsies based on elastography-targeted biopsy results.

Cochlin et al [15] and König et al [16] conducted the first of such studies on 100 and 404 patients, respectively with TRUS-guided biopsies as the reference standard. There were mixed findings with poor sensitivity. Elastography-guided prostate biopsy was compared directly to systematic biopsy in 230 screening volunteers [17]. Up to five targeted biopsies from the peripheral zone were performed by an investigator and subsequently, another investigator blind to the

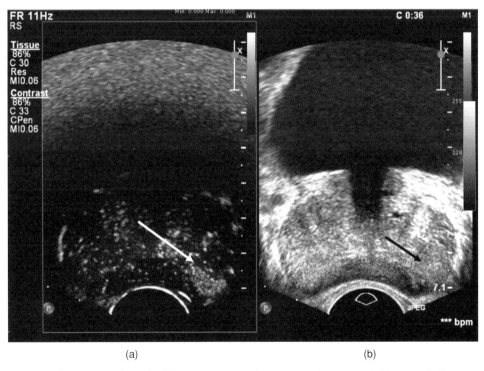

(a)                (b)

**Fig 9.1** CE-US (a) and conventional TRUS of the prostate in the same patient with prostate cancer (b). The suspicious lesion is depicted as a hypoechoic area (black arrow) in conventional TRUS. A much larger lesion is depicted by contrast enhancement (white arrow). Contrast agents may facilitate the detection of cancer providing additional information on tumor size.

Table 9.2 Elasticity imaging in the detection of prostate cancer.

| Reference | Patients | Reference standard | Imaging modalities compared | | Main study results |
|-----------|----------|--------------------|-----------------------------|---|--------------------|
| Taylor, 2005 [7][a] | 19 | RPS | 3D-SE | 3D-US | 3D-SE performs considerably better for tumors with volumes $\geq 1$ cm$^3$ |
| Miyanaga, 2006 [8] | 29[b] | PB | E | TRUS/DRE | E performs significantly better: Detection rates: E (93%), TRUS (55%), DRE (59%) |
| | | | | | The two patients missed had well-differentiated PCa |
| | 11[c] | | | | Similar detection rates for all modalities:[c] E (55%), TRUS (55%), DRE (64%) |
| Pallwein, 2007 [9] | 15 | RPS | E | – | Accuracy 92%, Best sensitivity at the appex-mid gland |
| Tsutsumi, 2007 [10] | 51 | RPS | E | TRUS | Detection rates: E (84%), TRUS (31%), combination of modalities (100%) |
| | | | | | Excellent detection rate for anterior tumors. Lower detection rate for higher grade tumors |
| Sumura, 2007 [11] | 17 | RPS | E | TRUS/DRE | Detection rate: E (74.1%), TRUS (48.1%), DRE (33.3%), CD (55.6%), MRI (47.4%) |
| | | | | CD/MRI | Detection rates similar at anterior-posterior gland, higher for higher Gleason scores or tumor volumes |
| Pallwein, 2008 [12] | 492 | PB | E | TRUS | E accurately detects PCa. Promising results especially in the apex |
| Salomon, 2008 [13] | 109 | RPS | E | – | E accuracy (76%). E findings correlate best in the apex. |
| | | | | | Higher detection rates for higher Gleason score (up to 93% for scores >7) |
| Eggert, 2008[d] [14] | 351 | PB | E | TRUS | E does not improve detection rate |

3D-SE, three-dimensional sonoelastography, CD, color Doppler, DRE, digital rectal examination, E, elastography, MRI, magnetic resonance imaging, Pca, prostate cancer, RPS, radical prostatectomy specimens, TRUS, conventional transrectal ultrasonography, US, gray-scale ultrasonography.

[a]Imaging performed in vitro.

[b]Previously untreated patients.

[c]Patients treated previously with hormone therapy. Elastography detection rate dropped possibly due to lesion softer-rendered consistency by treatment.

[d]Randomized clinical trial, conventional TRUS-guided 10-core biopsy offered to both arms. One arm was additionally offered elastography prior to biopsy.

previous results, performed 10 conventional gray-scale TRUS-guided systematic biopsies. Prostate cancer was detected in 35% of the population. The number of men with prostate cancer detected by the two strategies did not differ significantly (targeted vs. systematic: 30% vs. 25%, respectively). However, the difference in detection rates per core was significant (targeted vs. systematic: 12.7% vs. 5.6%). The targeted biopsy protocol in any one patient with prostate cancer was found to be 2.9-fold more likely to detect the tumor. Therefore, targeted biopsy protocols seemed to detect more cases of cancer with fewer than half the number of cores. No significant differences were detected regarding the distribution of Gleason scores. In addition, the detection rate for targeted biopsy was slightly better in the apical areas. This study may have overestimated the benefit of conventional TRUS-guided biopsy as the second investigator will have been able to see the tracts formed by the targeted biopsies.

In a further study, targeted biopsies guided by conventional gray-scale TRUS, CD-US, and elastography were obtained along with systematic sextant biopsies in 137 patients, in order to compare the detection of prostate cancer and distribution of Gleason scores [18]. Targeted biopsies were more likely to detect cancer than systematic cores. Positive results on CD-US and elastography were strongly associated with high-grade and moderate- to high-grade cancers, respectively. It was concluded that CD-US and elastography are encouraging adjuncts to improve prostate cancer detection, although targeted biopsy alone was not sufficient to replace the sextant biopsy technique.

Kamoi et al [19] compared elastography with conventional TRUS and PD-US in107 men. All underwent transperineal systematic 8-core biopsies plus up to four biopsies based on suspicious findings of each modality. Patient analysis showed that TRUS had a significantly lower sensitivity (50%) compared to the other two modalities (PD-US: 70%, elastography: 68%), but the specificities were similar. Accuracies were comparable, ranging from 72% (TRUS) to 76% (elastography). The diagnostic performances did not differ significantly. The diagnostic performances of pair-wise or all-three modalities combinations were also similar. It was concluded that elastography should complement conventional TRUS for minimizing the number of missed cancers.

Based on the above data, it seems that elastography combined with TRUS represents a simple, non-invasive, relatively cheap technique that can be used for targeted biopsies and may reduce the number of biopsy cores per patient. Nevertheless, further clinical trials are still needed to better define the advantages and the exact role of this relatively novel technique in the diagnosis of prostate cancer.

*Contrast-enhanced ultrasound*
CE-US may potentially facilitate the detection of prostate cancer by providing additional information on tumor size and possibly aggressiveness. A multicenter study was carried out in four European countries during the period 2002–2006 (CONTRAST, QLRT-2001–2174) in order to determine the value of CE-US in the detection, localization, and treatment follow-up of prostate cancer. Recently, the results based on 3746 patients have been reported and compared to published data [2]. The individual studies employed various contrast agents imaged by, (a) CD-US [20], (b) 3D-PD-US [21], and (c) novel nonlinear imaging techniques (CPS).

It appears that technical improvements led to an increased sensitivity for the detection of perfusion patterns as demonstrated by correlation of histological findings in radical prostatectomy specimens with pre-operative CE-US images. Both 3D-CE-PD- and CE-CD-US could visualize lesions with an increased microvascular density. It was found that 3D-CE-PD-US was a better diagnostic tool than digital rectal examination, PSA, gray-scale, or PD-US; and that the combination of 3D-CE-PD-US and PSA was the most predictive for Prostate cancer. It was shown that CE-US based on wide-band harmonic imaging improved the sensitivity for prostate cancer detection, but also demonstrated false positives in the form of focal enhancement in areas of benign hyperplasia. Nevertheless, accurate detection of localized tumors was reported in up to 78% of patients with 3D-CE-PD-US [21]. In a larger group of 70 patients evaluated with the same technique, diagnosis by imaging alone was improved from 61% (standard detection and staging investigations) to an average of 86% of tumors with detection of foci $\geq 5$ mm in 68–79% [22]. In another small series, all tumors with extracapsular extension could be identified using microvascular imaging [2].

The clinical value of these promising results should be tested in a diagnostic setting. The effect of

CE-US on the prostate biopsy protocol and the detection rate has been extensively investigated. The European collaboration described above concluded that a clear association exists between prostate contrast enhancement and diagnosis of clinically significant prostate cancer. In addition, to the increased sensitivity of CE-US targeted biopsy, fewer biopsies are needed with the tumors detected by targeted biopsies a higher Gleason score than TRUS-guided biopsies which are subject to random error [2].

These findings are in accordance with results from studies outside the European multicenter study. By employing various CE-US methods including novel nonlinear imaging techniques (intermittent harmonic imaging, flash-replenishment, CPS), these studies either directly compared gray-scale ultrasound-guided systemic with CE-targeted biopsy protocols [23] (Table 9.3) or investigated the contribution of CE-US on systematic biopsy protocols [24] and its value in predicting the nature of hypoechoic lesions [25].

Currently, CE-US enables visualization of prostate cancer, and the detection rate is increased by the application of targeted biopsies upon a random protocol. However, sensitivity and specificity are still not high enough to warrant the abandonment of systematic random biopsies. The ability of CE-US to image prostate perfusion might enable visualization of minimal invasive or medical treatment effects that influence the perfusion of the organ (HIFU/cryoablation, hormone therapy) in prostate cancer and identify patients with early relapse using the presence or absence of blood signals as an indicator [26].

### Three-dimensional and four-dimensional imaging

Early work on prostate imaging identified several advantages of 3D over 2D TRUS with an improved diagnostic capacity, accurate diagnosis of extraprostatic tumor extension, and staging of localized prostate cancer [27]. The 4D technique has been used during TRUS-guided prostate biopsies improving diagnostic accuracy. Further clinical applications of 3D TRUS include treatment mapping for brachytherapy radioactive seeds placement and guidance for cryoablation of localized prostate cancer.

### Tissue characterization

Recently, a novel computer-aided ultrasound technology based on tissue characterization algorithms (HistoScanning™, Advanced Medical Diagnostics, Waterloo, Belgium) has been introduced as a tool with the potential to detect prostate cancer. HistoScanning is a tissue differentiation, visualization, and quantification imaging tool that identifies specific changes in solid organ morphology by extracting and quantifying statistical features from 3D backscattered ultrasound data. The geometric accuracy of the system facilitates identification of minimal, localized tissue structures. The characterization algorithms exploit the specific physical changes to sound waves that result from their interaction with the tumor and can be applied in discrete regions of interest in the prostate to ascertain the presence of cancer. HistoScanning™ can spatially orientate cancer foci within the gland, enabling both determination of their location and volume. It has been reported that foci of $\geq 0.50$ mL can be accurately detected [28], and it has been proposed as a potential triage test for men deemed to be at risk of prostate cancer who wish to avoid biopsy.

### Kidney cancer

#### Contrast-enhanced ultrasound

CE-US has been the major improvement in ultrasound technology applied to the diagnosis and staging of RCC. It has focused mainly on the diagnosis of complex renal masses (Figure 9.2) and on the evaluation of tumor vascularity to characterize a lesion as benign or malignant (Figures 9.3 and 9.4). CE-US can play an important role in differentiating and characterizing solid lesions and complex cystic masses of the kidney. Tamai et al [29] assessed the value of CE-US as a diagnostic tool for solid renal tumors in comparison to contrast CT. CE-US was more sensitive in the detection of small amounts of tumor blood flow as well as a useful tool in the preoperative diagnosis of hypovascular malignant renal tumors.

CE-US was compared with triple-phase helical CT in the classification of complex renal cysts using the Bosniak system. A complete concordance was found regarding the differentiation of surgical and nonsurgical complex cysts with a high interobserver agreement. In a similar study, Park et al [30] compared CE-US with CT. The difference between the diagnostic accuracies of the two modalities was statistically insignificant, although CE-US had greater accuracy rates. CE-US might better visualize septa number, septa and wall

**Table 9.3** Diagnostic performance of contrast-enhanced targeted compared to systematic gray-scale ultrasound guided biopsies of the prostate.

| | | Patient analysis | | | | | Biopsy core analysis | | | | | | |
| --- | --- | --- | --- | --- | --- | --- | --- | --- | --- | --- | --- | --- | --- |
| | | PCa (%) | | | | | PCa (%) | | | | | | |
| | | | | | | TB vs. SB | | | | | | TB vs. SB | |
| | Reference | Total | TB | SB | TB+SB | P value | Total | TB | Total | TB | SB | OR (95% CI) | P value |
| ERCP | Frauscher, 2002 [31] | 230 | 24.4 | 22.6 | 30.0 | n.s. | 3439 | 1139 | 7.0 | 10.4 | 5.3 | 2.6 (1.9–3.5) | <0.001 |
| | Pelzer, 2005 [32] | 380 | 27.4 | 27.6 | 37.6 | n.s. | 5700 | 1900 | 8.6 | 32.6[a] | 17.9[a] | 3.1 (n. a) | <0.01 |
| | Mitterberger, 2007 [33][b] | 690 | 26.1 | 24.1 | 32.0 | n.s. | 10317 | 3417 | 7.6 | 11.1 | 5.8 | n.a | <0.001 |
| | Mitterberger, 2007 [34][c] | 100 | 32.0 | 26.0 | 29.0 | 0.04 | 750 | 250 | 9.7 | 15.6 | 6.8 | n.a | <0.001 |
| | Mitterberger, 2008 [35][d] | 36 | 33.3 | 16.7 | 33.3 | 0.04 | 540 | 180 | 12.2 | 17.0 | 10.0 | 2 (n.a) | 0.027 |
| | Pallwein, 2008 [36] | 20 | 40.0 | 25.0 | 40.0 | n.s. | n.a | n.a | n.a | n.a | n.a | n.a | n.a |
| | Frauscher, 2001 [37] | 84 | 27.4 | 20.2 | 28.6 | 0.034 | 1249 | 409 | 7.7 | 13.4 | 4.9 | 4.3 (2.6–7.1) | <0.001 |
| | Halpern, 2005 [38] | 301 | 27.6 | 30.9 | 34.6 | n.s. | 2939 | 1133 | 363 | 15.4 | 10.4 | 2.0 (n.a.) | <0.001 |
| | Linden, 2007 [39] | 60 | 21.7 | 26.7 | 30 | n.s. | 825 | 225 | 9.6 | 12.9 | 8.3 | 2.0 (n.a.) | 0.034 |
| | Colleselli, 2007 [40] | 345 | 77.4 | 73.0 | n.a. | n.s.[e] | 5175 | 1725 | n.a | n.a | n.a | n.a | n.a |

CI, confidence interval; ERCP, European Research Coordination Program, n.a., not available, n.s., not signidficant, OR, odds ratio, Pca, prostate cancer, SB, systematic biopsy, TB, targeted biopsy.

[a] Detection rate based on number of positive cores per total number of cores in the 143 men with PCa detected by combined approach.

[b] TB detected significantly higher Gleason scores and may allow for identification of more aggressive tumors.

[c] The only randomized clinical trial to date (randomization 1:1).

[d] The short-term (14 days) application of dutasteride may improve cancer detection by contrast-enhanced targeted ultrasound-guided biopsies due to blood flow reduction in benign prostatic tissue.

[e] A statistically significant difference in PCa detection rate in favor of contrast-enhanced ultrasound was detected only in small prostate glands (69% vs. 88.1% and 70.4% vs. 80.8% for prostate volumes of <20 mL and 20–30 mL, respectively).

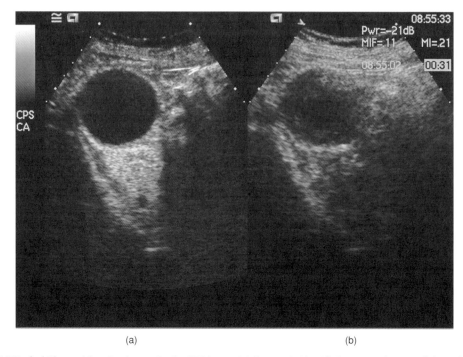

(a)                        (b)

**Fig 9.2** CE-US of a kidney with a simple cyst. In the CPS image (a) the cyst is identified as a simple one, while in the conventional B-mode image (b) it appears as a complex one.

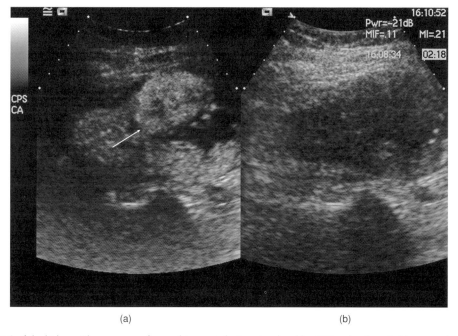

(a)                        (b)

**Fig 9.3** CE-US of the kidney. The presence of a renal tumor is better visualized by CPS technology (white arrow) compared to the conventional B-mode imaging.

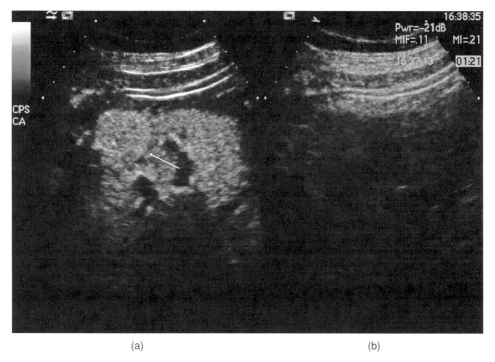

(a)                                                                                              (b)

**Fig 9.4** CE-US of the kidney. The presence of a renal tumor is imaged by CPS technology (white arrow), but it is missed on the conventional B-mode.

thickness, solid components, and the enhancement of some renal cystic masses; resulting in upgrading of the Bosniak category assigned by CT and thus a change in the treatment plan (Figure 9.5).

It has been reported that CE-CD-US achieves better results compared to conventional CD-US in the detection of tumor vascularity and discrimination between benign and malignant small renal masses [41]. The detection rate of intra- and/or peritumor vessels with the use of contrast agents was twice that achieved without their use. The characteristics of renal tumor perfusion detected by CE-US based on CPS technology was investigated and compared to clinical diagnoses and histological findings [42]. It was reported that CPS may have a role in determining perfusion patterns in kidney tumors. The same technique was also evaluated in the diagnosis of small renal masses (<4 cm) [43]. Similar diagnostic accuracy to MD-CT was shown for renal masses of 2–4 cm, while it was reported that CE-US was superior for lesions smaller than 2 cm.

*Other techniques*

Elasticity imaging for visualization of renal masses has only recently been investigated in vivo. Fahey et al [44] evaluated acoustic radiation force impulse imaging for real-time visualization of abdominal malignancies including two renal masses. They concluded that acoustic radiation force impulse imaging improves the visualization of kidney malignancies compared to the sole use of conventional ultrasound. In addition, imaging with 3D/4D-US may have several applications, such as evaluation and follow-up of renal lesions, execution of renal/adrenal biopsies, and percutaneous ablative procedures.

## Bladder cancer

Cystoscopy still remains an invasive procedure with drawbacks and limitations, such as failure to evaluate adjacent structures, risk of urinary tract infection, patient discomfort and anxiety, and iatrogenic injury of the lower urinary tract [45]. Nevertheless, the advent

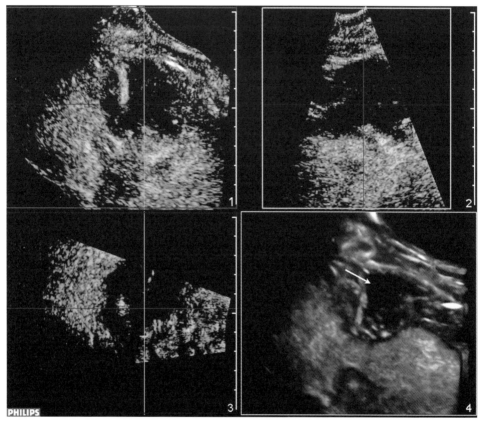

**Fig 9.5** CPS 3D reconstruction of a complex renal cyst. 1, 2 and are the different space planes of the lesion which is viewed in 4 as a 3D reconstruction.

of flexible instruments and digital chip technology has significantly increased its tolerability. Recently, efforts have centered on the development of new noninvasive techniques for the evaluation of the bladder. 3D- versus 2D-US of the bladder has been recently evaluated in 42 patients with hematuria [46]. 3D-US showed a better diagnostic performance with an overall correct diagnosis in 86% of the cases. The sensitivity for the detection of malignant and benign bladder lesions was 100% and 71%, respectively.

In a similar study, virtual cystoscopy based on 3D-US data was evaluated for the detection of bladder tumors [47]. The sensitivity, specificity, positive, and negative predictive values were 96.2%, 70.6%, 93.9%, and 80%, respectively. When combined with gray-scale multiplanar reconstruction, the sensitivity, specificity, positive, and negative predictive values in-

creased to 96.4%, 88.8%, 97.6%, and 84.2%, respectively.

### Testicular cancer

Testicular tumors are usually diagnosed clinically by physical examination and pathologically after orchidectomy. Imaging of the testis with ultrasound is used to confirm the presence of an intratesticular mass or in case of uncertainty about the clinical findings or to examine the contralateral testis to detect the presence of bilateral synchronous tumors. In current practice, high-resolution ultrasound combining gray scale and colour techniques (CD, PD) represents an extension and supplement to clinical evaluation. It is considered irreplaceable in the diagnostic work-up and the imaging modality of choice in patients with testicular cancer [48]. Ultrasound can be performed with minimal patient discomfort, at low-cost and without posing any risks. Despite its indisputable value in diagnosis; it has no role in staging with CT remaining the imaging technique of choice for this.

Recent technological advances such as the introduction of high frequency probes, have significantly improved the diagnostic performance, providing information on the normal anatomy, the morphological features, as well as relevant data on the vascular supply of the lesions. Despite its high sensitivity, ultrasound is not wholly sufficient for differentiating between benign and malignant solid lesions [49]. However, it can differentiate between intratesticular and extratesticular masses and determine their nature (cystic, solid, or complex). It is especially helpful in cases of clinical uncertainty, such as cases of impalpable tumors, suspicion of an occult primary testicular lesion, or in examining the contralateral testis to identify bilateral synchronous masses.

CD/PD-US cannot determine the type of a testicular tumor since the detection of vascularity depends upon the size rather than the histology. Tumors smaller than 1.6 cm tend to be hypovascular, while larger tumors are hypervascular [50]. Nevertheless, ultrasound color techniques may help in the visualization of a subtle small tumor and differentiate an avascular intratesticular hematoma from a vascular tumor. This is very important in patients presenting with a history of trauma. CD-US cannot be used to separate a focal inflammatory testicular mass from a tumor since hypervascular neoplasms have a similar appearance to inflammation. The sonographic features of the various types of testicular tumors are summarized as follows (Figure 9.6):

a Seminomas are well marginated, but can be ill-defined, round to oval-shaped. They are hypoechoic in comparison to the echotexture of the adjacent normal parenchyma. They contain diffuse low-level echoes without cystic areas or calcified foci. They can be multifocal and less commonly present a diffusely infiltrative pattern.

b Embryonal cell carcinomas are inhomogeneous, poorly marginated, and produce a lobulated testis outline due to invasion of the tunica albuginea. Cystic areas are common and foci of increased echogenicity with acoustic shadowing may be present.

c Teratomas are well-defined but have an inhomogeneous echo texture due to the presence of cystic areas and calcified foci (calcifications within areas of cartilage, bone, and fibrous tissue), which produce acoustic shadowing.

d Choriocarcinoma exhibits a complex echo pattern due to the presence of hemorrhage, necrosis, and calcification. Patients can present with metastatic choriocarcinoma without any evidence of a mass in the testis.

e Stromal tumors can appear hypoechoic when small, while larger tumors are more complex due to the presence of necrotic and hemorrhagic areas.

f Metastatic tumors are most commonly non-Hodgkin lymphoma. Lymphoma is the most common cause of bilateral testicular masses. The tumor is hypoechoic and may present as a focal well-defined mass or as a diffuse infiltrating process that replaces some or most of the parenchyma and enlarges the testis. CD demonstrates hypervascularity. Areas of necrosis, hemorrhage, and calcifications are rarely seen. Leukemia has a similar sonographic appearance to lymphoma and is often bilateral as well.

## Computed tomography

CT constitutes an integral part of the daily urological practice. CT technology has progressed rapidly since the introduction of the first helical scanners in the early 1990s, revolutionizing the value of this imaging modality in urology. The earliest helical CT devices allowed continuous data acquisition as a patient was advanced through the scanner. A thin beam with a single row of detectors was used providing high resolution only in the primary axial slice orientation. During the last years, additional rows of detectors have been added and the beam shape has been widened to simultaneously expose many rows of detectors (up to 256 currently in development) permitting a true volume acquisition. This latest CT technology, referred to as MD-CT has reduced acquisition times, and has offered higher resolution images through the entire abdomen in a single breath-hold, transforming CT from a transaxial cross-sectional technique into a true 3D imaging modality that allows for arbitrary cut planes as well as excellent 3D displays of the data volume. Advantages and disadvantages of MD-CT are presented in Table 9.4 [51] (Figure 9.7).

A major application of 3D CT in urology is CT-urography (CTU) because it provides a complete evaluation of the urinary collecting system. MD-CTU

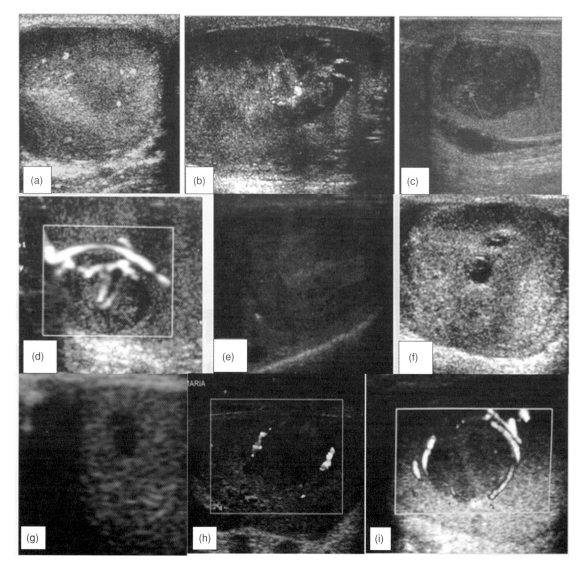

**Fig 9.6** Nine different ultrasound testicular images confirmed by pathological report. (a) classic seminoma, (b) mixed germ cell tumour with calcifications (white arrow), (c) Leydig cell tumour with calcifications (white arrow), (d) mixed germ cell tumour, (e) classic seminoma with solid component, (f) complex seminoma with hypoechoic compound, (g) Leydig cell tumour (anechoic lesion with posterior reinforcement) mimicking a cystic lesion, (h) testicular infarction, (i) Embryonal carcinoma, mimicking infarction (in both cases CD-US signal is around the lesion but not inside).

may be defined as the examination of the urinary tract by MD-CT in the excretory phase, following intravenous contrast administration [52]. A variety of protocols are used at different centers whereas the range of indications has rapidly expanded. (Figure 9.8) Table 9.5.

## Renal cell carcinoma

CT is an excellent imaging modality for the evaluation of a renal mass providing additional information on the function and morphology of the contralateral kidney. A dedicated imaging protocol is necessary, which

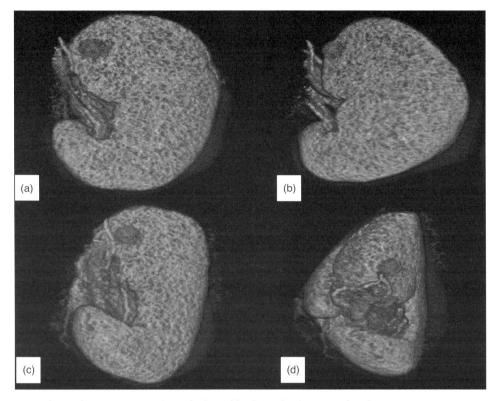

**Fig 9.7** MDCT of a renal tumor. Surgery plan is facilitated by this technology. *See also plate 9.7.*

**Table 9.4** Advantages and disadvantages of Multidetector Computed Tomography.

| Advantages | Clinical implication |
| --- | --- |
| Improved temporal resolution | Reliable image quality with minimal motion artifacts |
| Improved spatial resolution | Improve resolution in the z axis leads to increasing diagnostic accuracy |
| Increased concentration of intravascular contrast material due to faster scanning | Improved conspicuity of arteries and veins |
| Efficient x-ray tube use due to faster scanning | Diminished x-ray tube heating and less delay for x-ray tube cooling |
| Simultaneous registration of multiple sections during each rotation, and increased gantry rotation speed | Longer anatomic coverage, thanks to multiple detectors scanning |

| Disadvantages | Clinical implication |
| --- | --- |
| Increased data load | Time-consuming for the radiologist |
| Increased radiation dose due to multiphase, thin-section imaging | Increased exposure (consideration especially for younger population under follow-up) |

Table 9.5 The role of CT in diagnosis and staging of urological cancer.

|  | Diagnosis | Staging |
|---|---|---|
| Prostate | No role | Limited |
| Renal Cell Carcinoma | Reference standard | High performance in T- and M-staging Poor in N-staging. |
| Bladder Cancer | Limited | Recommended |
| Upper TCC | Method of choice | Recommended |
| Penile cancer | No role | Limited only where indicated |
| Testicular cancer | No role | Recommended but limited in small volume lymphadenopathy |

includes three imaging series performed during breath-hold: precontrast imaging, corticomedullary phase, and late nephrographic/early excretory phase [53].

High accuracy (sensitivity up to 100%, specificity up to 95%) has been reported in the detection of RCC using a triple-phase technique [54]. The key features in distinguishing a renal lesion on CT include char-acterization of the mass as cystic or solid, enhance-ment (attenuation change from the noncontrast to the contrast-enhanced images), presence and type of cal-cification, and presence of fat.

Several studies have been published on the dif-ferentiation of benign from malignant cystic masses of the kidney. CT provides information by assessing

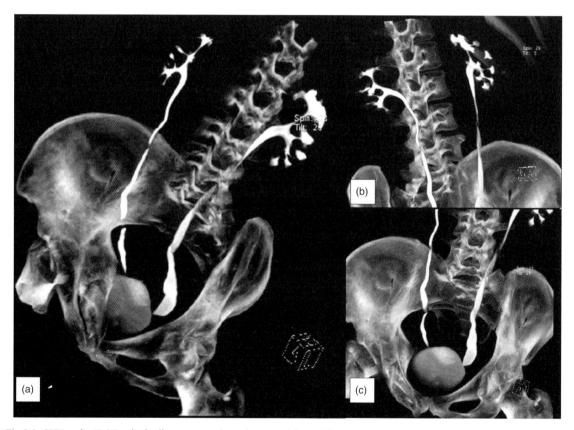

Fig 9.8 CTU and MDCT, which allows urography to be viewed form different angles.

wall thickness, presence and thickness of septa, calcifications, cyst attenuation, and foci of enhancement. The Bosniak classification system (Grade I to IV) grades the cystic renal masses for the likelihood of malignancy [55] based on the presence of enhancing soft tissue (either as mural nodule or thickened cystic wall/septation) and shows the highest sensitivity for predicting malignancy.

On the other hand, limited research has been performed on the differentiation of solid renal tumors based on CT findings. In principle, the presence of calcifications in a solid renal mass indicates possible malignancy, while the presence of fat on the precontrast images is suggestive of angiomyolipoma (AML). RCC rarely contains fat or lacks calcifications [56]. It is recommended that renal masses containing both fat and calcification should be considered malignant.

It is well accepted that the most consistent and important imaging criterion for the characterization of renal tumor subtype is probably the degree of enhancement. Clear cell RCCs and oncocytomas enhance avidly, chromophobe carcinomas and lipid poor angiomyolipomas enhance moderately, whereas papillary tumors enhance the least during the parenchymal phase [57]. In addition, the vast majority of clear cell RCCs are hypervascular and demonstrate a heterogeneous enhancing pattern of mixed solid soft-tissue components and low-attenuation areas that may represent cystic or necrotic changes. Chromophobe tumors are less hypervascular than clear cell tumors, and are more variable in their degree of enhancement with a more peripheral pattern of enhancement. However, their appearance is not sufficiently characteristic to allow them to be reliably differentiated from papillary lesions [57]. Papillary RCCs are typically hypovascular, and most commonly demonstrate a homogeneous or peripheral enhancement pattern. Since these lesions accumulate contrast material more slowly, delayed images may be helpful in confirming enhancement. A low tumor-to-aorta or tumor-to-normal renal parenchyma enhancement ratio is highly indicative of papillary RCC. Finally, oncocytomas cannot be reliably differentiated from RCCs on the basis of imaging features and degree of enhancement.

Studies have shown that CT has a staging accuracy of up to 91% making it the imaging method of choice in most cases [58]. The European Association of Urology (EAU) guidelines indicate that abdominal CT can detect extrarenal tumor spread providing information on venous, locoregional lymph node, adrenal gland, and liver involvement [59]. However, one of the main limitations is the correct identification of perirenal fat invasion, to distinguish T2 and T3a lesions. Perirenal stranding is found in about half of the patients with localized (T1 and T2) tumors, and it does not reliably indicate tumor spread. It may be caused by edema, vascular engorgement, or previous inflammation. It seems that CT-based distinction between confinement of RCC to the true renal capsule and extension into the perirenal fat is currently not fully reliable.

The imaging assessment of renal veins and the inferior vena cava (IVC) is crucial in the evaluation of patients with RCC, as these features impact on the optimal surgical approach. The presence of a thrombus in the renal vein or IVC may represent tumor thrombus, blood clot, or both. The presence of enhancement within the thrombus indicates tumor thrombus. Current CT techniques have reported sensitivities and specificities of 85% and 98%, respectively for detecting renal vein thrombus [60]. However, the imaging of the superior extent of tumor thrombus remains a problem even for MD-CT. On CT, it is difficult to accurately obtain optimal venous opacification, and there are some limitations in distinguishing bland thrombus from tumor thrombus and invasive from noninvasive tumor with respect to the vessel wall.

With respect to lymph node staging, the sensitivity of CT for detection of regional lymph node metastases has been found to be as high as 95% using a cut-off value of 1 cm for short-axis nodal size [61]. Overall accuracies of 83% and 89% have been reported [61,62]. However, enlarged nodes are not necessarily metastatic rather reactive so false-positive findings up to 58% have also been reported [61]. Chest CT is the most accurate investigation for chest staging, but at the very least routine chest radiography, albeit a less accurate alternative must be done for metastatic evaluation.

### Transitional cell cancer of the bladder

Cystoscopy remains the gold standard for evaluation of the bladder and detection of transitional cell cancer (TCC) of the bladder. Imaging is a useful supplement to cystoscopy. A standard CT protocol for patients with known or suspected bladder cancer consists of a noncontrast followed by a contrast-enhanced CT scan. This can be valuable in distinguishing a blood clot, wall edema, or tissue debris from a mass based on its enhancement characteristics [63]. Bladder cancer may show various patterns of tumor growth along the bladder wall, including papillary, sessile, infiltrating, mixed, or flat intraepithelial growth while calcifications may also be present [64]. MD-CT improves the accuracy of CT offering greater speed, improved spatial resolution, and wider coverage. High-quality multi-planar reconstructions with MD-CT have improved the sensitivity of CT in the detection of bladder tumors, especially those located at the base or dome. Cancers less than 1 cm can now be routinely detected.

CT scan is unable to differentiate between stages Ta to T3a, since it does not depict the individual layers of the bladder wall. For this reason, CT is not recommended for staging noninvasive bladder cancer (Ta and T1 disease). It can however distinguish T3a from T3b or higher stage tumors. CT features that suggest perivesical invasion include loss of the clear interface between the bladder wall and the adjacent fat, and irregularity or stranding in the perivesical fat. MD-CT offers excellent inherent contrast between the bladder and extraperitoneal fat, which helps in the detection of extravesical spread and allows evaluation of multiple organs in the abdomen for metastatic disease and for complications such as hydronephrosis. Adjacent organ invasion can be excluded if a clear plane of separation is preserved, although the presence or absence of the fat plane is not completely reliable for determination of microscopic invasion.

The assessment of nodal metastasis based simply on size is limited by the inability of CT to identify metastases in normal sized or minimally enlarged nodes. Similar to the evaluation of nodal status of other organs, pelvic and abdominal nodes with a maximum short axis diameter greater than 8 mm and 10 mm, respectively should be considered enlarged [65]. The specificity is low as nodal enlargement may be due to benign pathology, the sensitivity ranging from 48% to 87% [65].

The overall reported CT accuracy in detecting and staging bladder cancer varies between 64% to 97%, whereas that for perivesical invasion and for lymph node metastases ranges from 83% to 93% and 73% to 92%, respectively [66]. In addition, the sensitivity and specificity of MD-CTU for the diagnosis of perivesical invasion is 89% and 95%, respectively (Figure 9.9).

Other considerations regarding the use of CT for bladder cancer staging include the need for an adequately distended bladder for accurate interpretation,

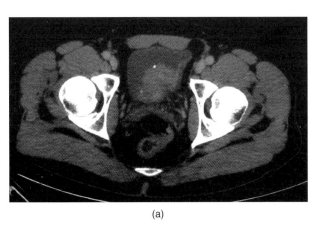

(a)

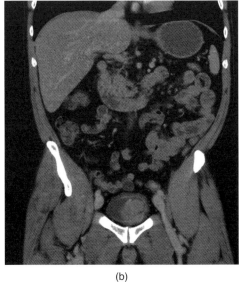

(b)

**Fig 9.9** Staging MDCT of an invasive bladder tumor. (a) Transversal view showing a big bladder tumor (left bladder wall) with retraction of the perivesical fat (white arrow), suggestive of tumour invasion (T3-T4), (b) Coronal view allowing a better localization of the tumor.

and optimal timing for the performance of CT. Overdistension of the bladder may result in underestimation of the bladder wall thickness and effacement of fat planes between the bladder and the adjacent structures. Overstaging may result from misinterpretation of normal fat planes between the posterior bladder wall and the seminal vesicles. In a study of 65 patients assigned to four groups (less than or equal to T1, T2-T3a, T3b, or T4 disease), the accuracy was reported to be 90.5% for contrast-distended bladder images, 95% for air-distended bladder images, and 87% in noncontrast studies [67]. In addition, early postoperative CT, may also lead to inaccurate staging. Recent transurethral resection of bladder tumor frequently causes linear or focal enhancement along the bladder mucosa or wall, bladder wall thickening, perivesical fat stranding, or fibrosis, limiting the specificity of CT. This can be avoided by performing the examination after an adequate time interval postoperatively or ideally before any intervention to avoid over-staging due to perivesical fibrosis. Kim et al found that sensitivity and specificity for perivesical invasion detection by CT were 92% and 98%, respectively, when performed 7 or more days after the resection. Sensitivity and specificity were 89% and 95%, respectively, in a cohort of 67 patients without a postoperative CT delay [66].

For patients with confirmed muscle-invasive bladder cancer, MD-CT of the chest, abdomen, and pelvis is the optimal form of staging, including MD-CTU for complete examination of the upper urinary tract. Metastases to bones or brain at presentation of invasive bladder cancer are rare.

## Transitional cell cancer of the upper urinary tract

In many centers, CTU is used as an alternative to conventional intravenous urography (IVU). Recent studies have also shown higher detection rates for upper and lower tract urothelial malignancies with CTU over IVU. In addition, CTU requires a shorter examination time, allows more detailed evaluation of the renal parenchyma and perirenal tissues and permits a better evaluation of obstructed collecting systems. EAU guidelines indicate that CTU is more informative than IVU in invasive tumors of the upper tract, and consider MD-CTU the technique of choice for the diagnosis of upper urinary tract urothelial cancer [65]. It is also suggested that MD-CTU should be incorporated

into the CT staging protocol to rule out extravesical carcinoma.

CT is well established in the preoperative staging and assessment of upper tract TCC, although sensitivity limitations of this modality have been reported [68]. The introduction of CTU offers single breath hold coverage of the entire urinary tract, improved resolution, and the ability to capture multiple phases of contrast material excretion. Upper tract urothelial neoplasms commonly present as a single or as multiple irregular filling defects on CTU. Recent studies evaluating the ability of MD-CTU to detect urothelial tumors in the renal collecting system or in the ureter have reported very promising results. It has been shown that MD-CTU can detect urothelial tumors in up to 89% [69]. Fritz et al found that MD-CTU is an accurate means for detection and staging of upper urinary tract TCC, with accuracy for tumor detection and overall staging of 100% and 87.8%, respectively [70]. In addition, organ-confined disease was correctly staged in 28/29 tumors (96.6%) while stage locally advanced tumors were correctly classified in 8/12 patients (66.6%) [70].

Considerations regarding the use of CTU include the need for adequate distension and opacification of the ureter for the detection of small upper tract lesions and the increased radiation exposure [71]. Therefore, different protocols and techniques have been developed to overcome these limitations. Currently, the diagnosis of nodal metastases with CTU is based on anatomic size criteria. Therefore, CTU has the same limitations as the other CT phases in the detection of normal-sized lymph nodes with metastatic involvement or in differentiating enlarged nodes due to a benign process.

## Prostate cancer

There is virtually no place for CT in the detection or local primary tumor staging of prostate cancer. This is due to the fact that the margins of the prostate are poorly defined on CT, and that intraprostatic anatomy is not well demonstrated. However, because of the increased temporal resolution, MD-CT more clearly depicts intraprostatic anatomy.

The major role of CT, especially with the multislice technique, is in nodal staging. Typically, the criterion used to identify a metastatic node is a short-axis measurement greater than 10 mm. However, since

**157**

nodal metastases are often microscopic, CT cannot be used to reliably detect all cases. In addition, the majority of patients with newly diagnosed localized prostate cancer are at low risk for metastasis, and the diagnostic yield of the CT is low. In a subgroup of such patients with a serum PSA level of less than 20 ng/mL, the likelihood of positive findings on abdominal/pelvic CT is extremely low (<1%) [72]. Therefore, CT may be warranted only in patients with a very high risk of harbouring lymph node metastases since the specificity of a positive scan is high (93–96%) [73]. The American College of Radiology recommends the use of CT for patients with a PSA level greater than 10.0 ng/mL and a biopsy Gleason score greater than 6 [74].

The best available evidence regarding the diagnostic accuracy of preoperative CT in the diagnosis of lymph node metastases in prostate cancer is derived from a recent meta-analysis [75]. A total of 1024 patients with CT data from 18 studies were included and results were compared to those obtained with magnetic resonance imaging (MRI) [75]. Sensitivity and specificity of CT in individual studies ranged from 5% to 94% and 59% to 99%, respectively; while the respective pooled sensitivity and specificity was 42% (95% CI: 20–56%) and 82% (95% CI: 80–83%), respectively. Studies showed variability regarding the reported diagnostic odds ratios (0.07 to 92.48). In addition, the average prevalence of lymph node metastasis in this patient population was 0.17 for CT and when this was used as a pretest probability, the post-test probabilities of a positive and negative test were 0.31 (95% CI: 0.23–0.4) and 0.12 (95% CI: 0.1–0.16), respectively. The authors concluded that both CT and MRI have an equally poor diagnostic performance regarding the detection of lymph node metastases in prostate cancer, and that the reliance on their results misdirects the therapeutic strategies offered to patients. It is therefore clear to see why EAU guidelines on prostate cancer indicate that accurate lymph node staging can only be determined by operative lymphadenectomy [74]. CT has also been used to monitor bone metastases, but bone scan and MRI have been reported to be superior to CT in the diagnosis of bone metastases [76].

### Testicular cancer

CT has no role in the diagnosis of testicular tumors, but it remains the imaging technique of choice in staging testicular germ cell tumors (GCT). EAU guidelines suggest that retroperitoneal and mediastinal lymph nodes are best assessed with CT scan, whereas the supraclavicular nodes are best assessed by physical examination [77]. Lymph node metastases may vary in size from a single small-volume node of 10 mm in diameter to huge intra-abdominal retroperitoneal masses. Large volume seminomatous disease usually exhibits a soft-tissue density, but occasionally may present with a central low-density area secondary to necrosis. In large volume nonseminomatous (NSGCT) disease, complex cysts associated with foci of soft tissue may be seen. Large-volume NSGCT masses are frequently heterogeneous in density, being composed of multiloculated complex cystic areas as well as soft-tissue elements. The diagnosis of large-volume disease is easily made on CT, but the diagnosis of small volume lymphadenopathy may prove to be very difficult and represents the main limitation of CT imaging. The overall sensitivity of abdomino-pelvic CT scanning has been reported to be between 70% and 80% with the accuracy dependent on the size of the nodes [77].

Several studies have been performed to assess the diagnostic value of different lymph node size thresholds. In general, by reducing the lymph node size accepted as normal, the likelihood of detecting positive nodes increases, but the specificity of the test decreases. For practical purposes a 10 mm cut-off is used to differentiate between normal and abnormal lymph nodes. Nodes measuring between 8 mm and 10 mm are considered suspicious. A parameter that should also be taken into account is that normal nodes in the superior retroperitoneum are smaller than those in the inferior retroperitoneum on CT. However, occult microscopic metastases are present in 25–30% of patients with testicular cancer, and they cannot be detected by CT [77,78]. False-negative results are therefore inevitable, but the number of false-negative examinations can be minimized by eliminating observer error and recognizing the limitations of imaging. The differentiation of nodal enlargement from bowel loops or vascular abnormalities can be facilitated using a modern MD-CT unit with multiplanar reformations (Figure 9.10).

Diagnosis of small-volume metastatic disease is crucial for patient management since it can alter therapeutic decisions. For this reason, new imaging modalities including PET and MRI with lymphotrophic

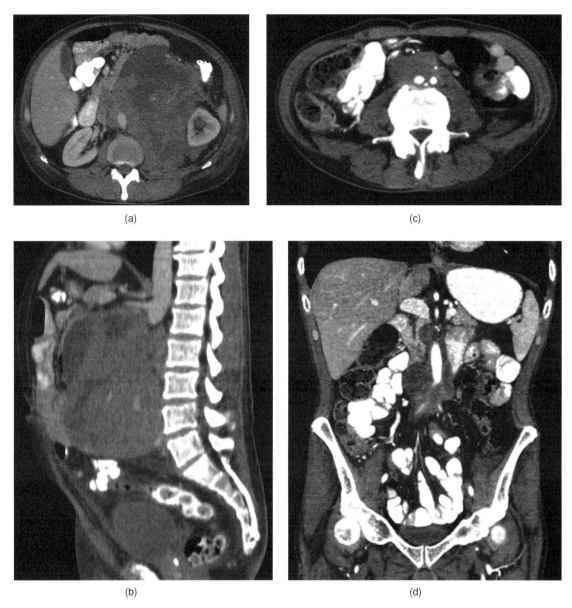

(a)

(c)

(b)

(d)

**Fig 9.10** MDCT of a testicular tumour in a patient with NSGCT. a-b: at diagnosis, (a) transversal view of the retroperitoneum, in which a huge mass is observed, (b) sagital view allows better visualization of tumour size. c-d: after chemotherapy, (c) transversal view of the retroperitoneum, in which down sizing of the lesion can be seen, (d) coronal view of the residual mass.

nanoparticles have been developed to improve diagnosis of involved lymph nodes. A chest CT is mandatory in all patients with NSGCT, as up to 10% can present with small subpleural nodes that are not radiologi-cally visible, in seminoma and those with a positive abdominopelvic CT scan [77]. Chest MD-CT has not been shown to increase nodule detection compared to single-slice CT for slice thicknesses of 5 mm.

Penile cancer

The presence and extent of primary tumor and lymph node metastasis represent significant prognostic factors in penile cancer with important treatment implications. The role of CT in staging (both locoregional and distant) is limited. Physical examination can estimate the extent of the primary lesion that determines its T-stage [79]. Imaging modalities including ultrasound or MRI have been used in order to identify the depth of tumor invasion, particularly with regard to corpora cavernosa infiltration [80]. On the other hand, CT seems to be inferior to MRI in the evaluation of primary penile cancer due to the superior soft-tissue contrast resolution of MRI.

There is no indication for imaging or histological examination if the inguinal nodes are impalpable [79]. Since CT differentiates lymph nodes based on their size and shape, and lymph nodes frequently undergo reactive enlargement in penile cancer, a relatively high rate of false-positive lymph node findings has been reported [80]. In addition, occult metastases in normal-sized lymph nodes will go undetected.

The use of pelvic/abdominal CT is recommended in patients with proven inguinal lymph node metastasis in order to identify deep pelvic and retroperitoneal lymph nodes as well as more distant sites of metastasis. Zhu et al evaluated the role of CT in the prediction of pelvic lymph node metastases in comparison to the state of Cloquet's node, and to the disease burden of inguinal lymph nodes [81]. It was found that pelvic CT was of limited use (sensitivity 37.5%, specificity 100%), in contrast to the pathological characteristics of inguinal lymph nodes, which were significantly associated with pelvic lymph node metastases [82].

## Positron emission tomography

PET is a diagnostic tool, which provides, by means of a radiotracer, morphologic evidence (visualization) of certain metabolic activity of tissue. The radiotracer is composed of a radionuclide and a transport substance with special affinity for specific tissues, as a result of which the radiotracer is accumulated within the tissue of interest. The radioisotope (included in the radiotracer) reaches the tissues and releases positrons. Each positron crashes with an electron from the closest nucleus. The collision destroys both masses and produces two photons with an energy of 511KeV according to the equation $E = mc^2$, which travel through the body in opposite directions at light speed. These photons are simultaneously received by two opposite photon detectors (photomultiplicator tubes), allowing the scanner to verify the line of positron destruction and the exact location of the radiotracer within the body (Figure 9.11).

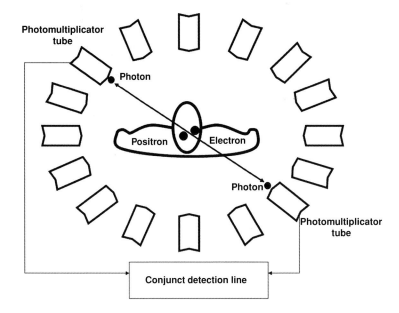

Fig 9.11 Schematic representation of photon detection and the principle of anatomic body location. Photons produced by a collision are detected by two opposite photomultiplicator tubes allowing the location of the collision site.

The injection of a proper radiotracer dose into a given patient results in thousands of crashes per second, which can be detected by means of a ring of photomultiplicator tubes, for a mathematical and statistical reconstruction of the image. As the photons travel through the body, some of them are absorbed by the tissues and some are scattered. This obvious loss of photons is not a precise illustration of in vivo radioactivity. The PET can compensate for this loss of photons by means of a proper attenuation correction of the tissue activity.

PET has the ability to deliver simultaneous dynamic tomographic pictures of a certain volume, due to the design and placement of several detector rings through the scanner. The employment of mathematical techniques used for tissue perfusion estimation or metabolic ranges requires a fast acquisition structure, in such a way that the dynamic changes of the radioactivity in the blood and tissue can be represented as a tissue radioactivity related to time curves. The combination with cross-sectional imaging allows PET to model and quantify the physiological biochemical process in vivo, since the radiotracer tissue concentration can be transformed on an image.

The analysis of the PET images can be carried out qualitatively and quantitatively using the semi-quantitative-uptake index (SUV), which is related to the activity of the radiotracer in a certain area, depending on the dose employed and the weight of the patient. The higher the metabolic activity is, the higher is the SUV.

In recent years, the combination of morphological imaging (CT) and metabolic (PET) images has been achieved. This integration results in a very useful tool, referred to as PET-CT, which overcomes the limitations of the constituent imaging techniques and allows a precise location of the lesion with a functional registry. This feature is important for correct pretreatment staging, including bone and lymph nodes, and for assessment of treatment response or biochemical progression, especially when as the functional changes can precede the anatomical ones. PET-CT can be visualized either as a CT or a PET scan, through a fusion spectrum with different weights for each technique providing volumetric data; it has the advantage of being able to be presented in any plane (Figure 9.12).

## Radiotracers

Radionuclides used in PET scanning are typically isotopes with short half-lives, such as carbon-11 (~20 minutes), nitrogen-13 (~10 minutes), oxygen-15 (~2 minutes), and fluorine-18 (~110 minutes). They are incorporated either into compounds normally used by the body such as glucose (or glucose analogues), or into molecules that bind to receptors or other sites of drug action. Due to the short half-lives of most radioisotopes, the radiotracers must be produced using a cyclotron and radiochemistry laboratory that are in close proximity to the PET imaging facility.

An ideal radiotracer for oncological use is one that posses an intrinsic affinity for the tumor. The most widely used radiotracer in oncology is fluorodeoxyglucose (2-fluoro-2-deoxy-D-glucose [FDG]), a glucose analogue. The fluorine in the FDG molecule is chosen to be the positron-emitting radioactive isotope fluorine-18, to produce $^{18}$F-FDG. After FDG is injected into a patient, a PET scanner can form images of its distribution around the body (FDG-PET). FDG-PET can be used for the diagnosis, staging, and

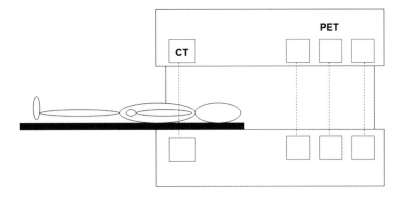

Fig 9.12 Diagram showing the principle of fusion imaging in PET-CT. The same device posses two systems that perform at the same time both studies, resulting in a more precise image. Image correction is performed by means of CT (X-rays) opposite to the PET, where they were performed by means of Germanio sources transmission mechanism. Exploration time is considerably reduced.

monitoring of treatment of various cancers, including among others thyroid cancer, breast, lymphoma, lung, head and neck, and colorectal.

FDG is taken up by high-glucose-using cells such cancer cells, where phosphorylation prevents the glucose from being released intact. The 2-oxygen in glucose is needed for further glycolysis, so that FDG cannot be further metabolized in cells, and therefore the FDG-6-phosphate formed does not undergo glycolysis before radioactive decay. As a result, the distribution of $^{18}$F-FDG is a good reflection of the distribution of glucose uptake and phosphorylation by cells in the body. Before FDG decays, it is inhibited from metabolic degradation or use because of the fluorine at the 2′ position in the molecule. It is, therefore, accumulated and images can be taken [83]. However, after FDG decays radioactively, its fluorine is converted to $^{18}$O, and after picking up an H$^+$ from the environment, it becomes glucose-6-phosphate labeled with harmless nonradioactive "heavy oxygen" (oxygen-18) at the 2′ position, and is thereafter metabolized normally in the same way as ordinary glucose.

Unfortunately $^{18}$F-FDG is not the ideal radiotracer for use in urology due to its urinary elimination, which prevents the proper visualization of the bladder and surroundings. To minimize this limitation, the studies are performed under bladder catheterization and the use of diuretics. The limitation of FDG urinary elimination led to other radiotracers that use different metabolic pathways and are not excreted in the urine. The radiotracers employed in uro-oncology are summarised in Table 9.6.

## Prostate cancer

Since the introduction of PET for the investigation of prostate pathology by Inaba [84], who discovered an increased blood flow in malignant compared to benign hyperplastic prostate tissue, several studies have been performed to establish the exact role of this technique in the work-up of prostate cancer patients.

### Primary diagnosis and staging
The information regarding lymph node status is of key importance for the appropriate treatment planning in patients with newly diagnosed prostate cancer. Although the incidence of lymph node metastasis has significantly dropped in the PSA era; it may still range from 1% to 26% depending on the patient popula-

tion studied, the extent of lymph node dissection, and the quality of the histopathological analysis [85]. $^{18}$F-FDG PET has a limited role in the primary diagnosis or staging due to the fact that prostate cancer often lacks an increased glucose metabolism in contrast to many other tumors.

During recent years, studies using $^{11}$C- or $^{18}$F-choline have shown promising results [83,86]. The results of a number of series have been summarised in Table 9.7 [87–94].

Studies on other radiotracers ($^{11}$C-acetate and $^{11}$C-methionine PET) are scarce. It has been reported that they are more sensitive than $^{18}$F-FDG in primary prostate cancer detection and the detection of regional lymph node or bone metastases [95].

In conclusion, $^{11}$C-choline, $^{11}$C-acetate, and $^{11}$C-methionine, seem to be superior to $^{18}$F-FDG for primary staging due to better biodistribution pattern. Most of the studies have compared one of these radiotracers with $^{18}$F-FDG. Only one study compared $^{11}$C-choline with $^{11}$C-acetate and found a similar performance. However, more studies are needed to determine which of these tracers performs best [96].

### Follow-up
Until 1999, $^{18}$F-FDG has been the most commonly used radiotracer. However, It has been clearly demonstrated that its ability to detect lymph node involvement in organ-confined tumors is low and therefore it stopped being recommended in clinical practice. Larson et al [97] retrospectively evaluated the $^{18}$F-FDG PET images performed between 1997 and 2003 at their institution and calculated the PSA level and PSA velocity cut-offs for best clinical performance to be 2.4 ng/mL and 1.3 ng/mL/year. The use of these "best" cut-offs resulted in a sensitivity of 80% and 73%, respectively, and a specificity of 71% and 77%, respectively. Several studies have shown the diagnostic advantages of $^{11}$C-choline against $^{18}$F-FDG, in restaging patients after radical treatment and biochemical failure [98] (Figure 9.13).

One of the most difficult clinical problems faced is assessing recurrence at the time of biochemical relapse after radical treatment, and whether to treat by means of local salvage surgery or ablation or systemic therapy. $^{11}$C-choline PET-CT has been evaluated for its utility in this process. Reske et al [99] assessed the value of $^{11}$C-choline PET-CT for detecting occult relapse after radical prostatectomy in 49 patients. In

**Table 9.6** Most employed radiotracers in urology, their function and their application in urology oncology.

| Radiotracer | Biologic analogue | Function | Measured effect | Tumors |
|---|---|---|---|---|
| $^{18}$F-2-fluoro-2-deoxy-D-glucose (FDG) | Glucose | Glycolysis | Aerobic and anaerobic glycolysis, Glucose consumption | Prostate (advanced), Invasive Bladder, Testis (Seminoma), Kidney cancer |
| $^{11}$C-choline | Choline | Choline kinase | Cellmembrane metabolism, tumor proliferation | Prostate and bladder cancer |
| $^{18}$F-choline | Choline | Choline kinase | Cellmembrane metabolism, tumor proliferation | Prostate cancer |
| $^{11}$C-Acetate | Acetate | Fatty acid synthase | Lipid synthesis | Prostate cancer |
| $^{11}$C-Metionine | Methionine | a-a transport | Protein synthesis | Prostate cancer |
| $^{124}$I-cG250 | NA | Ab-Ca IX | Ab-ag reaction Recognices and joint to Ca IX | Kidney cancer |
| $^{131}$I-cG250 | NA | Ab-Ca IX | Ab-ag reaction recognizs and joint to Ca IX | Kidney cancer |
| $^{18}$F-Fluoromisonidazole ($^{18}$F-FIMSO) | NA | Measure hipoxia | Tumor hipoxia | Kidney cancer |
| 1-Amino-3–18-F-Fluorocyclobutane-1-Carboxyl (FACBC) | | a-a transport | | Prostate cancer |
| $^{18}$F (18-ß-(18)F)-Fluoro-5$\alpha$-dihydrotestosterona ($^{18}$F-FDHT) | Testosterone | Androgen receptor | Measures androgen receptor | Prostate cancer |
| $^{18}$F-NaF | Fluor | Bone mineralization | Measures the bone status | Metastatic prostate, bladder, and renal cancer |

patients with biochemical relapse (mean PSA 2.0 ng/mL, range: 0.3–12.1 ng/mL) PET-CT showed true positive (with histological confirmation) lesions with increased $^{11}$C-choline uptake in the prostatic fossa in 70% of the cases. Similar results were achieved by [100] external radiotherapy, and interstitial brachytherapy. The same group of investigators studied the diagnostic value $^{11}$C-choline PET-CT for targeted salvage lymph node dissection in biochemical relapse after primary curative therapy [101]. A positive histology was reported in 8/15 patients, only one patient had PSA nadir <0.1 ng/mL after salvage surgery, three patients developed metastases during follow-up, and one had stable disease with a PSA of 0.5 ng/mL. Krause et al [102] assessed the relationship

between the detection rate of $^{11}$C-choline PET-CT and serum PSA level in biochemical failure. The detection rate was 36% for a PSA value of 1 ng/mL, 43% for a PSA value of 1 ng/mL to 2 ng/mL, 62% for a PSA value of 2 ng/mL to 3 ng/mL, and 73% for a PSA value of 3 ng/mL or more.

According to Scattoni et al [103] $^{11}$C-choline PET-CT should be used as a diagnostic tool for the detection of lymph node metastases in recurrent prostate cancer. This group evaluated 25 patients who had a mean PSA of 1.98 ng/mL. Of four patients with a negative $^{11}$C-choline PET-CT and positive MRI, none had nodal metastases. Nineteen of the 21 patients (90%) with positive $^{11}$C-choline PET-CT had nodal involvement.

**Table 9.7** Summary of the PET studies on prostate cancer.

| Author and radiotracer | Sensitivity | Specificity | Comments |
|---|---|---|---|
| **(a) Primary diagnosis and staging** | | | |
| De Jong IJ [11]C-Choline | 80% | 96% | Median PSA pre surgery 130 ng/mL |
| Häcker A [18]F-Choline | 10% | | Mean PSA 28.4, Compared with sentinel node (80% sensibility) |
| Scher B [11]C-Choline | 86.5% | 61.9% | For primary tumor detection |
| Scher B [11]C-Choline | 81.8% | 100% | For metastases spread detection |
| Testa C [11]C-Choline | 55% | 86% | Comparison between MRI, MR Spectroscopy, and PET/CT |
| Husarik DB [18]F-Choline | 33.3% | 100% | For detecting positive lymph nodes prior surgery. Mean PSA = 11.58 ng/mL |
| Rinnab L [11]C-Choline | 36% | | Local staging, data referring for detecting pT3-pT4 disease |
| Schiavina R [11]C-Choline | 60% 41.4% | 97.6% 99.8% | Detecting lymph nodes, and per lymph node analysis |
| Nunez R [11]C- Methionine | 72.1% 48% (FDG) | | Compares [11]C Methionine with [18]FDG with conventional imaging as standard reference |
| Giovanchi [11]C-Choline | 72% | 43% | Nagative correlation between uptake (SUVmax) and androgenic therapy |
| **(b) Restaging, follow-up, and progression** | | | |
| Larson SM [18]F-FDG | 80% 73% | 71% 77% | For a PSA 2.4 ng/mL For a PSA velocity of 1.3 ng/mL/year |
| Picchio [11]C-Choline vs. [18]F-FDG | | | Abnormal focal increases were noted in 47% of patients on [11]C-Choline -PET and in 27% on [18]F-FDG -PET. No positive PSA ≤5 ng/mL |
| Jong IJ [11]C-Choline | 38.4% 77.7% | 100% 100% | For surgery patients For external bean radiation |
| Reske SN [11]C-Choline | 63.8% | 92.3% | PSA relapse after biochemical recurrence. Mean PSA positive studies 2.6 ng/mL |
| Rinnab L [11]C-Choline | 91% | 50% | For detecting recurrence after primary treatment, with surgery or radiation. Data for PSA<2.5 ng/mL |
| Rinnab L [11]C-Choline | 34.7% | | For salvage lymphadenectomy after primary treatment |
| Pelosi E [18]F-Choline | 20% 40% 88,8% | | PSA≤ 1 ng/mL PSA>1 ng/mL ≥5 ng/mL PSA< 5 ng/mL |
| Nunez [11]C-Methionine vs. [18]F-FDG | Soft tissue 70% vs. 48% Bone 70% vs. 34% | | |
| Scattoni [11]C-Choline | 64% | 90% | Detection of lymph node metastases of recurrent prostate cancer |
| **(c) Progressive metastatic disease** | | | |
| Nunez [11]C-Methionine vs. [18]F-FDG | 72% vs. 48% | | 95% of metabolically active [11]C-Methionine while only 65% metabolize [18]F-FDG |

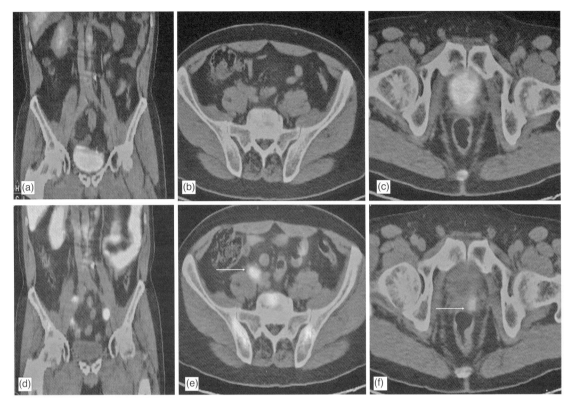

**Fig 9.13** Comparison of $^{18}$F-FDG (a, b, c) with $^{11}$C-choline PET (d, e, f) in a patient with PCa and biochemical failure (PSA = 2.1 ng/mL) after external beam radiotherapy. No pathological uptake was seen on $^{18}$F-FDG PET. Metastatic uptake was observed in the seminal vesicle as well as in both external iliac and right ilio-obturator lymph nodes on $^{11}$C-choline PET. *See also plate 9.13.*

$^{18}$F-choline has also been used for studying recurrence after primary curative treatment. Heinisch et al [104] evaluated the role of $^{18}$F-choline for restaging patients with biochemical failure after radical treatment. When the PSA cut-off point was set at 5 ng/mL, 41% of the examinations were true positive. Therefore, $^{18}$F-choline PET-CT should not be restricted to patients with PSA >5 ng/mL. Moreover, Vess et al [105] assessed the value of $^{18}$F-choline and $^{11}$C-acetate PET-CT for residual or recurrent tumor after radical prostatectomy in 20 consecutive patients with a mean PSA value of 0.33 ng/mL (range 0.08–0.76 ng/mL). PET-CT detected residual or recurrent disease in about half of the patients with PSA <1 ng/mL. Recently, Pelosi et al [106] reported that the detection rate in patients with biochemical failure after radical prostatectomy was related to the PSA level, with a sensitivity of 20%, 44%, and 88.8% for PSA ≤1 ng/mL, 1 ng/mL< PSA ≤5 ng/mL, and PSA >5 ng/mL, respectively.

Albercht et al [107] studied $^{11}$C-acetate PET in the diagnosis of prostate cancer recurrence after radiotherapy (17 patients, median PSA 6 ng/mL) or radical surgery (15 patients, median PSA 0.4 ng/mL). In all postradiotherapy patients (n = 6) in whom biopsies were obtained, histology confirmed the local recurrence. In the postsurgical group, $^{11}$C-acetate PET was positive or equivocal for local recurrence in nine of 15.

Only a very limited number of reports are available for the use of $^{11}$C-methionine. Nilsson and coworkers [108] reported $^{11}$C-methionine uptake in most of the lesions in patients with androgen-independent prostate cancer. In another study, Nunez and coworkers [95] compared the diagnostic yield of $^{11}$C-methionine and $^{18}$F-FDG in patients with a rising

**165**

PSA. They reported that [11]C-methionine not only detected more lesions than[18]F-FDG, but also the intensity of methionine uptake in these lesions was significantly higher than [18]F-FDG. The sensitivity of [11]C-methionine for the detection of soft-tissue and bone metastases was equal (70%), while [18]F-FDG showed a sensitivity of 48% and 34%, respectively.

Recently, anti1-amino-3–18 F-fluorocyclobutane-carboxylic acid (anti-[18]F-FACBC) has shown promising results [109]. Fifteen patients with a recent diagnosis of prostate cancer ($n = 9$) or suspected recurrence ($n = 6$) and a mean PSA of 15 ng/mL were included in this study. Anti-[18]F-FACBC PET-CT images were compared with clinical details, conventional images, and pathological follow-up. In the newly diagnosed prostate cancer, [18]F-FACBC correctly identified malignancy in 40/48 prostate sextants. Pelvic node metastases were identified in seven out of nine patients and were undetermined in two out of nine. In all four patients who had proven recurrence anti-[18]F-FACBC identified malignancy.

*Progressive metastatic disease* The correct staging of metastatic prostate cancer is of high value in order to monitor treatment response and disease progression (Figure 9.14). Conventional imaging techniques (namely scintigraphy, CT, or MRI), are usually used in this respect. Nunez et al [95] compared [18]F-FDG, [11]C-methionine PET, and conventional imaging techniques. The respective sensitivities were 48%, 72%, and 100%.

In this group of patients, it is important if a test is going to change disease management. Tuncel et al [110] demonstrated that [11]C-choline PET-CT is a very useful tool whether for staging and restaging patients with advanced prostate cancer and changed disease management in 24% of the patients. In order to evaluate the best modality for detection of bone metastases, Beheshti et al [111] performed a study comparing [18]F-choline and [18]F-fluoride PET-CT. It was concluded that [18]F-choline PET-CT may be superior for early detection (bone marrow involvement) of metastatic disease, while [18]F-fluoride PET-CT seemed to be superior in the diagnosis of sclerotic lesions.

[18]F-FDG has little accuracy for diagnosing or staging prostate cancer. However, increased lipid metabolism and biosysnthesis of cell membranes, and their association with increased uptake of [11]C-acetate or [11]C-choline radiotracers seems to demonstrate promise. [11]C-choline, [18]F-choline have been successfully applied for staging primary and recurrent disease. [18]F-fluoride seems to have encouraging

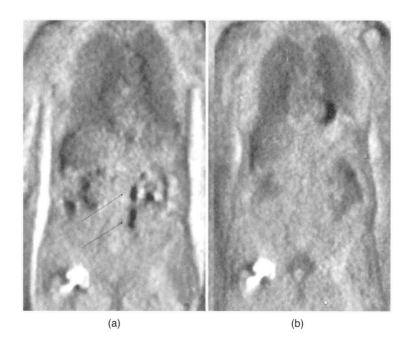

(a)                    (b)

Fig 9.14 [18]F-FDG PET in an advanced PCa patient. (a) evidence of retroperitoneal metastases (arrows), (b) Metastases have disappeared after radiotherapy.

results in evaluation of bone disease. Other radiotracers, such as [11]C-metionine, anti-[18]F-FACBC, and [18]F-dihydrotestosterone await further testing (Table 9.7).

Kidney cancer

*Initial diagnosis and staging*
The detection of RCC with PET is often hampered because most radiotracers are excreted through the kidneys. [18]F-FDG PET has not been useful in the primary diagnosis of RCC, but is more effective for the detection of distant metastases. The role of [18]F-FDG PET in metastatic RCC might be even more important as it might change the therapeutic decision. Dilhuydy et al [112] showed that a positive, [18]FDG PET may modify the decision made in up to 20% of the patients, while a negative result should not modify the decision-making especially for surgery. Another radiotracer that has been studied for RCC is [11]C-acetate. Sherve et al [113] reported that RCC accumulates more [11]C-acetate than normal kidney parenchyma, but this observation was not confirmed by Kotzerke et al [114] who reported the opposite.

Preoperative identification of tumor type could have important implications for the choice of treatment for RCC. In this field several radiotracers have been studied. Nitroimdizoles, which have emerged as a noninvasive technique to measure tumor hypoxia, have been studied in RCC since RCC is resistant to chemo- and radiotherapy, behaving as a hypoxic tumor. [18]F-Fluoromisonidazole has been explored as a potential tool for staging RCC by Lawrentschuck et al [115] who showed that seven of eleven tumors showed mild uptake. The antibody cG250 reacts against carbonic anhydrase-IX, which is overexpressed in clear cell carcinomas. The value of [124]I-cG250 in predicting this type of RCC has been recently investigated in a phase I trial [116]. Twenty six patients with renal masses scheduled for surgery underwent [124]I-cG250 PET-CT. Fifteen of 16 clear cell carcinomas were identified accurately by the antibody PET. The sensitivity of [124]I-cG250 PET-CT was 94% and the specificity was 100%.

Radioimmunotherapy is based on the use of a radiotracer, which instead of $\gamma$-photons, uses $\beta$ particles that destroy cellular DNA rather than providing images. RCC has been targeted with [131]I-G250 [117]. Although only modest, the results were promising in predicting who might respond to treatment with fractionated radiolabeled G250. Nevertheless, it should be noted that the study was performed before the use of PET-CT and thus the location of the deposits was not ideal.

[18]F-Fluorothymidine is a radiolabeled compound based on the nucleic acid thymidine. It has emerged as an important radiotracer that mirrors cellular proliferation in PET. Early studies in human tumors are promising.

*Follow-up*
[18]F-FDG PET has been more successful in monitoring RCC progression. Safei et al [118] used this modality for restaging advanced RCC. [18]F-FDG PET correctly staged 32/36 patients (89%), and missed 4 (11%) giving an overall 87% sensitivity and 100% specificity. The accuracy of PET for classifying lesions that were biopsied was also investigated. PET correctly classified 21/25 lesions biopsied with 88% sensitivity and 75% specificity. Ramdave et al [119], also showed the superiority of [18]F-FDG PET over CT in the evaluation of suspected RCC recurrence (accuracy 100% vs. 88%).

A recent meta-analysis investigated the role of [18]FDG PET in RCC [120] and concluded that [18]FDG PET is able to restage and diagnose metastatic lesions with a sensitivity of 87% (95% CI: 75–95%) and a specificity of 93% (95% CI: 86–97%) (Figure 9.15). The usefulness of PET in RCC remains unclear. In the local staging there is no evidence to support its use, but novel radiotracers are showing promising results regarding the identification of RCC prior to surgery. In monitoring and restaging advanced disease PET has already showed good results, which leads to a potential role for this technique within the targeted therapy era.

Testicular cancer

PET remains a promising tool in testicular cancer because the three major diagnostic problems, namely correct staging of patients classified as stage I, evaluation of residual masses after chemotherapy, and evaluation of rising levels of tumor markers without evidence of clinical disease remain unsolved by conventional techniques.

To date [18]F-FDG is the only radiotracer used for imaging GCT. Several clinical studies have

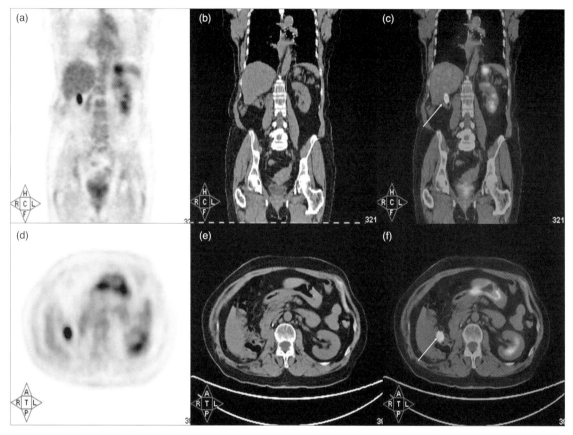

**Fig 9.15** Coronal (a, b, c) and axial images (d, e, f) of $^{18}$F-FDG PET (a, d), CT (b, e), and fusion images (c, f) of a patient with a history of right radical nephrectomy due to RCC (one year postoperatively). PET-CT was performed due to the suspicion of recurrence. A hypermetabolic deposit compatible with local recurrence is visualized (arrow) at the site of the previous operation. *See also plate 9.15.*

investigated the clinical role of $^{18}$F-FDG PET in primary tumor staging and in the monitoring of therapy either in seminomatous GCT or NSGCT. $^{18}$F-FDG PET has several major limitations. Inflammatory and granulomatous tissues also show extensive $^{18}$F-FDG uptake, lesions <1 cm can often be overlooked, and mature teratoma is indistinguishable from normal and necrotic tissue [121].

*Nonseminomatous germ cell tumors*
There has been a lot of controversy regarding the usefulness of this technique in the evaluation and staging of NSGCT until Huddart et al published their results [122]. They investigated whether the $^{18}$F-FDG could identify patients without occult metastatic disease for whom surveillance is an attractive option. In this multicenter study, 111 high-risk patients with NSGCT underwent $^{18}$F-FDG PET within 8 weeks after orchiectomy or marker normalization. Positive scans were excluded from the study while negative scans were observed in a surveillance program. Of the 88 PET-negative patients, one requested adjuvant chemotherapy, while 87 proceeded to surveillance. Within a median follow-up of 12 months, 33 of the 87 patients on the surveillance relapsed. The trial was prematurely stopped in 2005 due to an unacceptably high-relapse rate in PET-negative patients. The authors concluded that although $^{18}$F-FDG PET identified some patients with disease not detected by CT, the relapse rate among PET-negative scans remains

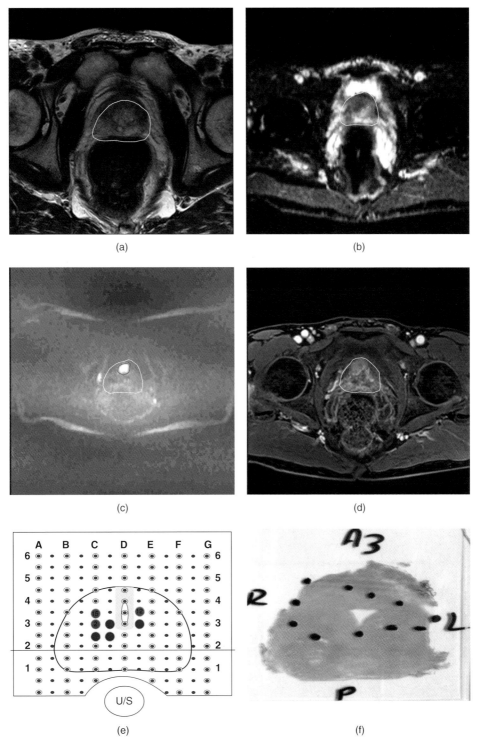

(a)

(b)

(c)

(d)

(e)

(f)

**Plate 1.3** Multiparametric MRI in a man with two previous negative prostate transrectal biopsies on a background of a rising PSA (3.6 ng/mL to 5.8 ng/mL) and a positive family history. (a–d) All MRI sequences (T2W, ADC map and high *b*-value diffusion weighted, dynamic contrast enhancement) on a 1.5 T scanner demonstrate an anterior tumor. (e) This was confirmed on transperineal template biopsies (circles with lines and the circle with dots; numbers representing maximum cancer core length involvement). (f) The patient subsequently had surgery in which the tumor was again shown to be in the anterior transition zone. (Images provided courtesy of Hashim U Ahmed, University College London, UK.)

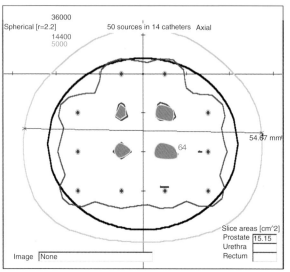
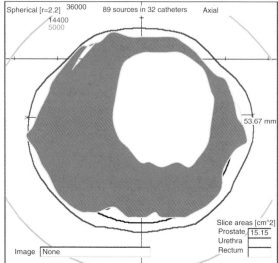

**Plate 2.3** Pure uniform loading (a) and pure peripheral loading (b).

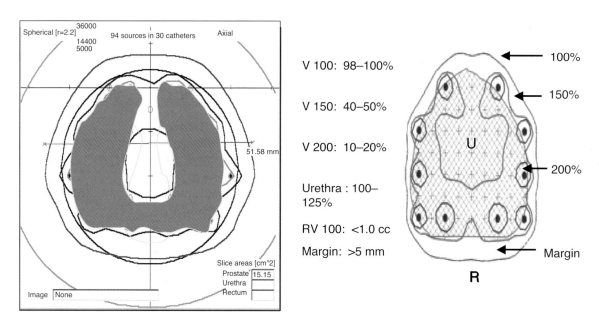

V 100: 98–100%

V 150: 40–50%

V 200: 10–20%

Urethra : 100–125%

RV 100: <1.0 cc

Margin: >5 mm

**Plate 2.4** Modified uniform loading (a) and Seattle model (b).

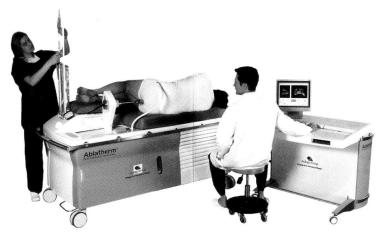

**Plate 3.3** Ablatherm HIFU system. Treatment module (left). Control module (right). (Reproduced with permission from Focus Surgery, Inc.)

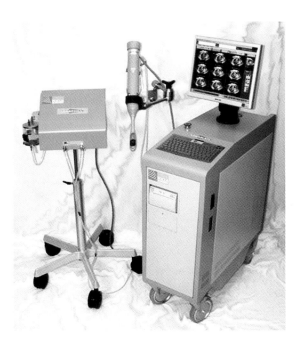

**Plate 3.4** Sonablate 500 HIFU system. Console (left). Cooling device (right). HIFU probe with articulated arm (Top right). (Reproduced with permission from Focus Surgery, Inc.)

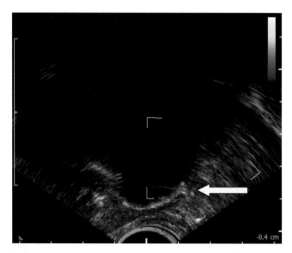

**Plate 4.1** Doppler Ultrasound demonstrating the edge of iceball and proximity of neurovascular bundles (arrow) after focal cryotherapy.

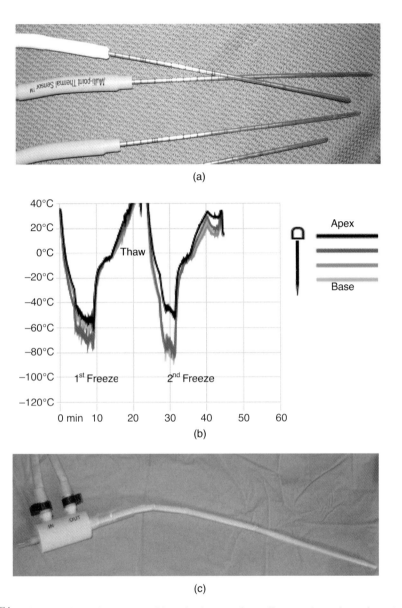

**Plate 4.2** (a) MTS$^{TM}$ Multipoint thermal sensors (Galil Medical Inc, Arden Hill, MN); (b) isothermal monitoring of freezing process using MTS; (c) Urethral warming catheter.

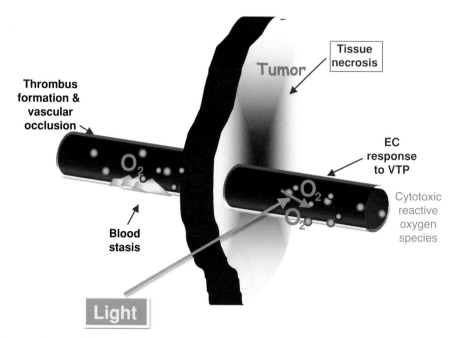

**Plate 6.1** Schematic diagram of the reactions that occur with photodynamic therapy.

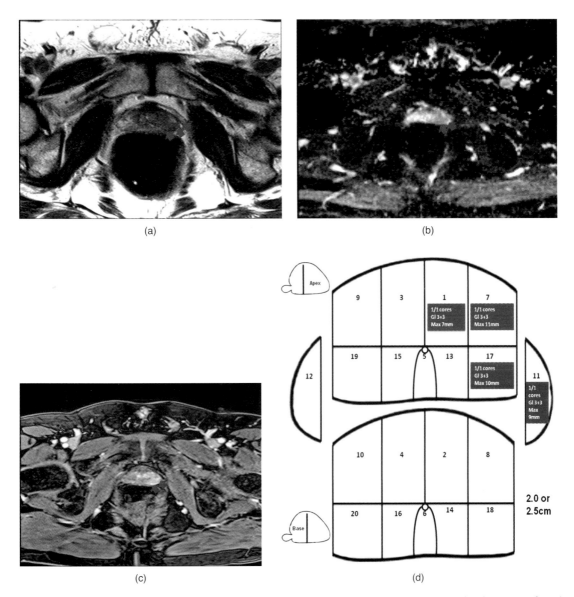

(a)

(b)

(c)

(d)

**Plate 8.6** Multiparametric MRI in a man who has bio-chemical recurrence after primary external beam radiation therapy a number of years prior. Apical disease on the right side is not visible on axial T2W images, (a) but obvious on coronal T2W images (b) as well as on diffusion (c) and dynamic contrast-enhanced scans (d). This was confirmed histologically on template mapping biopsies (e) (green and yellow zones). (Courtesy of Hashim U Ahmed, University College London.)

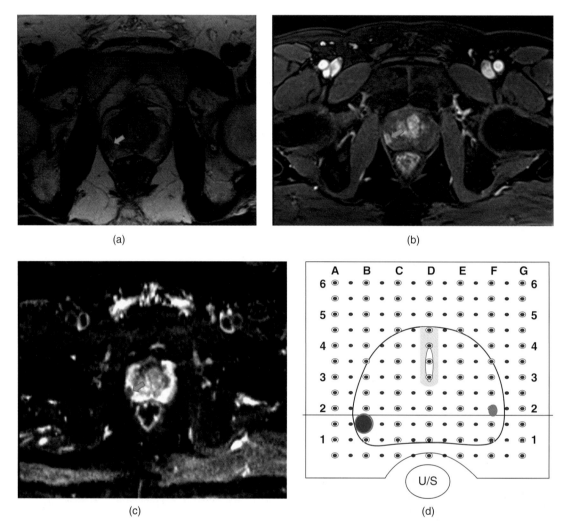

(a)

(b)

(c)

(d)

**Plate 8.7** Axial images taken on a 1.5 Tesla MRI using a pelvic phased-array coil in a man with intermediate-risk prostate cancer on TRUS-guided biopsies. (a) T2-weighted image shows a low-signal area in the left lobe, although not clear. (b) Dynamic contrast-enhanced image shows enhancement in the left lobe consistent with cancer. (c) Diffusion-weighted image confirms the same area has poor signal on ADC map (arrows). (d) The man underwent template transperineal mapping biopsies using a 5-mm sampling frame, which confirmed the area on the MRI in the left lobe (red areas). A total of 24 cores were taken. (Courtesy of Hashim U Ahmed, University College London.)

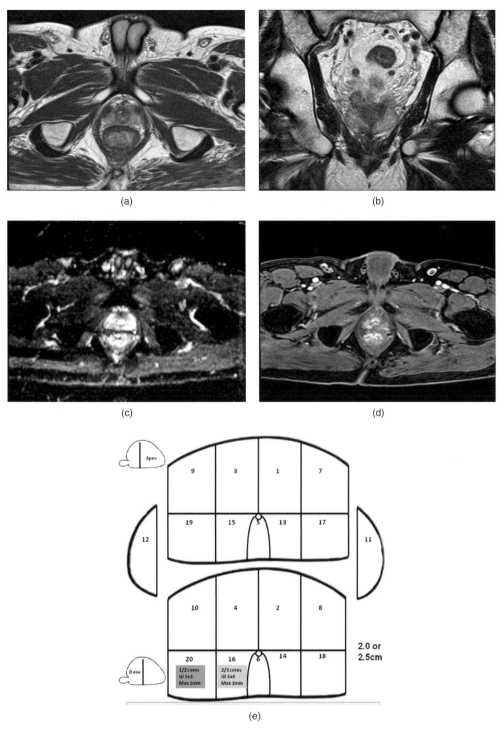

(a)

(b)

(c)

(d)

(e)

**Plate 8.8** Axial images taken on a 1.5 Tesla MRI using a pelvic phased-array coil in a man with a PSA of 6.5 ng/mL. (a) T2-weighted image shows a low-signal area in the right-peripheral zone although this is far from clear. (b) Dynamic contrast-enhanced image shows enhancement in the right-peripheral zone lesion consistent with cancer. (c) Diffusion-weighted image confirms the same area has poor signal on ADC map. (d) The man underwent template transperineal mapping biopsies using a 5-mm sampling frame rather than transrectal biopsies (arrows). The template biopsies confirmed the area on the MRI in the right-peripheral zone (red) with 2 cores positive for Gleason score 4 + 3 3 mm and 5-mm cancer core length. A smaller, presumed insignificant area was also shown on the left (blue) with 1 mm of Gleason 6 cancer. A total of 66 cores were taken. (Courtesy of Hashim U Ahmed, University College London.)

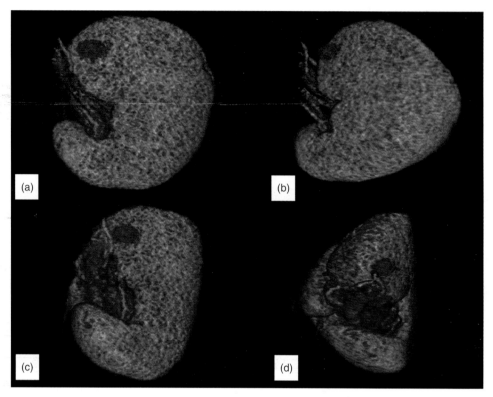

**Plate 9.7** MDCT of a renal tumor. Surgery plan is facilitated by this technology.

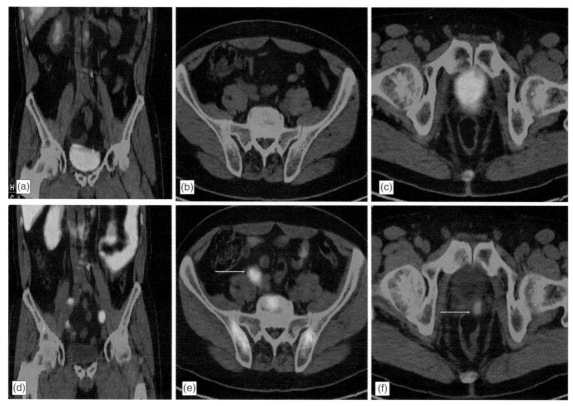

**Plate 9.13** Comparison of $^{18}$F-FDG (a, b, c) with $^{11}$C-choline PET (d, e, f) in a patient with PCa and biochemical failure (PSA = 2.1 ng/mL) after external beam radiotherapy. No pathological uptake was seen on $^{18}$F-FDG PET. Metastatic uptake was observed in the seminal vesicle as well as in both external iliac and right ilio-obturator lymph nodes on $^{11}$C-choline PET.

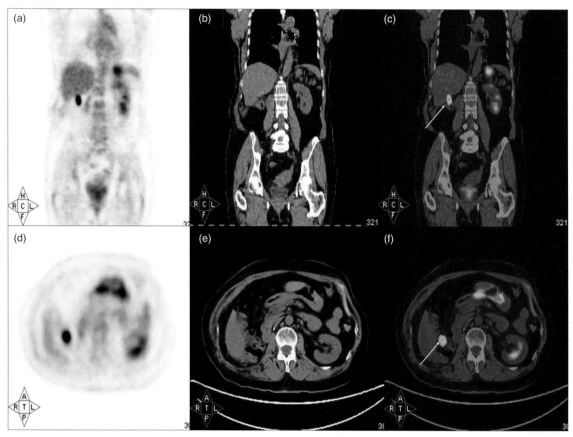

**Plate 9.15** Coronal (a, b, c) and axial images (d, e, f) of $^{18}$F-FDG PET (a, d), CT (b, e), and fusion images (c, f) of a patient with a history of right radical nephrectomy due to RCC (one year postoperatively). PET-CT was performed due to the suspicion of recurrence. A hypermetabolic deposit compatible with local recurrence is visualized (arrow) at the site of the previous operation.

high, and that [18]F-FDG PET is not sufficiently sensitive to identify patients at low risk of relapse to guide management.

*Seminomatous germ cell tumors*
Several studies assessing the role of [18]F-FDG PET in seminomatous GCT suggested that the technique has a place as a standard tool in evaluating residual tissue postchemotherapy for seminoma. De Santis et al [123] studied 56 patients with metastatic pure seminoma who either had the histology of the resected lesion or the clinical outcome documented by CT, tumor markers, and/or physical examination during follow-up. The size of the residual lesions on CT, either >3 cm or ≤3 cm, was correlated with the presence or absence of viable residual tumor. The specificity, sensitivity, positive predictive value, and negative predictive value of [18]F-FDG PET was 100% (95% CI, 92–100%), 80% (95% CI, 44–95%), 100%, and

96%, respectively, versus 74% (95% CI, 58–85%), 70% (95% CI, 34–90%), 37%, and 92%, respectively, for CT discrimination of the residual tumor by size (>3 cm/≤3 cm) These results confirm that [18]F-FDG PET is the best predictor of viable residual tumor in post-chemotherapy seminoma residual tissue, and should be used as a standard tool for clinical decision making in this patient group. The above results were reproduced by Becherer et al [124] corroborating that [18]F-FDG PET contributes to the management of residual seminoma lesions, especially in terms of avoiding unnecessary additional surgery for patients with lesions ≥3 cm. (Figure 9.16)

PET seems to be one of the most promising tools in the work-up of patients with testicular tumors. However, the results of Huddart et al [122] showed that PET results are poor and should not be considered in identifying low-risk patients that may be suitable for surveillance strategies. However, the only

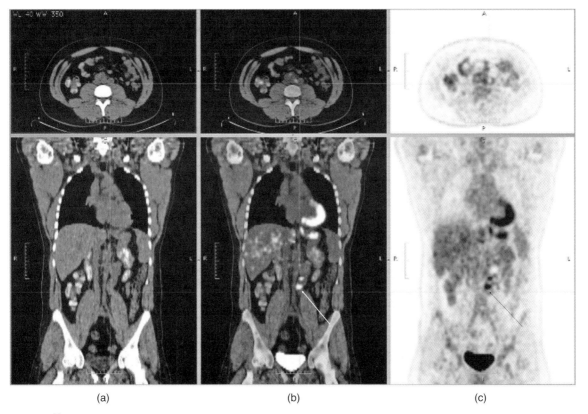

(a)                              (b)                              (c)

**Fig 9.16** [18]F-FDG PET in a patient with seminoma. A suspicious lesion was initially observed in the CT scan. The PET was performed to visualize the activity of the lesion confirming the presence of an active tumor.

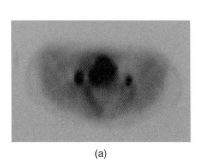

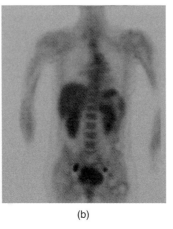

(a)                                        (b)

Fig 9.17 Images of a patient with an invasive bladder cancer and a suspicious iliac lymph node on the preoperative CT scan. $^{18}$F-FDG PET ensured the diagnosis (a: coronal view, b: axial view), which was confirmed in the pathology specimen after the radical cystectomy and an extended lymph node resection.

established role for PET in uro-oncology is the monitoring of seminomas.

## Bladder cancer

Invasive bladder cancer confined to the pelvis is treated by means of radical cystectomy and pelvic lymph node resection. Preoperative accurate staging is needed to identify patients at high risk for extraperitoneal spread in whom a combined treatment may be offered. CT and MRI are widely used for preoperative staging. However, these imaging modalities have limitations. Bladder cancer metastases frequently replace normal nodes, causing little if any enlargement and false-negative rates are therefore significant. Thus, there is

a need for a noninvasive imaging modality that has greater accuracy for bladder cancer staging.

### Local disease and staging

The role of $^{18}$F-FDG PET for the detection of localized disease is limited due to the urinary excretion of $^{18}$F-FDG. On the other hand, $^{18}$F-FDG PET may have a role in identifying locoregional lymph node and other distant metastases (Figures 9.17 and 9.18). Drieskens et al [125] evaluated the preoperative use of $^{18}$F-FDG PET for detecting lymph node and distant metastasis in 55 patients with bladder cancer. For the diagnosis of metastatic disease the sensitivity, specificity and accuracy of $^{18}$F-FDG PET was 60%, 88%, and 78%, respectively. Liu et al [126] investigated the

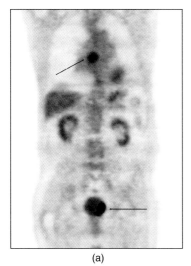

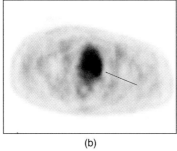

(a)                                        (b)

Fig 9.18 Preoperative PET scan of a patient with a suspicious lesion on the chest CT, compatible with metastasis. The result was confirmed on biopsy. (a) the metastasis is clearly visible in the chest (axial view), (b) coronal view of the tumor at the level of the bladder on the left side.

value of [18]F-FDG PET for detecting metastatic disease in 46 patients. The investigators reported 76.9% sensitivity in 36 patients who received no prior systematic chemotherapy. However, in 10 who were imaged after receiving chemotherapy, sensitivity decreased to 50%. The group recommended that [18]F-FDG PET should be interpreted with caution in patients who have received prior chemotherapy.

Trying to avoid the urinary elimination of [18]F-FDG, in order to improve PET results, some authors have tried with different radiotracers. Ahlstrom et al [127] reported [11]C-methionine to be superior to [18]F-FDG, however the sensitivity was only 78%. de Jong et al [128] used [11]C-choline PET in 18 patients to evaluate bladder cancer. Normal bladder wall tracer uptake was low and in 10 patient's tumor was detected correctly by [11]C-choline PET. Gofrit et al [129] evaluated [11]C-choline PET for preoperative staging in 18 patients. They noted that [11]C-choline PET was highly positive for primary and metastatic bladder cancer, and in all primary transitional cell carcinomas [11]C-choline uptake was found. Picchio et al [130] reported that [11]C-choline PET was comparable to CT for detecting residual cancer after transurethral bladder cancer resection but it appeared to be superior for detecting lymph node metastasis.

## Future directions

The introduction of MRI and PET scan in urological oncology has challenged the position of CT. However, with progress in CT technology and the application of 3D rendering, this imaging modality has reinforced its position. The current role of CT in the diagnosis and staging of urological cancers is summarized in Table 9.5.

In the future, further technological advances are expected. Multiplanar reformatted and 3D volume-rendered presentations of the obtained images will offer better visualization of the relationships of structures and in combination with CT angiography will provide all the critical information for accurate staging. This has the potential to improve surgical planning (i.e., in the setting of a nephron-sparing procedure), and eventually to simulate each procedure preoperatively on an individual basis.

Virtual cystoscopy, obtained by manipulating CTU data acquired through the contrast-filled bladder during the excretory phase has been introduced with promising results for detecting bladder mucosal lesions. Further research on virtual cystoscopy and virtual navigation in the upper urinary tract is awaited.

The advantage of PET stems from its ability to track radio-labeled biomarkers with a detection sensitivity below the picomolar range for functional imaging, whereas MRI and CT provide high-resolution anatomic information. Thus, the combination of two or more imaging modalities in order to get complementary information, such as morphology and function, is a worthwhile goal.

Although the combination of PET and CT has already been achieved in clinical and preclinical scanners, PET-CT has many limitations. Its major drawback is that the imaging is performed sequentially rather than simultaneously. In preclinical studies, this adds considerable time for studying the subjects and eliminates any temporal correlation between the two modalities, such as CT perfusion measurements and PET tracer kinetics. Furthermore, CT has limited soft-tissue contrast. Hence, a preferred choice would be the PET-MRI combination, not only because of the absence of ionizing radiation but also for its excellent soft-tissue contrast, its flexible scan protocols and its capability to perform functional MRI parameters. The simultaneous acquisition of different functional parameters using PET and functional MRI in addition to high-resolution anatomic information, creates enormous possibilities and provides new opportunities to study pathology and biochemical processes in vivo [131] (Figure 9.19). PET-MRI provides a

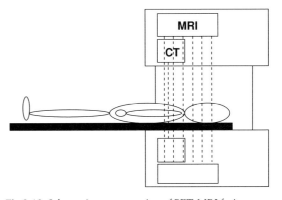

**Fig 9.19** Schematic representation of PET-MRI fusion, one of its major advantages is that both the functional image (PET) and the morphological image (MRI) are taken simultaneously rather than sequentially (like in the PET-CT).

powerful tool for studying biology and pathology in preclinical research and has great potential for clinical applications.

## Conclusions

[18]F-FDG PET is useful for identifying distant metastases due to increased [18]F-FDG uptake by the lesions but not by the primary tumor because of urinary excretion of [18]F-FDG, which interferes with local staging. [11]C-choline and [11]C-methionine may prove to be more effective than [18]F-FDG, but this remains unclear and further studies are needed to elucidate this issue in the future.

## References

1. Lassau N et al (2007) Dynamic contrast-enhanced ultrasonography (DCE-US) with quantification of tumor perfusion: a new diagnostic tool to evaluate the early effects of antiangiogenic treatment. Eur Radiol 17 (suppl. 6): F89–F98.
2. Wink M et al (2008) Contrast-enhanced ultrasound and prostate cancer; A multicentre European research coordination project. Eur Urol 54(5): 982–992.
3. Tang J et al (2008) Enhancement characteristics of benign and malignant focal peripheral nodules in the peripheral zone of the prostate gland studied using contrast enhanced transrectal ultrasound. Clin Radiol 63: 1086–1091.
4. Garra BS (2007) Imaging and estimation of tissue elasticity by ultrasound. Ultrasound Q 23: 255–268.
5. Salomon G et al (2008) Evaluation of prostate cancer detection with ultrasound real-time elastography: a comparison with step section pathological analysis after radical prostatectomy. Eur Urol 54(6): 1354–1362.
6. Eggert T et al (2008) Impact of elastography in clinical diagnosis of prostate cancer: a comparison of cancer detection between B-mode sonography and elastography-guided 10-core biopsies. Urologe A 47: 1212–1217.
7. Taylor LS, Rubens DJ, Porter BC, et al (2005) Prostate cancer: three-dimensional sonoelastography for in vitro detection. Radiology 237: 981–985.
8. Miyanaga N, Akaza H, Yamakawa M, et al (2006) Tissue elasticity imaging for diagnosis of prostate cancer: a preliminary report. Int J Urol 13: 1514–1518.
9. Pallwein L, Mitterberger M, Struve P, et al (2007) Real-time elastography for detecting prostate cancer: preliminary experience. BJU Int 100: 42–46.
10. Tsutsumi M, Miyagawa T, Matsumura T, et al (2007) The impact of real-time tissue elasticity imaging (elastography) on the detection of prostate cancer: clinicopathological analysis. Int J Clin Oncol 12: 250–255.
11. Sumura M, Shigeno K, Hyuga T, Yoneda T, Shiina H, Igawa M (2007) Initial evaluation of prostate cancer with real-time elastography based on step-section pathologic analysis after radical prostatectomy: a preliminary study. Int J Urol 14: 811–816.
12. Pallwein L, Mitterberger M, Pinggera G, et al (2008) Sonoelastography of the prostate: comparison with systematic biopsy findings in 492 patients. Eur J Radiol 65: 304–310.
13. Salomon G, Köllerman J, Thederan I, et al (2008) Evaluation of Prostate Cancer Detection with Ultrasound Real-Time Elastography: A Comparison with Step Section Pathological Analysis after Radical Prostatectomy. Eur Urol. 54(6): 1354–1362.
14. Eggert T, Khaled W, Wenske S, Ermert H, Noldus J (2008) Impact of elastography in clinical diagnosis of prostate cancer: A comparison of cancer detection between B-mode sonography and elastography-guided 10-core biopsies. Urologe A 47: 1212–1217.
15. Cochlin DL, Ganatra RH, Griffiths DF (2002) Elastography in the detection of prostatic cancer. Clin Radiol 57: 1014–1020.
16. König K et al (2005) Initial experiences with real-time elastography guided biopsies of the prostate. J Urol 174: 115–117.
17. Pallwein L et al (2007) Comparison of sonoelastography guided biopsy with systematic biopsy: impact on prostate cancer detection. Eur Radiol 17: 2278–2285.
18. Nelson ED et al (2007) Targeted biopsy of the prostate: the impact of color Doppler imaging and elastography on prostate cancer detection and Gleason score. Urology 70: 1136–1140.
19. Kamoi K et al (2008) The utility of transrectal real-time elastography in the diagnosis of prostate cancer. Ultrasound Med Biol 34: 1025–1032.
20. Mitterberger M et al (2007) A prospective randomized trial comparing contrast-enhanced targeted versus systematic ultrasound guided biopsies: impact on prostate cancer detection. Prostate 67: 1537–1542.
21. Goossen TE et al (2003) The value of dynamic contrast enhanced power Doppler ultrasound imaging in the localization of prostate cancer. Eur Urol 43: 124–131.
22. Sedelaar JP et al (2002) Value of contrast ultrasonography in the detection of significant prostate cancer: correlation with radical prostatectomy specimens. Prostate 53: 246–253.
23. Frauscher F et al (2001) Detection of prostate cancer with a microbubble ultrasound contrast agent. Lancet 357: 1849–1850.

24. Taymoorian K et al (2007) Transrectal broadband-Doppler sonography with intravenous contrast medium administration for prostate imaging and biopsy in men with an elevated PSA value and previous negative biopsies. Anticancer Res 27: 4315–4320.

25. Tang J et al (2007) Peripheral zone hypoechoic lesions of the prostate: evaluation with contrast-enhanced gray scale transrectal ultrasonography. J Ultrasound Med 26: 1671–1679.

26. Wondergem N, De La Rosette JJ (2007) HIFU and cryoablation-non or minimal touch techniques for the treatment of prostate cancer. Is there a role for contrast enhanced ultrasound? Minim Invasive Ther Allied Technol 16: 22–30.

27. Mitterberger M et al (2007) The value of threedimensional transrectal ultrasonography in staging prostate cancer. BJU Int 100: 47–50.

28. Braeckman J et al (2008) The accuracy of transrectal ultrasonography supplemented with computer-aided ultrasonography for detecting small prostate cancers. BJU Int 102(11): 1560–1565.

29. Tamai H et al (2005) Contrast-enhancerd ultrasonography in the diagnosis of solid renal tumors. J Ultasound Med 2412: 1635–1640.

30. Park BK et al (2007) Assessment of cystic renal masses based on Bosniak classification: comparison of CT and contrast-enhanced US. Eur J Radiol 612: 310–314.

31. Frauscher F, Klauser A, Volgger H, et al (2002) Comparison of contrast enhanced color Doppler targeted biopsy with conventional systematic biopsy: impact on prostate cancer detection. J Urol 167: 1648–1652.

32. Pelzer A, Bektic J, Berger AP, et al (2005) Prostate cancer detection in men with prostate specific antigen 4 to 10 ng/ml using a combined approach of contrast enhanced color Doppler targeted and systematic biopsy. J Urol 173: 1926–1929.

33. Mitterberger M, Pinggera GM, Horninger W, et al (2007) Comparison of contrast enhanced color Doppler targeted biopsy to conventional systematic biopsy: impact on Gleason score. J Urol 178: 464–468.

34. Mitterberger M, Horninger W, Pelzer A, et al (2007) A prospective randomized trial comparing contrast-enhanced targeted versus systematic ultrasound guided biopsies: impact on prostate cancer detection. Prostate 67: 1537–1542.

35. Mitterberger M, Pinggera G, Horninger W, et al (2008) Dutasteride prior to contrastenhanced colour Doppler ultrasound prostate biopsy increases prostate cancer detection. Eur Urol 53: 112–117.

36. Pallwein L, Mitterberger M, Pelzer A, et al (2008) Ultrasound of prostate cancer: recent advances. Eur Radiol 18: 707–715.

37. Frauscher F, Klauser A, Halpern EJ, Horninger W, Bartsch G. (2001) Detection of prostate cancer with a microbubble ultrasound contrast agent. Lancet 357: 1849–1850.

38. Halpern EJ, Ramey JR, Strup SE, Frauscher F, McCue P, Gomella LG. (2005) Detection of prostate carcinoma with contrast-enhanced sonography using intermittent harmonic imaging. Cancer. 104: 2373–2383.

39. Linden RA, Trabulsi EJ, Forsberg F, Gittens PR, Gomella LG, Halpern EJ. (2007) Contrast enhanced ultrasound flash replenishment method for directed prostate biopsies. J Urol 178: 2354–2358.

40. Colleselli D, Bektic J, Schaefer G, et al (2007) The influence of prostate volume on prostate cancer detection using a combined approach of contrast-enhanced ultrasonography-targeted and systematic grey-scale biopsy. BJU Int 100: 1264–1267.

41. Pallwein L et al (2007) Small renal masses: the value of contrast-enhanced colour Doppler imaging. BJU Int 1001: 47–50.

42. Wink MH et al (2007) Ultrasonography of renal masses using contrast pulse sequence imaging: a pilot study. J Endourol 21: 466–472.

43. Pallwein L et al (2008) Diagnostic evaluation of small renal masses: value of contrast-enhanced US in comparision to multidetector CT. J Urol 179(suppl.): 331.

44. Fahey BJ et al (2008) In vivo visualization of abdominal malignancies with acoustic radiation force Elastography. Phys Med Biol 531: 279–293.

45. Newhouse JH et al (2000) Radiologic investigation of patients with hematuria. American College of Radiology. ACR Appropriateness Criteria. Radiology 215(suppl.): 687-691.

46. Mitterberger M et al (2007) Three-dimensional ultrasonography of the urinary bladder: preliminary experience of assessment in patients with haematuria. BJU Int 99: 111–116.

47. Kocakoc E et al (2008) Detection of bladder tumors with 3-dimensional sonography and virtual sonographic cystoscopy. J Ultrasound Med 27: 45–53.

48. Andipa E, Liberopoulos K, Asvestis C (2004) Magnetic resonance imaging and ultrasound evaluation of penile and testicular masses. World J Urol 22: 382–391.

49. Carmignani L et al (2003) High incidence of benign testicular neoplasms diagnosed by ultrasound. J Urol 170: 1783–1786.

50. Horstman WG et al (1992) Testicular tumors: findings with color Doppler US. Radiology 185: 733–737.

51. Joudi FN, Kuehn DM, Williams RD (2006) Maximizing clinical information obtained by CT. Urol Clin N Am 33: 287–300.

52. O'Connor OJ, McSweeney SE, Maher MM (2008) Imaging of Hematuria. Radiol Clin N Am 46: 113–132.

53. Zhang J (2008) Recent advances in preoperative imaging of renal tumors. Curr Opin Urol 18: 111–115.

54. Kopka L et al (1997) Dual-phase helical CT of the kidney: value of the corticomedullary and nephrographic phase for evaluation of renal lesions and preoperative staging of renal cell carcinoma. AJR Am J Roentgenol 169: 1573–1578.

55. Bosniak MA (1986) The current radiological approach to renal cysts. Radiology 158(1): 1–10.

56. Schuster TG et al (2004) Papillary renal cell carcinoma containing fat without calcification mimicking angiomyolipoma on CT. Am J Roentgenol 183: 1402–1404.

57. Zhang J et al (2007) Differentiation of solid renal cortical tumors by CT. Radiology 244: 494–504.

58. Yoon J, Herts BR (2003) Staging renal cell carcinoma with helical CT: the revised 1997 AJCC and UICC TNM criteria. Crit Rev Comput Tomogr 44: 229–249.

59. Ljungberg B et al (2007) Renal cell carcinoma guidelines. Eur Urol 51: 1502–1510.

60. Welch TJ, LeRoy AJ (1997) Helical and electron beam CT scanning in the evaluation of renal vein involvement in patients with renal cell carcinoma. J Comput Assist Tomog 21: 467–471.

61. Studer UE et al (1990) Enlargement of regional lymph nodes in renal cell carcinoma is often not due to metastases. J Urol 144: 243–224.

62. Johnson CD et al (1987) Renal adenocarcinoma: CT staging of 100 tumors. AJR Am J Roentgenol 148: 59–63.

63. Beyersdorff D et al (2008) Bladder cancer: can imaging change patient management? Curr Opin Urol 18: 98–104.

64. Wong-You-Cheong JJ et al (2006) From the Archives of the AFIP: neoplasms of the urinary bladder: radiologic-pathologic correlation. Radiographics 26(2): 553–580.

65. Stenzl A et al (2009) The updated EAU guidelines on muscle-invasive and metastatic bladder cancer. Eur Urol 55(4): 815–825.

66. Kim JK et al (2004) Bladder cancer: analysis of multidetector row helical CT enhancement pattern and accuracy in tumor detection and perivesical staging. Radiology 231(3): 725–731.

67. Caterino M et al (2001) Primary cancer of the urinary bladder: CT evaluation of the T parameter with different techniques. Abdom Imaging 26(4): 433–438.

68. Scolieri MJ et al (2000) Limitations of computed tomography in the preoperative staging of upper tract urothelial carcinoma. Urology 56: 930–934.

69. Caoili EM et al (2005) MDCT urography of upper tract urothelial neoplasms. AJR Am J Roentgenol 184(6): 1873–1881.

70. Fritz GA et al (2006) Multiphasic multidetector-row CT (MDCT) in detection and staging of transitional cell carcinomas of the upper urinary tract. Eur Radiol 16: 1244–1252.

71. Anderson EM et al (2007) Multidetector computed tomography urography (MDCTU) for diagnosing urothelial malignancy. Clin Radiology 62: 324–332.

72. Browne RFJ et al (2005) Transitional cell carcinoma of the upper urinary tract: spectrum of imaging findings. RadioGraphics 25: 1609–1627.

73. Huncharek M, Muscat J (1996) Serum prostate-specific antigen as a predictor of staging abdominal/pelvic computed tomography in newly diagnosed prostate cancer. Abdom Imaging 21(4): 364–367.

74. Heidenreich A et al (2008) EAU guidelines on prostate cancer. Eur Urol 53(1): 68–80.

75. Amis ES Jr et al (2000) Pretreatment staging of clinically localized prostate cancer. Radiology 215(suppl.): 703–708.

76. Taoka T et al (2001) Factors influencing visualization of vertebral metastases on MR imaging versus bone scintigraphy. Am J Roentgenol 176: 1525–1530.

77. Albers P et al (2005) Guidelines on testicular cancer. Eur Urol 48(6): 885–894.

78. Hilton S et al (1997) CT detection of retroperitoneal lymph node metastases in patients with clinical stage I testicular nonseminomatous germ cell cancer: assessment of size and distribution criteria. AJR Am J Roentgenol 169: 521–525.

79. Solsona E et al (2004) EAU Guidelines on Penile Cancer. Eur Urol 46(1): 1–8.

80. Lont AP et al (2003) A comparison of physical examination and imaging in determining the extent of primary penile carcinoma. BJU Int 91: 493–495.

81. Hughes B et al (2008) Non-invasive and minimally invasive staging of regional lymph nodes in penile cancer. World J Urol 27(2): 197–203.

82. Zhu Y et al (2008) Predicting pelvic lymph node metastases in penile cancer patients: a comparison of computed tomography, Cloquet's node, and disease burden of inguinal lymph nodes. Onkologie 31: 37–41.

83. Jones S et al (1982) The radiation dosimetry of 2[f-18]fluoro-2-deoxy-D-glucose in man. J Nucl Med 28: 910.

84. Inaba T (1992) Quantitative measurements of prostatic blood flow and blood by positron emission tomography. J Urol 148: 1457.

85. Heidenreich A, Varga Z, Von Knobloch R (2002) Extended pelvic lymphadenectomy in patients undergoing radical prostatectomy: high incidence of lymph node metastases. J Urol 167: 1681–1686.

86. Powles T et al (2007) Molecular positron emission tomography and PET/CT imaging in urological malignancies. Eur Urol 51: 1511–1520.

87. De Jong IJ et al (2003) Preoperative staging o pelvic lymph node in prostate cancer by (11)C-Choline PET. J Nucl Med 44: 331–335.

88. Häcker A et al (2006) Detection of pelvic lymph node metastases with clinically localized prostate cancer: comparision of (18 F)-fluorocholine positron emission tomography-computerized tomography and laparoscopic radioisotope guided sentinel lymph node dissection. J Urol 176: 2014–2019.

89. Scher B et al (2007) Value of 11 C-Choline PET and PET/CT in patients with suspected prostate cancer. Eur J Nucl Med Mol Imaging 34: 45–53.

90. Testa C et al (2007) Prostate cancer: sextant localization with MR Imaging, MR spectroscopy, and 11 C-Choline PET/CT. Radiology 244: 797–806.

91. Husarik DB et al (2008) Evaluation of (18)F-Choline PET/CT for staging and restaging of prostate cancer. Eur J Nucl Med Mol Imaging 35: 253–263.

92. Rinnab L et al (2007) 11 C-choline positron emission tomography/computed tomography and transrectal ultrasonography for staging localized prostate cancer. BJU Int 99: 1421–1426.

93. Giovacchini G et al (2008) (11 C)Choline uptake with PET/CT for initial diagnosis of prostate cancer: relation to PSA levels, tumour stage and antiandrogenic therapy. Eur J Nucl Med Mol Imaging 35(6): 1065–1073.

94. Schiavina R et al (2008) (11)C-Choline positron emission tomography/computerized tomography for preoperative lymph-node staging in intermediate-risk and high risk prostate cancer: comparision with clinical staging nomograms. Eur Urol 54(2): 392–401.

95. Nunez R et al (2002) Combined 18 F-FDG and 11 C-methionine PET scans in patients with newly progressive metastatic prostate cancer. J Nucl Med 43: 46–55.

96. Jana SJ, Blaufox MD (2006) Nuclear medicine studies of the Prostate, Testes and Bladder. Semin Nucl Med 36(1): 51–72.

97. Larson SM, Schöder H (2008) Advances in positron emission tomography applications for urologic cancers. Curr Opin Urol 18: 65–70.

98. Jong IJ et al (2003) 11 C-Choline positron emission tomography for the evaluation after treatment of localized prostate cancer. Eur Urol 4: 32–39.

99. Reske SN, Blumstein NM, Glatting G (2008) (11)C-Choline PET/CT imaging in occult local relapse of prostate cancer after radical prostatectomy. Eur J Nucl Med Mol Imaging 35: 9–17.

100. Rinnab L et al (2007) Evaluation of (11)C-Choline positron emission tomography/computed tomography in patients with increasing prostate-specific antigen levels after primary treatment for prostate cancer. BJU Int 100: 786–793.

101. Rinnab L et al (2008) (11)C-CholinePET/CT for targete salvage lymp node dissection in patient with biochemical recurrence after primary curative therapy for prostate cancer. Preliminary results of a prospective study. Urol Int 81: 191–197.

102. Krause BJ et al (2008) The detection rate of (11 C) Choline PET/CT depends on the serum PSA-value in patients with biochemical recurrence of prostate cancer. Eur J Nucl Med Mol Imaging 35: 18–23.

103. Scattoni V et al (2007) Detection of lymph-node metastases with integrated [11 C]choline PET/CT in patients with PSA failure after radical retropubic prostatectomy: results confirmed by open pelvic-retroperitoneal lymphadenectomy. Eur Urol 52: 423.

104. Heinisch M et al (2006) Positron emission tomography/computed tomography with F-18-fluorocholine for restaging of prostate cancer patients: meaningful at PSA < 5 ng/ml? Mol Imaging Biol 8(1): 43–48.

105. Vees H et al (2007) 18 F-Choline and/or 11 C-Acetate positron emission tomography: detection of residual or progressive subclinical disease at very low prostate-specific antigen values (<1 ng/ml) after radical prostatectomy. BJU Int 99: 1415–1420.

106. Pelosi E et al (2008) Role of whole body (18)F-Choline PET/CT in disease detection in patients with biochemical relapse after radical Treatment for prostate cancer. Radiol Med 113(6): 895–904.

107. Albrecht S et al (2007) (11) Choline PET in the early evaluation of prostate cancer recurrence. Eur J Nucl Med Mol Imaging 34: 185–196.

108. Nilsson S, Kalner K, Ginman C (1995) C-11 methionine positron emission tomography in the management of prostatic carcinoma. Antibody Immunoconjug Radiopharm 8: 23–38.

109. Schuster DM et al (2007) Initial experience with the radiotracer anti-1-amino-3–18 F-fluorocyclobutane-1-carboxylic acid with PET/CT in prostate carcinoma. J Nucl Med 48: 56.

110. Tuncel M et al (2008) (11) Choline positron emission tomography/computed tomography for staging and restaging of patients with advanced prostate cancer. Nucl Med Biol 35: 689–695.

111. Beheshity M et al (2008) Detection of bone metastases in patients with prostate cancer by F-18 fluorocholine and F-18 fluoride PET-CT: a comparative study. Eur J Nucl Med Mol Imaging 35(10): 1766–1774.

112. Dilhuydy MS et al (2006) PET scans for decisión-making in metastatic renal cell carcinoma: a single-institution evaluation. Oncology 70: 339–344.

113. Sherve P et al (1995) Carbon-11-acetate PET imaging in renal disease. J Nucl Med 36: 1595–1601.

**175**

114. Kotzerke J et al (2007) (11-C) acetate uptake is not increased in renal cell carcinoma. Eur J Nucl Med Mol Imaging 34: 884–888.

115. Lawrenschuk N et al (2005) Assessing regional hypoxia in human renal tumours using 18 F-fluoromisonidazole positron emission tomography. BJU Int 96: 540–546.

116. Divgi CR et al (2007) Preoperative characterization of clear-cell renal carcinoma using iodine-124-labelled antibody chimeric G250 (124I-cG250) and PET in patients with renal masses: a phase I trial. Lancet Oncol 8: 304–310.

117. Divgi CR et al (2004) Phase I clinical trial with fractionated radioimmunotherapy using 131I-labeled chimeric G250 in metastatic renal cancer. J Nucl Med 45: 1412–1421.

118. Safaei A et al (2002) The usefulness of F-18 deoxyglucose whole-body positron emission tomography (PET) for re-staging of renal cell cancer. Clin Nephrol 57: 56.

119. Ramdave S et al (2001) Clinical role of F-18 fluorodeoxyglucose positron emission tomography for detection and management of renal cell carcinoma. J Urol 166: 825.

120. Martínez de Llano SR et al (2007) Meta-análisis sobre el rendimiento diagnóstico de la tomografía por emisión de positrones con 18 F-FDG en el carcinoma de células renales. Rev Esp Med Nucl 26: 19–29.

121. De Santis M, Pont J (2004) The role of positron emission tomography in germ cell cancer. World J Urol 22(1): 41–46.

122. Huddart RA et al (2007) 18fluorodeoxyglucose positron emission tomography in the prediction of relapse in patients with high-risk, clinical stage I nonseminomatous germ cell tumours: preliminary report of MRC Trial TE22–the NCRI Testis Tumour Clinical Study Group. J Clin Oncol 25(21): 3090–3095.

123. De Santis M et al (2004) 2–18fluoro-deoxy-D-glucose positron emission tomography is a reliable predictor for viable tumour in postchemotherapy seminoma: an update of the prospective multicentric SEMPET trial. J Clin Oncol 22(6): 1034–1039.

124. Becherer A et al (2005) FDG PET is superior to CT in the prediction of viable tumour in post-chemotherapy seminoma residuals. Eur J Radiol 54(2): 284–288.

125. Drieskens O et al (2005) FDG-PET for preoperative staging of bladder cancer. Eur J Nucl Med Mol Imaging 32: 1412.

126. Liu IJ et al (2006) Evaluation of fluorodeoxyglucose positron emission tomography imaging in metastatic transitional cell carcinoma with and without prior chemotherapy. Urol Int 77(1): 69–75.

127. Ahlström H et al (1996) Positron emission tomography in the diagnosis and staging of urinary bladder cancer. Acta Radiol 37(2): 180–185.

128. de Jong IJ et al (2002) Visualisation of bladder cancer using (11)C-choline PET: first clinical experience. Eur J Nucl Med Mol Imaging 29: 1283.

129. Gofrit ON et al (2006) Contribution of 11 C- choline positron emission tomography/computerized tomography to preoperative staging of advanced transitional cell carcinoma. J Urol 176: 940.

130. Picchio M ct al (2006) Value of 11 C-choline PET and contrast-enhanced CT for staging of bladder cancer: correlation with histopathologic findings. J Nucl Med 47: 938.

131. Judenhofer MS et al (2008) Simultaneous PET-MRI: a new approach for functional and morphological imaging. Nat Med 14(4): 459–465.

# 10 Imaging after minimally-invasive interventions in urological cancers

*Rowland Illing and Alex Kirkham*

Department of Specialist Imaging, University College Hospital, London, UK

## Introduction

The International Working Group on Image-guided Tumor Ablation have recommended standardization of terminology and reporting criteria [1] to allow comparison between centers using different interventional techniques. The term "ablation zone" has been coined to describe the zone of induced treatment effect (i.e., the area of gross tumor destruction visualised at imaging). This should be used in place of the term "lesion," which could either refer to the "ablation zone" or the underlying tumor. The zone of cell-death at pathological examination is referred to as "coagulation" or "coagulation necrosis." These terms are recommended so as to avoid the term "necrosis" or "coagulative necrosis," both of which have well-defined histological features, which may be found in tumors that have not been ablated.

The precise distinction between imaging appearances and histological appearances is stressed because although in many cases there is good overlap between radiological and pathological findings, this is not always the case [2]. Postprocedure imaging can only ever be an approximate guide to the success of ablative therapy with accuracy currently limited by contrast and spatial resolution to approximately 2–3 mm depending upon the modality. Thus, microscopic foci of residual or recurrent disease may not be identified.

The timing of imaging is important. In the acute postablation period the zone of ablation may lack the classic, well-defined histological appearance of coagulation necrosis surrounded by a thin rim of granulation tissue. Thus, in the acute setting neither contrast-enhanced CT nor ultrasound may be reliable in determining the true ablation zone.

The term "ablation margin" is directly analogous to the "surgical margin" in open or laparoscopic oncological surgery. Methods to create an "ablation margin" of 0.5–1.0 cm around a tumor have been proposed, but this may not be ideal when dealing with renal tumors in patients with little renal reserve or who have a high risk of forming more tumors (such as von Hippel Lindau disease), or in the prostate where the neurovascular bundles are closely associated with the capsule.

For vascular organs the "ablation zone" is generally of low attenuation on CT, mixed signal on MRI, and has absent perfusion on contrast-enhanced imaging. Increased attenuation occurs in low-density tissues, such as fat or lung parenchyma, where "groundglass" shadowing is used to describe the periablation zone. It is recognized that in some organ sites, specifically the kidney, apparent minimal contrast enhancement (<20 Hounsfield units [HU] for CT) may be seen after ablation in tissue, which at pathological analysis is shown to be completely necrotic.

"Benign periablation enhancement" is a transient finding that may last up to six months post treatment. It usually manifests as a smooth uniform rim of peripheral enhancement up to 5 mm in early scans,

*Interventional Techniques in Uro-oncology*, First Edition. Edited by Hashim Uddin Ahmed, Manit Arya, Peter T. Scardino & Mark Emberton.  © 2011 Blackwell Publishing Ltd. Published 2011 by Blackwell Publishing Ltd.

**Table 10.1** Categorization of renal tumors by size in ablation reporting, from Goldberg et al [2].

| Size (short axis diameter) | Category |
| --- | --- |
| 3 cm or less | Small |
| 3–5 cm | Intermediate |
| More than 5 cm | Large |

which occurs on the arterial phase and which may persist on delayed phase imaging. This represents the benign physiological process of hyperemia and subsequent granulation and healing around the ablation zone. This is in contrast to "irregular peripheral enhancement," which is the result of residual tumor at the treatment margin, often best appreciated on delayed phase imaging.

Involution of the ablation zone occurs over time, and is the favored term over either "shrinkage" or "regression." Lack of involution does not imply treatment failure. In the reporting of tumor and ablation sizes, the term "index tumor" is preferred for the tumor target. For both the index tumor and the resulting zone of ablation reporting the size along all three axes is recommended, with the short-axis diameter given as a minimum. For renal tumors, size categorization may be used as in Table 10.1.

## Defining success on imaging

It is important that different investigators use the same language to describe outcomes; therefore the above terms have been coined to describe different endpoints. "Technical success" is the term used to describe whether in any given session the tumor was treated according to protocol and covered completely. This is often based on real-time imaging during, or immediately after, the treatment process and is important for defining the population in whom treatment has been technically possible.

"Technique effectiveness" is the complete absence of macroscopic tumor (by a defined imaging modality) at a given time point. It is reasonable to assume therefore that it may require several "technically successful" treatment sessions over a given period of time before an assessment of "technique effectiveness" can be made.

## Renal cancer

### Imaging after radiofrequency ablation

As discussed in Chapter 5, placement of radiofrequency probes may be performed under ultrasound, CT, or MR guidance. However, none of these modalities permit accurate, real-time monitoring of the ablation zone. MR-temperature mapping holds the potential for this, but the technology is not commercially available and hyper-acute imaging may not necessarily be accurate in assessing the response to ablation since the RF-ablative effect can develop over a period of weeks. Contrast-enhanced computed tomography (CE-CT) has been shown to correlate well with the histological zone of ablation, with the ablated tumor showing a complete absence of contrast enhancement [3]. However, in the acute setting circumferential "benign periablation enhancement" described in the preceding paragraphs may be observed, lasting up to two weeks. Thus, authors have recommended waiting up to a week until the first, postablation imaging [4].

At our institution we perform an initial CT one week post treatment to assess technical success, with subsequent CT assessment at 6 monthly intervals. This involves unenhanced and arterial phase imaging through the tumor followed by images of the chest, abdomen, and pelvis in the portal venous phase after the administration of 100-mL iodinated contrast media (300 mg/mL) at a rate of 4 mL/s.

The time taken for the zones of ablation to involute varies widely 6 months to three months. Over time, as the treated region involutes, fat may interpose between the zone of ablation and the adjacent normal renal tissue (Figure 10.1).

Although it is possible that completely ablated tissue may appear to enhance by up to 20HU on CT, largely due to the phenomenon of pseudoenhancement, any enhancement more than 10HU in the ablation zone is considered suspicious. As RF energy is deposited in a spherical manner, residual tumor is usually seen as an enhancing, nonuniform crescent at the periphery of the ablation zone ('irregular peripheral enhancement'). Late arterial-phase imaging may be useful to maximize the avid differential enhancement of vascular tumors.

Hematoma is a well-known complication of needle-ablative therapy, so that noncontrast CT is useful in the post-treatment setting to differentiate high

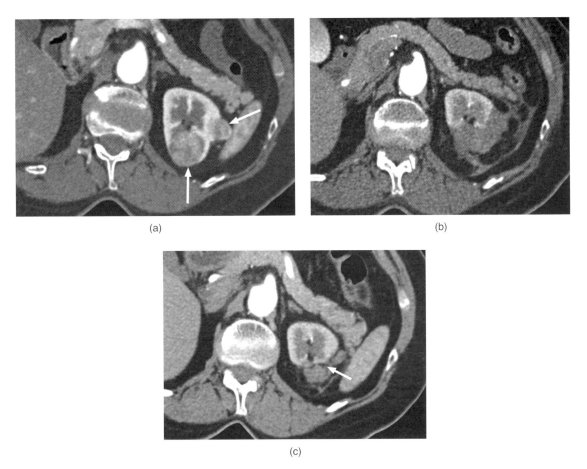

(a)

(b)

(c)

**Fig 10.1** Axial CTs 35s after iv contrast showing (a) two tumors in the left kidney before treatment (*arrows*), (b) the appearance of nonenhancing, ablated tissue at 1 month after RFA, and (c) shows the appearance at 5 months: fat interposition is seen (*arrow*) between viable kidney and ablated renal tumor. (Courtesy of Dr Alice Gillams.)

attenuation degraded blood products from tumor enhancement. A postablation "halo" is also well described as a non-enhancing fibrotic ring lying parallel to the zone of ablation, which may represent the demarcation of the inflammatory reaction with the surrounding fat (Figure 10.2). Segmental arterial thrombosis may occur either within or adjacent to the treatment zone resulting in a cortical wedge-shaped infarction (Figure 10.3).

Post-treatment imaging is also useful for monitoring complications of treatment. The full range of complications encountered during any nephron-sparing surgery may be observed such as pelvicalyceal injury resulting in perforation or stricture, pneumothorax, perirenal collection, or metastasis within the surgical track.

There remains limited experience in the follow-up of ablated lesions with magnetic resonance imaging (MRI), although most findings seen on CT are replicated [5]. There is predominantly high signal on T1 and low signal on T2-weighted imaging of the ablation zone, with absent enhancement post gadolinium. Again any residual, asymmetric enhancement is considered to indicate either incomplete ablation or tumor recurrence, not to be confused with a thin rim of "benign periablation enhancement" that may also be seen on the postcontrast T1-weighted images. The peritumor "halo" is low signal on both

**179**

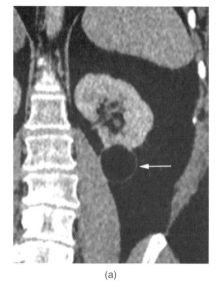

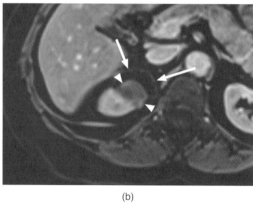

(a)

(b)

**Fig 10.2** (a): Coronal contrast-enhanced CT through a renal tumor six months post RFA demonstrating typical post RFA "halo" artifact (*arrow*) *(courtesy of Dr David Breen)*, (b) is a postcontrast gradient echo image in a different patient 5 months after RFA , showing a halo (*arrows*) and persisting but nonenhancing soft tissue in the position of the tumor (*arrowhead*) (Courtesy of Dr Alice Gillams.)

T1 and T1-weighted images, consistent with a fibrotic band.

The appearances of the ablation zone on ultrasound are nonspecific and difficult to interpret. Contrast-enhanced ultrasound holds some promise in the immediate postablation setting, but remains experimental.

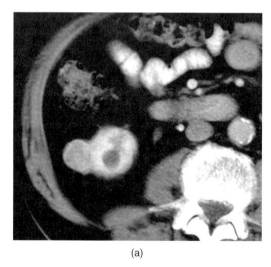

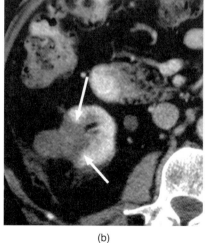

(a)

(b)

**Fig 10.3** Axial contrast enhanced CT scans (a) before RFA and (b) two weeks after RFA showing subjacent "wedge" cortical infarct confirming complete treatment (*arrows*) (Courtesy of Dr David Breen.)

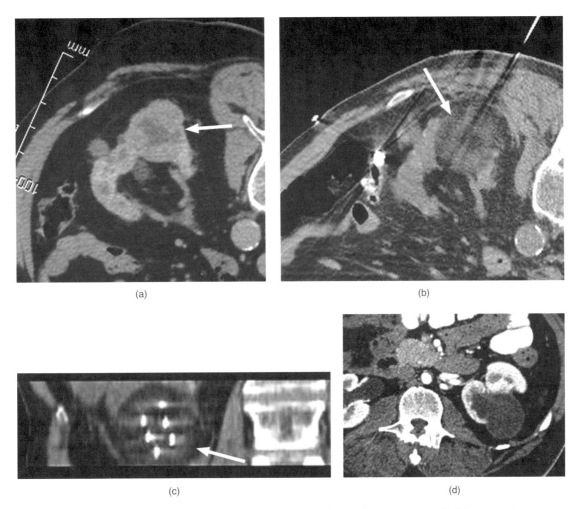

(a)

(b)

(c)

(d)

**Fig 10.4** Contrast-enhanced CT scan of 55 mm inter-polar renal cell carcinoma. Axial image (a) before RFA (the arrow shows the tumor), (b) is an unenhanced axial image, and (c) a coronal reconstruction during 6 probe cryotherapy demonstrating ice-ball formation (*arrow*). A contras-enhanced axial image (d) four weeks after cryotherapy shows lack of contrast uptake in the treated region (Courtesy of Dr David Breen.)

## Imaging after cryotherapy

Renal lesions treated with cryotherapy have a similar imaging natural history to those treated with RFA. Lack of contrast enhancement on both CT and MR imaging corresponds with ablation [6] (Figure 10.4). Benign periablation enhancement is not uncommon and is noted more frequently in those studies using MRI follow-up [7] than CT [8]. In the former, the enhancement has been noted to last up to 14 months from the time of treatment. The zones of ablation also show varying degrees of involution over time: between 19% and 94% reduction in size at 12 months have been reported [9]. Calcification has also been identified in some of the ablation zones both on CT and histologically [8].

## Imaging after extracorporeal high-intensity focused ultrasound

Thus far there are only limited data regarding the imaging appearances following renal HIFU. One group used color Doppler ultrasound to assess target

**181**

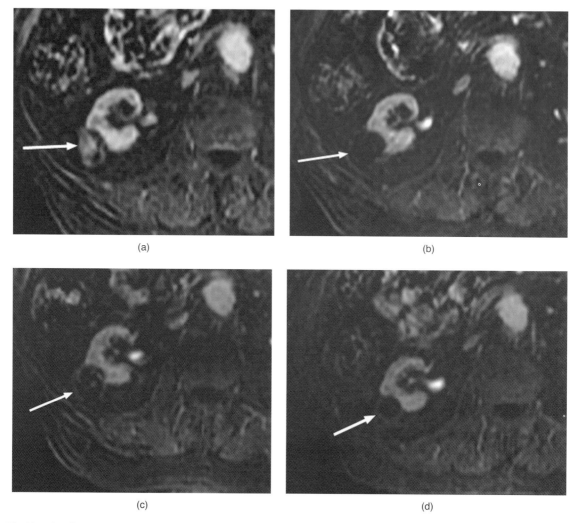

(a)

(b)

(c)

(d)

**Fig 10.5** Axial T1 postcontrast subtraction images of a right renal tumor (a) before HIFU (*arrow*), (b) 12 days after HIFU, demonstrating lack of contrast uptake (c) 6 months after HIFU, and (d) 1 year after HIFU, with a persistent fibrotic "halo" (*arrow*) (Courtesy of Dr David Breen.)

lesion size before and after HIFU, noting a mean reduction in size of 58% at 1 year [10]. Unenhanced MRI changes are inconsistent, with mixed signal changes on both T1 and T2-weighted imaging. Contrast-enhanced MRI provides evidence of no persistent perfusion within the ablation zones [11] up to one year post treatment, which has been shown to correlate with complete tissue destruction on histological examination. Similarities with RFA are noted,

with the formation of a "fibrotic halo" around some treated lesions (Figure 10.5).

It is likely that all of the ablative modalities will to some extent demonstrate similar post-treatment imaging findings. However, there are some anecdotal reports that early post-treatment imaging differs subtly between RFA and cryotherapy. RFA leads to instantaneous coagulation necrosis, thus early loss of contrast uptake would be expected; on the other hand, there is preservation of the cellular architecture following cryotherapy with a more delayed vascular insult resulting from sloughing of the endothelium. As a result, early peripheral contrast uptake following cryotherapy may not indicate treatment failure, and more delayed imaging is required before the treatment is considered to have been unsuccessful.

## Prostate cancer

All ablation is a compromise between the achievement of complete coagulative necrosis and damage to surrounding structures. Although cryotherapy and HIFU have the advantage that the composition of the treated tissue has only a small effect on the response to heating or cooling, there is some evidence that vascularity can affect completeness of treatment with HIFU; and certainly large vessels have heat-sink effects with cryotherapy, in particular at the margin. In addition, the operator often has some control over the parameters of the ablative technique [12].

At the time of the procedure, the operator is trying to achieve complete coagulative necrosis, and to determine how successful he/she has been, feedback about the location and completeness of ablation is important. Such feedback becomes even more important in the era of focal therapy [13]. Focal ablation is by necessity image-directed, and although the primary way of mapping the disease has been transperineal template biopsy [14], it is likely that MRI will play an increasing role in defining the tumor and planning the treatment [15]. In the longer term, the emphasis shifts from the need to define the treated volume to the need to detect residual disease, and, particularly in focal therapy, to detect new, significant cancers in the remaining prostate.

### Techniques for real- or near-time feedback

The difficulty of assessing perfusion in real time over a treatment lasting several hours means that real-time feedback for the time being has been achieved by the measurement of parameters that predict complete necrosis – in particular the temperature of the treated tissue, and, with less sensitivity, the presence of flowing blood on doppler ultrasound. These real time techniques will be examined in detail before discussing the use of intravenous contrast enhancement.

### Monitoring heat on MRI

HIFU produces coagulative necrosis in small, well-defined volumes, by rapid heating. In contrast, radiofrequency, laser, and microwave techniques produce larger volumes of heating for a longer time. This makes HIFU a particularly exacting test of imaging techniques for measuring tissue temperature: not only is the peak temperature short-lived (of the order of a second), but the treated volume is built up from a series of small ablations little larger than a grain of rice, making demands on both temporal and spatial resolution, two imaging parameters that are as a rule traded off against each other.

There are several parameters on MRI that vary with temperature, including spin-lattice relaxation time (T1), proton resonance frequency (spectroscopy), and diffusion. With these techniques spatial resolution of 0.5–1 mm can be achieved, with a temperature resolution of $2°C$, and scan times of the order of a second, although there is an inevitable trade off between all of these parameters. One commercial system that makes use of real-time proton diffusion-based thermometry in a closed loop to modulate the intensity of HIFU energy delivery is available; and has shown promise in the treatment of fibroids, with similar systems under development for the prostate [16]. Considerable problems remain with motion artifact (including that produced by ultrasound, and in particular cavitation) and absolute temperature measurement (important in HIFU systems where there is reectal cooling). Therefore, we are not yet at the stage where the short, intense bursts of heating currently used with HIFU can be accurately monitored. However, techniques such as RFA or microwave ablation, where a more prolonged change in temperature is produced, are easier to measure and monitor [17].

### Monitoring cold on MRI

Although the ice ball produced by cryotherapy is visible on both ultrasound, MRI, and CT; it has been known for some time that freezing does not equate to kill, and that the zone of certain necrosis lies around 3 mm inside the edge of the ice ball, although the exact zone depends on nadir temperature, rate of freezing, and rate of thawing. Thermometry of frozen tissue is possible in the prostate using R2* weighted imaging and has been demonstrated in dogs, although the resolution is of the order of several millimeters [18]. It is considerably easier to image the ice ball on conventional T2-weighted MRI sequences, where it appears as a volume of relative signal dropout, and at the moment this has a much higher resolution than thermometry.

Ultrasound can be used for real-time monitoring of ablation in several ways. First, and most importantly, it can be used to monitor the treatment zone: in cryotherapy by imaging the edge of the ice ball, in HIFU by observing grayscale changes due to cavitation and boiling [19], and, less successfully, in RFA or microwave treatment by observing microbubbles at the edge of the treated zone. The second potential use is in the real-time monitoring of tissue vascularity, which is feasible in the gaps between HIFU ablations, although is probably not of sufficient resolution to confirm necrosis. The third is measurement of elastic properties, which show promise in vitro, but again have not yet been shown to have sufficient resolution to monitor necrosis.

### Near-time monitoring: assessment of necrosis

Although changes with perfusion have been studied extensively, necrotic tissue also changes in elasticity and shows altered proton diffusion. Both MRI and ultrasound can be used to measure tissue elasticity and delineate the hardening effect of heating, but there is currently no evidence that they can delineate areas of necrosis in a clinically useful way. Similarly, consistent changes have been shown in the diffusion properties of the prostate both after cryoablation and HIFU, with the results of each ablation very similar, but the spatial resolution of this technique limits its utility.

There is little doubt that the best techniques for assessing necrosis in the prostate rely on the delineation of a perfusion defect. CT, MRI, and ultrasound can be used to delineate the lack of perfusion that is a fundamental property of necrotic tissue, and is the final common outcome with all ablative techniques.

CT has often been used to delineate necrosis in renal and liver tumors for several reasons. First, the contrast between the normal surrounding tissue and the necrotic treated zone is sufficiently high to delineate the necrosis. Second, imaging can be performed in a breath hold. In the prostate, contrast enhancement with CT has been disappointing for the detection of tumors, and the same holds for delineating necrosis.

For this reason, MRI is clearly superior for the prostate and is not significantly affected by respiratory motion.

### Ultrasound to delineate necrosis

Ultrasound is alone among the three modalities in that it can image blood flow using the doppler shift without the need for contrast. However, to accurately delineate perfusion, it is probably necessary to increase the sensitivity and contrast resolution of the technique by using microbubble- contrast agents. This has been done with some success after HIFU in the prostate, with a high correlation between ultrasound-estimated necrosis and pathological hemorrhagic necrosis [20]. Recent work with histological correlation in pigs has shown that in necrosis induced by radiofrequency ablation of the liver, contrast-enhanced ultrasound is of comparable accuracy to CT and MRI in delineating the zone of necrosis [21], but there is no work directly comparing ultrasound and MRI in the prostate. Even if ultrasound and MRI are of similar sensitivity for perfusion, comparison with the position of tumor on old scans (a vital part of the assessment of treatment) is in our experience far easier with the consistent planar images produced by MRI.

### MRI to delineate necrosis: imaging protocol

Although there are changes on T1 and T2-weighted sequences after prostate ablation, they have never been shown to accurately delineate coagulative necrosis without enhancement. Conversely, contrast-enhanced MRI, with gadolinium-based agents, is a sensitive method for demonstrating prostate perfusion, and has been examined in several studies with histological correlation. Before discussing this correlation in detail, we will describe our imaging protocol and the MR appearances soon after ablation.

We are strong advocates of the routine use of prostate MRI soon after ablation to provide feedback to the operator for quality control of ablative *dosimetry*. For this to be acceptable to the patient, both in terms of cost and inconvenience, the scanning protocol should be restricted to the essential sequences: there is little point in looking for residual tumor or subtle changes in diffusion or spectroscopy at this stage because there is much more marked abnormality from the hemorrhagic necrosis. We have found a pelvic phased-array coil adequate, and although

Table 10.2 MRI sequences used for prostate imaging.

| | TR | TE | Flip angle/ degrees | Plane | Slice thickness (gap) | Matrix size | Field of view /mm | Time for scan |
|---|---|---|---|---|---|---|---|---|
| 1. T2 TSE | 7500 | 92 | 180 | axial | 3 mm | 230 × 256 | 180 × 180 | 6 min 24 s |
| 2. T1 TSE | 749 | 13 | 150 | axial | 3 mm | 230 × 256 | 180 × 180 | 7 min 14 s |
| 3. T1 TSE (post contrast, fat suppressed) | 461 | 19 | 60 | axial +/− sagittal, coronal | 3 mm | 192 × 256 | 200 × 200 | 6 min 6 s |
| 4. T1 VIBE | 5.31 | 2.5 | 15 | axial | 3 mm | 159 × 256 | 260 × 260 | 7 min (26 acquisitions, 16s each) |
| 5. Diffusion | 2200 | 98 | | axial | 5 mm | 172 × 100 *b* values: 0, 150, 500, 1000 | 260 × 260 | 5 min 44 s (16 averages) |

We always perform sequence 1. Either sequence 4 or sequences 2 and 3 will adequately delineate necrosis. Contrast used is 20 mL gadoteric acid (Dotarem®; Guerbet, Villepinte, France), given intravenously at 3 mL/s. Sequences 4 and 5 are used for scans at 6 months or later to detect residual tumor.
FLASH, Fast low-angle shot; TSE, turbo spin echo.

perineal discomfort is mild after most ablations, the endorectal coil is never a pleasant experience for the patient.

There are three essential sequences in the imaging protocol (Table 10.2). Firstly, a high-resolution T2-weighted axial sequence is essential for delineating the margins of the prostate. After this there are two options for assessing enhancement: either a gradient-echo dynamic acquisition, or pre- and postcontrast spin echo T1-weighted sequences.

Although one group has suggested (in a study of the thigh muscle of rabbits) that calculated parameters, such as $K^{trans}$ and extracellular volume fraction may delineate subtle areas of necrosis not well seen with simple visual inspection [22], the time resolution necessary for the calculation will result in a trade-off in spatial resolution and at the moment is of uncertain clinical benefit. Gradient and spin echo sequences give very similar results, although the spatial resolution with the latter may be a little better. However they are derived, the axial postcontrast sequences can if necessary be followed by sequences in the sagittal (and less usefully) coronal planes to better delineate extraprostatic necrosis and the external sphincter.

The optimal timing for the post-treatment MRI has not yet been determined, but is likely to be less than 5 days after treatment: the volume of nonenhancing tissue can decline by around 50% in the first month as involution of necrotic tissue takes place. In our experience, the appearances are increasingly difficult to interpret after 3–4 weeks.

### MRI to delineate necrosis: early appearances

HIFU: On all sequences the prostate swells during and soon after treatment, by up to 60% (78), and after a focal treatment this is seen as a localized expansion of the treated zone. The T2-weighted changes after ablation are frequently confusing. Zonal anatomy is often lost in whole-gland treatments and the T2 signal may be reduced, but not in a predictable way that allows accurate delineation of necrosis [12]. T1-weighted sequences show variable high-signal hemorrhage.

After a successful ablation with HIFU there is usually a confluent volume of nonenhancing material surrounded by an enhancing rim measuring 2 to 8 mm in diameter [12]. Extraprostatic necrosis is well shown, and in our experience is common at the anterolateral aspect of the prostate, abutting the levator. In fact, such a feature seems almost inevitable after a good treatment. In some patients, there is intense enhancement of the periosteum of the pubic bone, together with increased enhancement in the bone marrow, which usually resolves spontaneously. Posteriorly, the nonenhancing zone may extend outside the prostate and involve a segment of the rectum, with either the muscularis or, much less commonly, the whole width of the wall involved, although a reactive *increase* in rectal wall enhancement is much more common. The contrast between treated tissue and its surroundings on MRI (Figure 10.6) is much higher than with necrosis seen on CT (Figure 10.7). Figure 10.8 shows microbubble-enhanced images of the treated prostate and a postcontrast MRI for comparison: note the excellent contrast between apparently avascular and perfused tissue with ultrasound, but the inferior spatial resolution compared to MR.

After hemiablation or focal ablation the enhancing rim extends across the prostate and there is often residual, low-level enhancement in the untreated part of the gland, likely indicating inflammation. Figure 10.9 shows these changes, with a persisting focus of enhancement early after treatment in the ablated half of the gland that predicted residual tumor at 6 months.

Cryotherapy: There is usually a confluent volume of nonenhancing tissue, with reactive hyperemia in the adjacent tissues, and a "halo" or "penumbra" around the nonenhancing zone, although the enhancing rim has not been formally characterized. Residual enhancing prostatic tissue and extraprostatic necrosis are also common [23] (80) (Figure 10.10b).

Photodynamic therapy: has been described in Chapter 6. There is only one report on post treatment appearances on MRI [24]. As with HIFU, T2-weighted sequences cannot be used to define necrosis. After contrast most of the prostate tissue fell into two categories: either nonenhancing or enhancing similarly to pretreatment scans. Nonenhancing islands were often surrounded by relatively normal, enhancing tissue. We have found in many cases that the nonenhancing volume conforms remarkably to the outline of the prostate (Figure 10.10a). The enhancing rim

is still present, but the sloughing of necrotic material seen after HIFU (and reported by the patients as the passage of debris) does not generally occur. Extraprostatic necrosis is also seen, and occasionally there may be a "skip" lesion discrete from the main body of ablation.

Bracytherapy: MRI is often performed soon after brachtherapy to assess seed placement, and some studies have been done with dynamic contrast enhancement, although they have not described the acute effect on the tumor [25].

## Histological correlates of early appearances

The key question to be answered in MRI of necrosis is related to whether lack of enhancement implies nonviable, necrotic tissue. In addition, the significance of the hyperenhancing rim and how much viable tissue it is likely to contain requires evaluation. This rim is a constant finding in several tissues, including liver, kidney, and brain. In the liver it becomes gradually less conspicuous over six months, and is seen on both CT and MRI. Within the prostate it has been shown to occur after laser ablation of benign prostatic hyperplastic tissue as well as HIFU for malignant tumors [26].

Histological evidence in animal models – including rabbit and porcine liver – suggests that the enhancing rim corresponds to an area of inflammation and then fibrosis, with a variable amount of residual, viable tissue. How much of the rim will be viable after ablation of the prostate in humans remains uncertain. On the one hand, after HIFU biopsy shows "partial or complete necrosis" in the rim. On the other hand, after laser ablation of benign prostatic hyperplasia the volume of coagulative necrosis at histology correlates very well with the central nonenhancing region at MRI, not including the rim.

There is one study of a prototype rotating transurethral ultrasound ablative device in dog prostates, which has interesting and relevant results. In this study the necrosis at histology is complete centrally around the device in the urethra. A line drawn around the nonenhancing area at contrast-enhanced MRI lies *within* a line drawn at the junction of complete and incomplete necrosis on histology. In other words, the nonenhancing tissue always indicated complete necrosis [27]. The implication from this and other studies is likely to be that a variable amount of

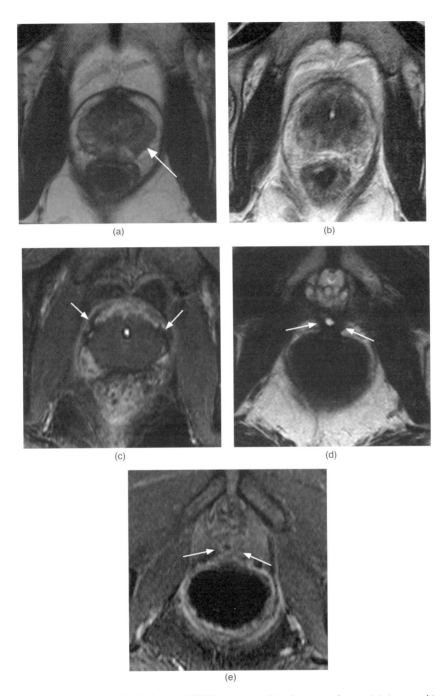

**Fig 10.6** A 59-year-old man treated with whole-gland HIFU (Sonablate 500). (a) is a T2-weighted image showing the low-signal tumor in the left peripheral zone (*arrow*), (b) and (c) are T2 weighted and T1 postcontrast images taken one month after treatment. The T2 weighted shows heterogeneous signal and does not accurately delineate the necrosis; the postcontrast image shows good contrast between the treated (and presumed necrotic) tissue and its surroundings, with a little anterolateral extraprostatic necrosis (*arrows*), (d) is a T2 image showing a small, fibrotic rim at 6 months (*arrow*). No foci of intense enhancement are seen on the gradient echo image after contrast (e)—there is no evidence of residual disease.

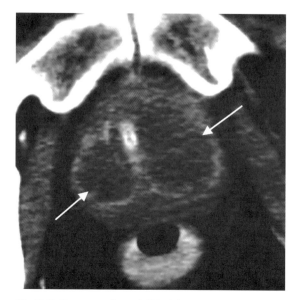

**Fig 10.7** Contrast-enhanced CT of the prostate in a 79-year-old man with bilateral transition zone necrosis (*arrows*). Although the lack of enhancement shows the necrotic are well, and a hyperenhancing rim, the contrast and spatial resolution is low.

the rim contains viable tissue depending on the organ being scanned, the nature of the treatment and the interval before the scan. The only area that can reliably be called necrotic area at MRI is that which does not enhance. Even this assumption seems questionable as small islands of enhancement that are beyond the resolution of MRI may exist. Studies correlating imaging findings with intermediate- and long- term outcomes are needed to see how reliably nonenhancement indicates true coagulative necrosis.

### Prognostic value of early MRI

There is a small amount of work correlating early MRI appearances with intermediate measures of outcome after cryotherapy and HIFU. Donnelly et al examined the appearance of the prostate at contrast-enhanced MRI three weeks after cryotherapy, and correlated it with PSA levels and the result of a transrectal biopsy at six months [28]. To their surprise, they found no significant correlation of imaging scores (related to persisting enhancing tissue) with the presence of viable prostate or tumor at future biopsy, although they did note a correlation between PSA level and the like-lihood of residual disease, which is far from surprising. In contrast, we have found different results in a small group of 13 patients who underwent contrast-enhanced MRI less than 1 month after whole-gland HIFU. Those with the most enhancing prostatic tissue on the early scan were most likely to have residual tumor at 6-month biopsy.

The significance of rectal wall necrosis depends critically on whether there has been previous radiotherapy. Rectal fistula is rare in primary treatment, and in our experience a segment of nonenhancing rectal wall, even if apparently complete, usually does not lead to fistula. However, in patients who have undergone external beam radiotherapy, the finding is more ominous. If there has been a combination of brachytherapy with external radiation, fistulation is likely, but often takes several months to occur [29].

### MRI after therapy: early changes (2 and 5 months)

The most consistent finding is a gradual reduction in the volume of nonenhancing tissue, although some usually persists. In patients having salvage treatment after radiotherapy, resorption of nonenhancing tissue is strikingly slower, and considerable necrotic tissue may still be seen at 1 year. The enhancing rim is still seen, and in many patients has a double configuration. The histological correlates of the inner- and outer-rings have yet to be determined.

At this stage several potential complications may be assessed on MRI. The earliest sign of rectal fistulation may be edema or fluid in the periprostatic fat, but in some cases a direct communication is seen, usually several months after the treatment (Figure 10.11) and usually seen best on a urethrogram (Figure 10.12). Although catheterization is the first step in dealing with this serious problem, it is rarely sufficient in previously irradiated pelvises, and reconstructive surgery is likely to be needed. Fistulation can also occur anteriorly, and track to the skin or involve the symphisis pubis (osteitis pubis). The more extensive the leak, the greater the danger of an accompanying oeteomyelitis.

At this stage recurrent disease is likely to be masked by the enhancing rim, but as on the immediate scan can be suspected if there is enhancing material at the location of the disease on pretreatment scan. This might prompt early reintervention, especially if the PSA is not falling as expected. Note, however, that it

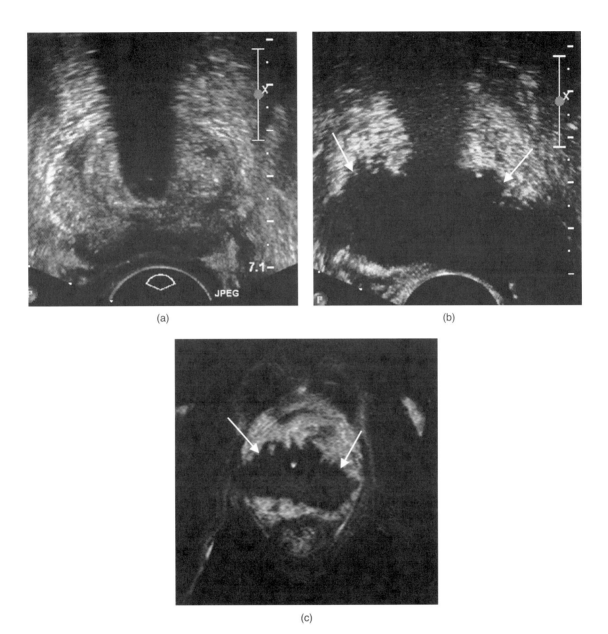

(a)

(b)

(c)

**Fig 10.8** Images from a 71-year-old man; one day after treatment of the whole prostate by HIFU (Ablatherm). (a) is a standard transrectal ultrasound image of the prostate, (b) an image after intravenous microbubble contrast (4.8 cc of Sonovue (Bracco, Italy)). Note the central shadowing from the catheter in the urethra. (c) is a postcontrast T1-weighted MRI image. Both (b) and (c) show the area of necrosis (*arrows*), with anterior sparing.(Images courtesy of Dr O Rouviere.)

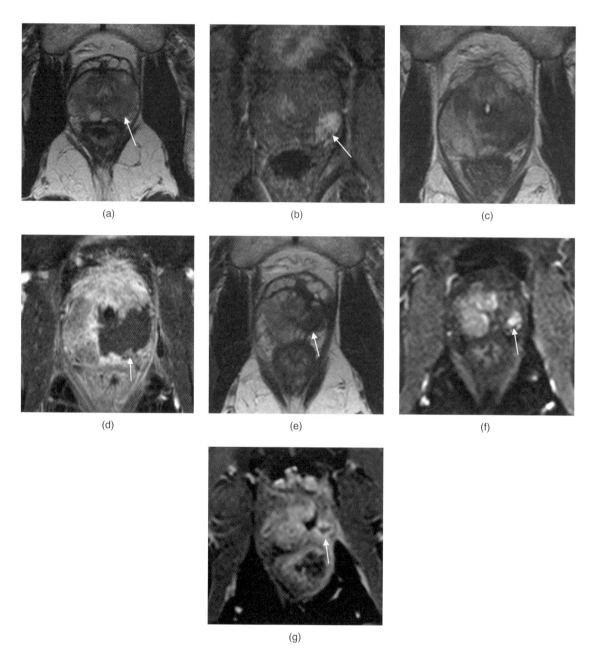

**Fig 10.9** Hemiablation of the prostate in a 68-year-old man. (a) and (b) are T2 and early dynamic contrast-enhanced image showing the tumor (*arrows*), (c) and (d) are T2 weighted and contrast-enhanced images one week after treatment. Note the small focus of persisting enhancement in the position of the tumor (*arrow*). (e) and (f) are 6 months after treatment; the left hemi-prostate has become predominantly atrophic and fibrotic on the T2-weighted image (e)(*arrow*), but a brightly enhancing focus (*arrow*) remains on the early postcontrast image (f), and was confirmed as tumor at biopsy. The patient was retreated, and (g) shows a rim of hyperenhancement around the treated volume, indicated by an arrow. A subsequent 6 month follow-up scan showed no residual tumor.

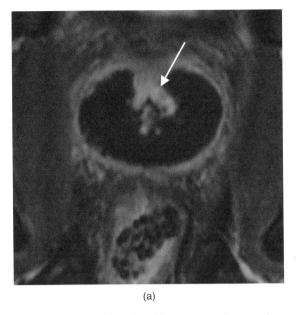

(a)

(b)

Fig 10.10 Early (less than 1 week) postcontrast images of the prostate after treatment with (a) photodynamic therapy (the arrow shows the persisting urethral enhancement—this area received a low-light dose) and (b) cryotherapy. Note that in each case the urethra remains predominantly enhancing and the hyperenhancing rim is a little less conspicuous than after HIFU (compare with Figures 10.6 and 10.8). The resorption and fibrosis that is the end result of treatment has a similar appearance to that after HIFU at 6 months. (Images courtesy of Dr Clare Allen and Dr Olivier Rouviere.)

may take 6 to 12 months after HIFU for the PSA nadir to be achieved.

## MRI after therapy: late changes (>6 months)

At six months we are in a position to detect residual tumor, which may be visible on T2-weighted sequences. However, because of the healing response this is often only revealed by contrast enhancement, although others have used diffusion-weighted imaging and spectroscopy [30].

In general PSA is a good test for recurrent disease after HIFU, but there are good reasons for also performing an MRI. First, if retreatment is considered, it may be more difficult to avoid damage to the external sphincter or rectum, so that accurate targeting of the recurrent disease is important. Second, in focal ablation, small rises in PSA are likely to be obscured by the persisting PSA from untreated prostate, and MRI becomes the primary modality for detecting small volumes of residual disease. Last, just as MRI can be used to target cancer at biopsy in a screening population [31]; it can also be used to target the biopsy to possible areas of recurrence after ablation.

At this stage, in both partial and complete ablations without previous radiotherapy, most or all of the necrosis has been resorbed. A variable amount of residual prostate remains. Some patients have virtually none, and the fibrosis that has replaced the prostate is of very low T2 signal, with faint, and often delayed, enhancement after intravenous contrast. At the other end of the spectrum, patients with very incomplete treatments may have persisting high-signal peripheral zone and preserved zonal anatomy (Figure 10.13). The same is true of hemi- or focal ablations: after a good treatment the targeted area should be of low volume and uniformly low in T2 signal.

Residual cancer has a similar appearance to pretreatment scans, but is more difficult to identify on all modalities because of the heterogeneous, distorted appearance of the surrounding prostate. The T2 signal of tumor is usually a little higher than surrounding

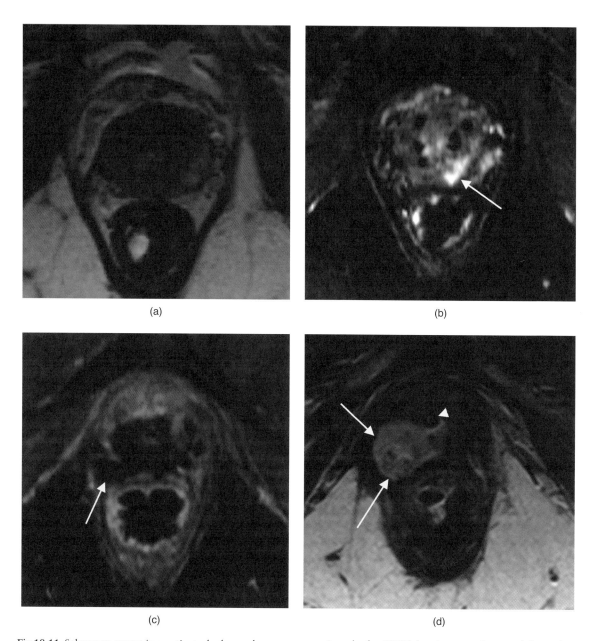

(a)

(b)

(c)

(d)

**Fig 10.11** Salvage treatment in a patient who has undergone brachytherapy and external-beam radiotherapy. (a) is a T2-weighted image showing the prostate, but not clearly outlining the tumor, (b) is a postcontrast gradient echo image showing early enhancement suggesting tumor (confirmed at biopsy)(*arrow*). (c) is a contrast-enhanced image 1 week after HIFU showing necrosis around the seeds and some extraprostatic necrosis on the left (*arrow*). At 6 months after contrast (d), this extraprostatic necrosis has become a cavity (*arrows*) communicating with the urethra (a urethral catheter is marked by arrowheads). A fistula between this cavity and the rectum developed later.

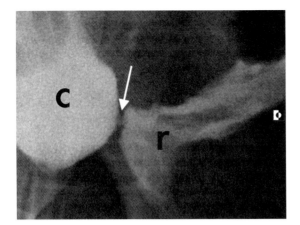

**Fig 10.12** Urethrogram outlining a capacious prostatic cavity (C) and leaking along a narrow track (*arrow*) to the rectum (r).

fibrosis, but lower than intact peripheral zone. It enhances early and intensely compared to fibrosis [30], and shows high signal on diffusion-weighted images with a b value of 1000 s/mm$^2$ and restriction on an apparent diffusion coefficient map.

In cryotherapy, MRI shows loss of zonal anatomy after a good treatment, with the formation of a "thick, fibrous capsule" around the prostate [23]. As with HIFU, recurrent cancer after cryotherapy is difficult to detect on T2 sequences alone, but has an elevated choline+creatanine/citrate ratio (similar to pretreatment scans) and that can be used to detect recurrent disease [23]. Postcryotherapy appearances with intravenous enhancement and diffusion-weighted imaging have not yet been described.

Little has been published on gland appearance and volume after RFA and photodynamic therapy, but we would expect a similar sequence of changes. There is one description of the T2 changes in the prostate after brachytherapy at 12 months, showing a diffuse loss of signal [32]— similar to after external-beam radiotherapy, where there is a reduction in gland size, reduced T2 signal throughout, and a variable loss of zonal anatomy (Figure 10.11).

### Prognostic value of late MRI

There are several published series examining the ability of MRI to detect residual disease after HIFU. The

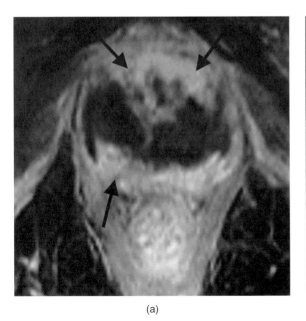

(a)

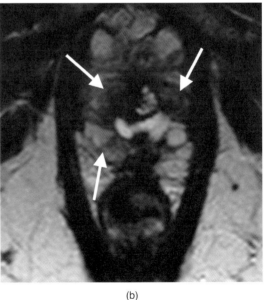

(b)

**Fig 10.13** Considerable undertreatment in a 50-year-old man. The gradient echo postcontrast (a) soon after HIFU shows considerable enhancement within the gland (*arrows*). At 6 months, the T2-weighted scan (b) shows persisting high-signal peripheral zone (*arrows*) and some zonal antomy.

**193**

largest is a series of 27 patients who had an MRI performed because of a PSA >1 ng/mL between 3 and 26 months after HIFU Therapy. Analyzed by sextant, the results of dynamic contrast-enhanced scans were compared with T2 and diffusion-weighted images. The dynamic contrast sequences showed better sensitivity (mean sensitivity 83%, specificity 66%) than the T2 and diffusion-weighted images, but the latter had better specificity (mean sensitivity 66%, specificity 76%) [30].

Our group has found that inexperienced observers can achieve a sensitivity of 75% and specificity of 76% for the detection of disease recurrence in the whole gland after HIFU [33], with an area under the receiver operating characteristic curve very similar to that for PSA. Consistent with the finding that MRI and PSA are of similar sensitivity, recent figures from an online registry of HIFU patients are comparable, showing sensitivity of 78% and specificity of 79% for detecting recurrent disease when using a cut-off of PSA nadir + 1.2 ng/mL [34]. Finally, recent evidence from Rouviere et al shows that biopsies targeted to areas of suspicion for recurrence on MRI are much more likely to be positive than standard cores [35].

The combination of T2-weighted sequences and spectroscopy has been examined in a group of 13 patients. Although the number is too small for meaningful estimates of sensitivity and specificity, an important finding was that magnetic resonance spectroscopy (MR spectroscopy) was suitable for analysis in only 3 of 10 patients who had partial necrosis [36].

Cryotherapy: Parivar et al have assessed the performance of MR spectroscopy for the detection of residual disease after cryothedrapy in a series of 25 patients, 5 of whom had an undetectable PSA several months after treatment [23]. MR spectroscopy correctly identified 8 patients with residual disease, but there were false positives (if biopsy was defined as the gold standard) in 5 out of 17 patients. There are currently no published data assessing the use of gadolinium-based contrast agents after cryotherapy.

Imaging after brachytherapy: No studies have assessed the ability to detect residual disease after brachytherapy, but recurrent tumor after external-beam radiotherapy can be detected with a sensitivity of 68% and specificity over 90% using T2 sequences alone, while the addition of spectroscopy improved sensitivity a little but at the cost of a marked increase in false positives [37]. Recent data have demonstrated a marked improvement in detection with contrast-enhanced MRI compared to T2 sequences (sensitivity and specificity 72% and 85% for contrast-enhanced MR compared to 38% and 80% for T2 sequences) [38].

Ultimately, there is no work directly comparing the performance of spectroscopy and contrast-enhanced scans after *any* ablative technique, and it is not clear whether the impressive results with spectroscopy in a small number of patients after cryotherapy [23] were in the context of a truly blinded study, and whether they will be reproduced in different groups. In all studies involving spectroscopy, there is a high proportion of voxels in which the signal to noise ratio is poor and accurate analysis is difficult [39], a problem that is likely to be worse after ablation, so that in our practice we rely on contrast enhancement to detect disease and target the post-treatment biopsy.

## Future directions

The routine role of imaging following ablation of renal and prostate cancer for image verification of treatment effect as well as surveillance after ablation is increasing. In the kidney, the principle is established and the practice widespread, but in the prostate it is not. This is likely due to the combination of skepticism about the value of MRI in the prostate in general, and the ability to assess and monitor treatment with PSA. However, the clear advantages of MRI—in particular anatomical feedback about treatment and the ability to localize recurrent disease—become even more important in the era of focal therapy.

Conventional positron emission scanning with (18)F-2-fluoro-D-deoxyglucose is of limited sensitivity and resolution for the detection of small volumes of residual or recurrent disease, and is currently clearly inferior to the MRI techniques that we have described [40]. The same is true of current monoclonal antibody imaging with the prostate specific membrane antigen antibody (111)In-capromab pendetide (ProstaScint®), although both may potentially have a role in the detection of lymph node metastases. However, new agents such as including (11)C and (18)F-choline and acetate have a potentially higher signal to noise ratio and have shown promise in the detection of cancer within the prostate, though they are still far from the performance of multiparametric MRI [41].

Much current research involves techniques for real-time feedback during ablation. Tissue elastography [42] and ultrasound thermometry [43] are in development but remain experimental. Magnetic resonance thermometry [44] is in clinical use, but MR scan time is expensive and the number of interventional scanners limited. Whether data obtained from real-time feedback will reduce the necessity for *near-time* feedback with contrast-enhanced imaging remains uncertain.

The link between verification scans soon after treatment and outcome will be a fertile area for clinical research over the next few years. It seems likely that techniques assessing completeness of necrosis will predict outcome, but it has so far been surprisingly difficult to show a good correlation in a large number of patients.

Finally, the advent of molecular imaging heralds a new era of functional as well as structural imaging [40, 45], and many of the new methods for the detection of renal, prostate, and bladder cancers will also be useful for the detection of recurrent disease after ablation.

## Conclusions

In the absence of techniques for accurately delineating necrosis in real time, we propose that limited contrast-enhanced MR should be performed soon after *all* ablative treatments in the prostate. It will enable the operator to optimize their technique, provide an early indication of the need for retreatment, give prognostic information to the patient and allow rapid optimization of new treatment parameters for any device.

In the longer term, complete ablation of the prostate can adequately be followed up by serial PSA measurements. MRI can be reserved for confirming and localizing suspected recurrent disease. However, in the era of focal therapy, PSA is likely to become a much less reliable tool, and contrast-enhanced MRI becomes an attractive, noninvasive method for monitoring for residual disease, targeting biopsy and planning retreatment. Whether spectroscopy and diffusion will *add* significant information in this context is uncertain.

## References

1. Goldberg SN et al (2005) Image-guided tumor ablation: standardization of terminology and reporting criteria. J Vasc Interv Radiol 16: 765–778.

2. Rendon RA et al (2002) The uncertainty of radio frequency treatment of renal cell carcinoma: findings at immediate and delayed nephrectomy. J Urol 167: 1587–1592.

3. Arzola J et al (2006) Computed tomography-guided, resistance-based, percutaneous radiofrequency ablation of renal malignancies under conscious sedation at two years of follow-up. Urology 68: 983–987.

4. Walther MC et al (2000) A phase 2 study of radio frequency interstitial tissue ablation of localized renal tumors. J Urol 163: 1424–1427.

5. Boss A et al (2006) Morphological, contrast-enhanced and spin labeling perfusion imaging for monitoring of relapse after RF ablation of renal cell carcinomas. Eur Radiol 16: 1226–1236.

6. Gill IS et al (2000) Laparoscopic renal cryoablation in 32 patients. Urology 56: 748–753.

7. Remer EM et al (2000) MR Imaging of the kidneys after laparoscopic cryoablation. AJR Am J Roentgenol 174: 635–640.

8. Beemster P et al (2008) Follow-up of renal masses after cryosurgery using computed tomography; enhancement patterns and cryolesion size. BJU Int 101: 1237–1242.

9. Gill IS et al (2005) Renal cryoablation: outcome at 3 years. J Urol 173: 1903–1907.

10. Wu T et al (2000) MR imaging of shear waves generated by focused ultrasound. Magn Reson Med 43: 111–115.

11. Illing RO et al (2005) The safety and feasibility of extracorporeal high-intensity focused ultrasound (HIFU) for the treatment of liver and kidney tumours in a Western population. Br J Cancer 93: 890–895.

12. Kirkham AP et al (2008) MR imaging of prostate after treatment with high-intensity focused ultrasound. Radiology 246: 833–844.

13. Polascik T, Mouraviev V (2008) Focal therapy for prostate cancer. Curr Opin Urol 18: 269–274.

14. Onik G (2004) The male lumpectomy: rationale for a cancer targeted approach for prostate cryoablation. A review. Technol Cancer Res Treat 3: 365–370.

15. Ahmed HU et al (2007) Will focal therapy become a standard of care for men with localized prostate cancer? Nat Clin Pract Oncol 4(11): 632–642.

16. Pauly KB et al (2006) Magnetic resonance-guided high-intensity ultrasound ablation of the prostate. Top Magn Reson Imaging 17: 195–207.

17. Chen JC et al (2000) Prostate cancer: MR imaging and thermometry during microwave thermal ablation-initial experience. Radiology 214: 290–297.

18. Wansapura J et al (2005) In vivo MR thermometry of frozen tissue using R2* and signal intensity1. Acad Radiol 12: 1080–1084.

19. Illing RO et al (2006) Visually directed high-intensity focused ultrasound for organ-confined prostate cancer:

a proposed standard for the conduct of therapy. BJU Int 98: 1187–1192.

20. Rouviere O et al (2009) Transrectal HIFU ablation of prostate cancer: assessment of tissue destruction with contrast-enhanced ultrasound. Eur Urol (suppl. 8): 356.

21. Vogt FM et al (2007) Morphologic and functional changes in nontumorous liver tissue after radiofrequency ablation in an in vivo model: comparison of 18 F-FDG PET/CT, MRI, ultrasound, and CT. J Nucl Med 48: 1836–1844.

22. Cheng HL et al (2003) Prediction of subtle thermal histopathological change using a novel analysis of Gd-DTPA kinetics. J Magn Reson Imaging 18: 585–598.

23. Parivar F et al (1996) Detection of locally recurrent prostate cancer after cryosurgery: evaluation by transrectal ultrasound, magnetic resonance imaging, and three-dimensional proton magnetic resonance spectroscopy. Urology 48: 594–599.

24. Haider MA et al (2007) Prostate gland: MR imaging appearance after vascular targeted photodynamic therapy with palladium-bacteriopheophorbide. Radiology 244: 196–204.

25. Bloch BN et al (2007) Prostate postbrachytherapy seed distribution: comparison of high-resolution, contrast-enhanced, T1- and T2-weighted endorectal magnetic resonance imaging versus computed tomography: initial experience. Int J Radiat Oncol Biol Phys 69: 70–78.

26. Rouviere O et al (2001) MRI appearance of prostate following transrectal HIFU ablation of localized cancer. Eur Urol 40: 265–274.

27. Boyes A et al (2007) Prostate tissue analysis immediately following magnetic resonance imaging guided transurethral ultrasound thermal therapy. J Urol 178: 1080–1085.

28. Donnelly SE et al (2004) Prostate cancer: gadolinium-enhanced MR imaging at 3 weeks compared with needle biopsy at 6 months after cryoablation. Radiology 232: 830–833.

29. Ahmed HU et al (2009) Rectal fistulae after salvage high-intensity focused ultrasound for recurrent prostate cancer after combined brachytherapy and external beam radiotherapy. BJU Int 103: 321–323.

30. Kim C et al (2008) MRI Techniques for prediction of local tumor progression after high-intensity focused ultrasonic ablation of prostate cancer. Am J Roentgenol 190: 1180–1186.

31. Kirkham A, Emberton M, Allen C (2006) How good is MRI at detecting and characterising cancer within the prostate? Eur Urol 50: 1163–1175.

32. Coakley FV et al (2001) Brachytherapy for prostate cancer: endorectal MR imaging of local treatment-related changes. Radiology 219: 817–821.

33. Kirkham A et al (2009) The value of magnetic resonance imaging and PSA in detecting recurrence after high intensity focused ultrasound. Eur Urol (suppl. 8): 322.

34. Blana A et al (2009) Defining biochemical failure following high intensity focused ultrasound of the prostate: The Stuttgart definition. Eur Urol (suppl. 8): 333.

35. Rouviere O et al (2009) Prostate cancer transrectal HIFU ablation: detection of local recurrences with MRI. Eur Urol (suppl. 8): 322.

36. Cirillo S et al (2008) Endorectal magnetic resonance imaging and magnetic resonance spectroscopy to monitor the prostate for residual disease or local cancer recurrence after transrectal high-intensity focused ultrasound. BJU Int 102: 452–458.

37. Pucar D et al (2005) Prostate cancer: correlation of MR imaging and MR spectroscopy with pathologic findings after radiation therapy-initial experience. Radiology 236: 545–553.

38. Haider MA et al (2008) Dynamic contrast-enhanced magnetic resonance imaging for localization of recurrent prostate cancer after external beam radiotherapy. Int J Radiat Oncol Biol Phys 70: 425–430.

39. Fütterer JJ et al (2006) Prostate cancer localization with dynamic contrast-enhanced MR imaging and proton MR spectroscopic imaging. Radiology 241: 449–458.

40. Pucar D, Sella T, Schoder H (2008) The role of imaging in the detection of prostate cancer local recurrence after radiation therapy and surgery. Curr Opin Urol 18: 87–97.

41. Giovacchini G et al (2008) [(11)C]choline uptake with PET/CT for the initial diagnosis of prostate cancer: relation to PSA levels, tumour stage and anti-androgenic therapy. Eur J Nucl Med Mol Imaging 35: 1065–1073.

42. Curiel L et al (2005) Elastography for the follow-up of high-intensity focused ultrasound prostate cancer treatment: initial comparison with MRI. Ultrasound Med Biol 31: 1461–1468.

43. Miller NR, Bograchev KM, Bamber JC (2005) Ultrasonic temperature imaging for guiding focused ultrasound surgery: effect of angle between imaging beam and therapy beam. Ultrasound Med Biol 31: 401–413.

44. Quesson B, de Zwart JA, Moonen CT (2000) Magnetic resonance temperature imaging for guidance of thermotherapy. J Magn Reson Imaging 12: 525–533.

45. Larson SM, Schoder H (2008) Advances in positron emission tomography applications for urologic cancers. Curr Opin Urol 18: 65–70.

# Index